HANDBOOK OF AIDS PSYCHIATRY

HANDBOOK OF AIDS PSYCHIATRY

Mary Ann Cohen
Harold W. Goforth
Joseph Z. Lux
Sharon M. Batista
Sami Khalife
Kelly L. Cozza
Jocelyn Soffer

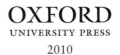

OXFORD
UNIVERSITY PRESS
2010

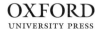

OXFORD
UNIVERSITY PRESS

Oxford University Press, Inc., publishes works that further Oxford University's
objective of excellence in research, scholarship, and education.

Oxford   New York

Auckland   Cape Town   Dar es Salaam   Hong Kong   Karachi
Kuala Lumpur   Madrid   Melbourne   Mexico City   Nairobi
New Delhi   Shanghai   Taipei   Toronto

With offices in
Argentina   Austria   Brazil   Chile   Czech Republic   France   Greece
Guatemala   Hungary   Italy   Japan   Poland   Portugal   Singapore
South Korea   Switzerland   Thailand   Turkey   Ukraine   Vietnam

Published by Oxford University Press, Inc.
198 Madison Avenue, New York, New York 10016

www.oup.com

Oxford is a registered trademark of Oxford University Press, Inc.

Library of Congress Cataloging-in-Publication Data

Handbook of AIDS psychiatry / Mary Ann Cohen ... [et al.].
p. ; cm.
Companion vol. to: Comprehensive textbook of AIDS psychiatry / edited by
Mary Ann Cohen and Jack M. Gorman. 2008.
Includes bibliographical references.
ISBN-13: 978-0-19-537257-1
ISBN-10: 0-19-537257-3
1. AIDS (Disease)—Psychological aspects—Handbooks, manuals, etc.
2. HIV infections—Psychological aspects—Handbooks, manuals, etc.
3. AIDS (Disease)—Patients—Mental health—Handbooks, manuals, etc.
4. HIV-positive persons—Mental health—Handbooks, manuals, etc.
I. Cohen, Mary Ann, 1941–   II. Comprehensive textbook of AIDS psychiatry.
[DNLM: 1. HIV Infections—psychology.   2. Acquired Immunodeficiency
Syndrome—complications.   3. Acquired Immunodeficiency Syndrome—psychology.
4. HIV Infections—complications.   5. Mental Disorders—complications.
6. Mental Disorders—therapy. WC 503.7 H236 2010]
RC606.63H36 2010
616.97′9206—dc22
2009030474

9 8 7 6 5 4 3 2 1

Printed in the United States of America
on acid-free paper

ACKNOWLEDGMENTS

We gratefully acknowledge all of the contributors to the *Comprehensive Textbook of AIDS Psychiatry*, which served as a source for this book. This handbook is a companion book that is a short and practical guide for clinicians. For more in-depth information, we refer the reader to the *Comprehensive Textbook*. Some of the *Textbook* chapters were adapted, updated, and rewritten for the *Handbook of AIDS Psychiatry*. The following chapters, from *Comprehensive Textbook of AIDS Psychiatry*, MA Cohen and JM Gorman (eds.), New York: Oxford University Press, 2008, are acknowledged with appreciation:

> Bialer P, Hoffman RG, and Ditzell J. Substance Use Disorders—The Special Role in HIV Transmission (pp. 85–96).
>
> Dickerman AL, Breitbart W, and Chochinov HM. Palliative and Spiritual Care of Persons with HIV and AIDS (pp. 417–437).
>
> Dorell K, Soffer J, and Gorman JM. Psychiatric Interventions (pp. 379–391).
>
> Ferrando SJ and Lyketsos CG. HIV-Associated Neurocognitive Disorders (pp. 109–120).
>
> Forstein M. Young Adulthood and Serodiscordant Couples (pp. 341–355).
>
> Gookin K and Stoff D. Older Age and HIV Infection (pp. 357–376).
>
> Pao M and Wiener L. Childhood and Adolescence Psychiatry (pp. 307–339).
>
> Ryan E and Byrd D. Neuropsychological Evaluation (pp. 73–84).
>
> Skapik J, Thompson A, Angelino A, and Treisman G. Psychotic Disorders and Severe Mental Illness (pp. 131–140).

PREFACE

The *Handbook of AIDS Psychiatry* is a practical guide for AIDS psychiatrists and other mental health professionals as well as other clinicians who work with persons with HIV and AIDS. It is a companion book to the *Comprehensive Textbook of AIDS Psychiatry* (MA Cohen and JM Gorman, Eds., Oxford University Press, 2008) from which some of its chapters were adapted. The *Handbook* offers insights into the dynamics of adherence to risk reduction and medical care in persons with HIV and AIDS. It also provides strategies to improve adherence using a biopsychosocial approach, as psychiatric factors both complicate and perpetuate the AIDS pandemic. When Joan Bossert, our editor at Oxford, suggested that we consider writing a handbook similar to others in the Oxford Handbook Series, we welcomed the idea because we realized that there was no short, practical guide that clinicians could consult to help diagnose and treat the psychological problems of persons with HIV and AIDS. Seven of the 72 contributors to the textbook took on the task of developing the *Handbook of AIDS Psychiatry*.

While there are psychiatric disorders linked directly and indirectly to risk behaviors and HIV infection, persons with HIV or AIDS may have no psychiatric disorder or any disorder described in the *Diagnostic and Statistical Manual of Mental Disorders, Fourth Edition (DSM-IV)*. In this handbook, we describe the psychiatric disorders most prevalent in persons with AIDS and most relevant for primary physicians, infectious disease specialists, and other caregivers. The impact of these disorders on health, adherence, behavior, and quality of life can be profound.

Psychiatric disorders may be the first and, at times, the only manifestation of HIV infection. Early diagnosis of central nervous system HIV-related abnormalities can lead to timely introduction of treatment with antiretroviral agents. In the literature, early neuropsychiatric disorders have been described, in addition to later manifestations of general psychopathology, dementia, psychosis, depression, and mania. These disorders can be a reaction to awareness of a diagnosis of HIV infection. Alternatively, psychopathology can be related to intrinsic involvement of the brain with HIV or opportunistic infections or cancers, such as toxoplasmosis, cryptococcosis, or lymphoma. In addition, antiretroviral therapies, treatments for opportunistic infections and cancers, and treatment for comorbid hepatitis C virus infection may have central nervous system side effects, including psychiatric symptoms. Multimorbid severe and complex medical conditions such as hepatic, renal, cardiac, neoplastic, endocrine, pulmonary, gastrointestinal, and other illnesses further complicate HIV and AIDS because of associated psychiatric manifestations.

Psychiatric disorders play a role in the transmission of HIV, and psychiatric factors also play a major role in the suffering endured by patients, their partners, families, and caregivers. Psychiatric disorders such as depression, addiction, mania, posttraumatic stress disorder, and cognitive disorders can worsen adherence, morbidity, prognosis and mortality. If psychiatric disorders go untreated, patients with HIV and AIDS have difficulty attending appointments and adhering to the complex medical treatments involved with care. Infectious disease specialists, primary physicians, nurses, social workers, case managers, other health care workers, and physicians in every specialty may find themselves frustrated that patients are not adhering to medical care and are getting ill in the same ways that patients did in the beginning of the pandemic, when few or no treatments were available and mortality was high. Now that perinatal HIV transmission can be prevented by antiretroviral protocols, obstetricians may find themselves stymied when pregnant women do not adhere to prenatal care and to antiretroviral treatment.

Persons with severe mental illness and substance use disorders have a higher prevalence of HIV infection than that in the general population. Persons with HIV infection, severe mental illness, and substance use disorder may also lack access to medical care and antiretroviral therapy. The course of HIV-related illness is very different in persons with severe mental illness who lack access to adequate medical care: they have a course similar to that of persons in the early years of the pandemic or of persons living in resource-limited areas of the United States or the rest of the world. This lack of access to care has led to a major disparity in the AIDS pandemic.

We describe the gaps in care and the entirely different HIV pandemics seen in persons with treated and untreated psychiatric disorders, and we provide strategies to close some of these gaps. We also address the chronic illness that AIDS has become for most persons with access to antiretroviral therapy. For example, we include a section on smoking cessation modalities, since more people with HIV who are treated with antiretroviral therapy will die of lung cancer, heart disease, emphysema, or complications of substance use disorders than will die of AIDS-related illness. We also cover the care and treatment of persons who lack access to care or are nonadherent to care. The *Handbook* has protocols for the evaluation and treatment of AIDS-related psychiatric disorders, as well as AIDS palliative psychiatry.

Because there is an ample body of evidence that psychiatric care can decrease transmission, diminish suffering, improve adherence, and decrease morbidity and mortality, we have aimed to provide insight into the interface between the psychiatric, medical, and social dimensions of HIV and AIDS in the chapters of this book. We hope that the *Handbook of AIDS Psychiatry*, as a practical guide to AIDS psychiatry, will help clinicians in a variety of clinical settings.

We are particularly grateful to Jack M. Gorman, co-editor, and all of the contributors to the *Comprehensive Textbook of AIDS Psychiatry* for the outstanding work that provided us with the basis for some of our chapters in this *Handbook*; to our editors and associate editors at Oxford University Press, Joan Bossert, Abby Gross, Nancy Wolitzer, and Aaron Van Dorn; and to our copy editor Jerri Hurlbutt, who made this work possible. We are especially grateful to our families and friends for their patience and support.

We dedicate this book to the courageous men, women, and children with HIV and AIDS, to their families and to their loved ones. We also dedicate the book to the compassionate and caring HIV clinicians who work with us to provide care and support for persons with HIV and AIDS.

Mary Ann Cohen
Harold W. Goforth
Joseph Z. Lux
Sharon M. Batista
Sami Khalife
Kelly L. Cozza
Jocelyn Soffer

CONTENTS

Authors

Sharon M. Batista, M.D.
Chief Resident
Department of Psychiatry
Mount Sinai School of Medicine
Mount Sinai Hospital
New York, New York

Mary Ann Cohen, M.D.
Clinical Professor of Psychiatry
Mount Sinai School of Medicine
Voluntary Attending Psychiatrist
Former Director, AIDS Psychiatry
Mount Sinai Medical Center
New York, New York

Kelly L. Cozza, M.D.
Associate Professor of Psychiatry
Uniformed Services University
Bethesda, Maryland
Consultant, Department of Psychiatry
Walter Reed Army Medical Center
Washington, D.C.

Harold W. Goforth, M.D.
Assistant Professor of Psychiatry and Behavioral Sciences
Duke University Medical Center
Durham, North Carolina

Co-director, Consultation Psychiatry Service and Attending Physician
GRECC—Division of Palliative Medicine
Durham Veterans Affairs Medical Center
Durham, North Carolina

Sami Khalife, M.D.
Attending Psychiatrist
Intensive Psychiatric Service
Manhattan Psychiatric Center
New York, New York

Joseph Z. Lux, M.D.
Attending Psychiatrist
Division of Consultation-Liaison Psychiaty
Bellevue Hospital Center
New York, New York

Jocelyn Soffer, M.D.
Child and Adolescent Psychiatry Resident
Department of Child and Adolescent Psychiatry
New York University
Clinical Instructor
New York University Child Study Center
New York, New York

Handbook of AIDS Psychiatry

1

SETTINGS AND MODELS OF AIDS PSYCHIATRIC CARE

Mary Ann Cohen, Harold W. Goforth, and Sami Khalife

From primary prevention to end-of-life care, AIDS psychiatry can make significant contributions to preventing risk behaviors and HIV transmission, mitigating suffering, and improving adherence to risk reduction and medical care. Early in the epidemic, stigma and discrimination magnified suffering and excluded persons known to have HIV and AIDS from many settings in the United States and throughout the world. Such treatment of persons with AIDS was described (Cohen, 1989) as a new form of discrimination called "AIDSism." As we approach the end of the third decade of the HIV pandemic, in most countries education, training, and experience have mitigated AIDSism, and persons with HIV and AIDS are now seen in varieties of medical and nonmedical settings. The multimorbid medical and psychiatric illnesses associated with HIV infection have complicated the care of persons with HIV and AIDS. A primary care guideline for the care of persons with HIV is available in print (Aberg et al., 2009) and online and is updated regularly at: http://www.journals.uchicago.edu/page/cid/IDSAguidelines.html.

AIDS psychiatrists, psychosomatic medicine psychiatrists, as well as child, adult, and geriatric psychiatrists and other mental health professionals are in a unique position to intervene and provide both preventive and treatment interventions for children, adolescents, and adults who are vulnerable to, infected with, or affected by HIV infection. Psychiatrists generally make long-term and trusting relationships with their patients and take complete histories including sexual histories and substance use histories. Primary physicians, pediatricians, obstetricians, and HIV specialists as well as parents and teachers may also have unique opportunities to intervene throughout the life cycle. In this chapter, we provide a list of settings where educational opportunities abound and can lead to an improved understanding of how to prevent HIV transmission. These settings are summarized in Table 1.1. Since a full description of every setting with potential for intervention is beyond the scope of this chapter, we provide more specific descriptions of settings where providing education and easy access to testing, condoms, and drug and alcohol treatment can be therapeutic and lifesaving.

Table 1.1 Settings for Potential HIV Prevention Interventions

Risk Prevention and AIDS Psychiatry

1. Parenting education for effective parenting and prevention of early-childhood trauma
   a. Providing effective parental role models
   b. Education about drugs and sex
   c. Providing adequate nurturing
   d. Prevention of emotional, physical, and sexual abuse
2. School interventions—introduction to risk-behavior prevention with age-appropriate sex education and programs for prevention of alcohol and other drug use
   a. Elementary
   b. Junior high school
   c. High school
   d. College
   e. Graduate school
3. Public service announcements
4. Alcohol and other drug prevention programs

Risk Reduction and AIDS Psychiatry—Education, HIV Testing Availability, Condom Distribution

1. Addiction treatment
   a. Methadone maintenance treatment programs—direct observation treatment (DOT) with antiretroviral therapy (ART) along with methaodone administration
   b. Drug rehabilitation programs—DOT availability
   c. Alcohol treatment programs—DOT availability
   d. 12-Step programs
   e. Naloxone and cardiopulmonary resuscitation (CPR) programs
   f. Needle exchange programs
   g. Supervised injection programs
2. Homeless outreach
3. Shelters
4. Soup kitchens
5. Correctional facilities with DOT availability
6. Acute care facilities—inpatient
   a. General care
   b. Urgent care
   c. Emergency room

    d. Psychiatric care
    e. Specialty care
    f. Obstetrics and gynecology
    g. Pediatrics and adolescent units
    h. Geriatric facilities
7. Ambulatory care
    a. Prenatal
    b. Medical clinic
    c. HIV clinic
    d. Chest clinic
    e. Dialysis unit
    f. Psychiatric clinics
    g. Geriatric clinics

Psychiatric and Other Mental Health Interventions

1. After HIV diagnosis
2. Mental health screening
    a. Mood disorders
    b. Cognitive disorders
    c. Substance abuse disorders
    d. Psychotic disorders
3. Treatment

Prevention of HIV in Older Adults

1. Geriatric facilities
2. Senior centers
3. Assisted living facilities

Long-Term Care Facilities—Education, HIV Testing Availability, Condom Distribution

1. Rehabilitation centers
2. Chronic care facilities
3. Nursing homes

PSYCHIATRIC FACILITIES

Persons with severe mental illness have a high prevalence of risky behaviors but may lack access to adequate medical care and access to HIV testing. Since early diagnosis and medical intervention are vital for survival, it is important to encourage persons with severe mental illness to get tested. Psychiatric facilities are ideal settings for HIV-related education and for initiating the process of testing and scheduling appointments for medical care for persons whose test results indicate HIV infection (see Table 1.2). Persons with HIV and AIDS who have multimorbid medical and

TABLE 1.2 Important Issues to Address in the Setting of Psychiatric Facilities

1. Awareness of risky behaviors
    a. The role of intimate partner violence
    b. Indiscriminate partner choice
    c. Intoxication with alcohol or other drugs can lead to risky sexual behaviors
    d. Exchange of sex for drugs
2. Risk reduction
    a. Use of barrier contraception such as condoms throughout the entire sexual act
    b. Use of sterile needles and drug paraphernalia in injecting drug use
    c. Introduction of the concept of "universal precautions" in sexual contact and injecting drug use, since some individuals may not be aware of or disclose their HIV seropositivity, while others may lie about it for sex or when exchanging sex for drugs
    d. Referral for alcohol or other drug abuse or dependence treatment
3. Condom availability—provide bowls of condoms with open access in psychiatric inpatient and outpatient facilities
4. Education about HIV, AIDS, and other blood-borne or sexually transmitted diseases such as hepatitis; readily available HIV and hepatitis B and C testing; information about hepatitis B vaccination

psychiatric disorders may lack access to medical care until their psychiatric disorders are treated.

Emergency rooms

Access to care through emergency evaluation can occur when a medical or a psychiatric complication occurs. Psychiatric emergencies affecting the HIV-positive individual can be associated with the direct effect of the virus on the brain, psychiatric symptoms secondary to medical illness, psychological distress related to the infection, or other factors such as substance abuse or homelessness (Lyketsos et al., 1995; Cunningham et al., 2005). The high frequency of multimorbid psychiatric symptoms in HIV-positive individuals often prompts psychiatric consultations when the patient presents for a medical emergency. The uncertain etiology of the presenting symptoms also requires a higher level of collaboration between the medical and psychiatric teams.

Patients who lack a regular source of medical care often gain access to care through emergency care settings (Swartz et al., 2003; Joyce et al., 2005). HIV status, drug use, and marginal housing have been associated with higher use of emergency services (Palepu et al., 1999; Kagay et al., 2004). Frequent use of emergency services has also been linked to higher mortality (Hansagi et al., 1990). In a large sample of drug users, Lundgren and colleagues (2005) found that use of the emergency room was strongly associated with mental health status and severity of drug use, whereas homelessness, HIV status, and sociodemographic factors were not.

Cunningham and colleagues (2005) evaluated utilization patterns of a highly marginalized population in New York City and found high levels of access to and use of ambulatory care services, along with high use of acute care services. Knowlton and colleagues (2005) found that persons with HIV and AIDS who had larger numbers of drug users in their support networks were more likely to have suboptimal emergency-room use than were persons with fewer drug users in their support systems. Enhancement of the support networks of HIV-positive individuals may lead to improvement in medical service utilization among underserved populations.

Leserman and colleagues (2005) found that patients with a history of trauma, recent stressful events, and posttraumatic stress disorder (PTSD) are more likely to require visits to the emergency room. Patients with a history of abuse had twice the risk of having an overnight stay in the hospital or an emergency-room visit compared to those without a history of abuse.

Despite availability for appropriate treatment, utilization of emergency care remains high, especially by populations struggling to maintain ongoing and stable treatment, such as active drug users and homeless persons. The development of case management teams in HIV clinics is likely to facilitate stability and continuity of care (Okin et al., 2000; Witbeck et al., 2000). Education for risk reduction is applicable here as well.

Psychiatric outpatient clinics

Psychiatrists and other mental health professionals are in an ideal position to prevent HIV transmission, encourage behavior change, and ensure adherence to care in persons with HIV and AIDS. Psychiatrists routinely take detailed and thorough substance use and sexual histories and thus may be able to recognize risky behaviors and encourage not only behavior change but also HIV testing. Psychiatrists also have long-term, trusting relationships with patients and routinely work with patients to identify and alter self-destructive behavior patterns. The ambulatory psychiatric setting may be an ideal place to provide education for prevention of transmission as well as adherence to medical care for persons with HIV and AIDS. The introduction of antiretroviral therapies has shifted most of the care for HIV-positive individuals from inpatient care to outpatient settings. There are several different models for delivery of HIV ambulatory medical and mental health care. Before discussing these models, however, it is important to discuss how conventional medical systems address the multiplicity of needs of persons with HIV and AIDS.

Because the HIV virus can affect every organ and every system in the human body, the expertise of a wide range of professionals is needed to address both the medical and the psychosocial needs of patients (Cohen, 1992). However, different treatment settings are often compartmentalized and isolated from each other, making a multidisciplinary approach difficult to achieve. Traditionally, mental health clinics, substance abuse clinics, and infectious disease or HIV clinics have been separate units and isolated from one another in general hospitals. Furthermore, specialized professionals often lack the ability to identify patients' needs that are not related to their particular expertise (Rosenheck and Lam, 1997).

Persons with HIV/AIDS and especially persons who are coinfected with hepatitis C often have multiple coexisting problems such as psychiatric and addictive disorders in addition to housing and financial instability that interfere with successful management of their care (Goldberg, 2005). Because these different issues are often addressed by different disciplines, fragmentation of care often leads to difficulty with entry into care, as well as easy disengagement. Although the fragmentation of care may occur with any combination of disabilities that cut across system boundaries, it is more likely to occur when psychiatric and substance use disorders are involved (Budin et al., 2004; Klinkenberg and Sacks, 2004). Psychiatric disorders cause disability in themselves, which, through effects on cognition, mood, and motivation, may have a disproportionate impact on the ability to negotiate a complex care system (Scheft and Fontenette, 2005; Willenbring, 2005).

Some innovative hospitals are able and willing to integrate medical, mental health, and substance abuse treatment within their programs. This integrated treatment approach enables staff to identify and treat individuals who often fall through the cracks in nonintegrated programs and therefore provide care to an even more impaired population (Batki, 1990; Gomez et al., 1999; American Psychiatric Association, 2000). Integrated care can be based in HIV clinics, infectious disease clinics, mental health centers, substance abuse treatment centers, or community-based centers. Integrated models vary in the degree and quality of the different services provided. These differences are often secondary to organizational constraints (Friedmann et al., 1999). The most common model in the United States is based in a medical clinic and uses a mental health case manager to identify needs and refer patients to psychiatric treatment (Gomez et al., 1999; Brunettte et al., 2003). More specialized centers offer psychiatric treatment within the medical clinic, identifying psychiatric and psychological needs at a very early stage. A different approach designates a psychiatrist in a mental health center as primary provider. Having a psychiatrist as the primary treatment provider can facilitate coordination of the medical and psychiatric care with the addiction treatment. In the United Kingdom, the National Health System designates a general practitioner to provide both medical and psychiatric care, with referral to specialist care provided only for the more complicated cases. Placing a medical provider in a mental health agency is another approach that may prove effective (Brunette et al., 2003).

While an integrated medical, psychiatric, and substance abuse treatment approach is crucial for basic care, integration of a fourth component, addressing community outreach, would engage the individuals who are not able to access the system and significantly optimize the care delivered to this population. Most evidence supporting integrated care is from observational data. Outcomes most often found to improve are process-of-care outcomes and patient satisfaction (Budin et al., 2004). Most randomized, controlled trials do not demonstrate the superiority of integrated care. The poor quality of available evidence may be a result of the difficulty in conceptualizing, planning, funding, and conducting large randomized, controlled trials for persons with HIV who are marginally domiciled or undomiciled and inconsistently adherent with medical care. However, preliminary results from available studies appear very promising (Taylor, 2005). Clearly, much more needs to be done to identify effective strategies for improving outcomes in these populations. Until this treatment modality is validated, integration may be desirable on a pragmatic basis alone (Willenbring, 2005).

Direct observation treatment

Directly observed therapy (DOT) has been historically used in the treatment of tuberculosis (TB), for which DOT programs have improved cure rates in hard-to-reach populations and have proved to be highly cost-effective (Gourevitch et al., 1998). HIV and TB are both infectious diseases that affect similar populations. Both populations may be poorly connected with the health system, thus it is very difficult to prevent, treat, and contain the spread of the infection. For both infections poor adherence increases the likelihood of the development of resistant strains, thus increasing the likelihood of the development of significant and resistant epidemics. As with TB, DOT may benefit HIV-infected people who have difficulty adhering to antiretroviral therapy (previously called highly active antiretroviral therapy, or HAART, and combination antiretroviral therapy, or CART, and now referred to as antiretroviral therapy, or ART). Directly observed therapy for management of HIV infection has been effective among prisoners and in pilot programs in Haiti, Rhode Island, and Florida (Mitty et al., 2002).

Many HIV-positive individuals are injection drug users who receive agonist treatment in methadone maintenance therapy programs. These programs require individuals to attend daily and receive methadone under direct observation. Such programs provide a unique opportunity to administer ART to HIV-infected persons in conjunction with their methadone therapy (Clarke et al., 2002).

Directly observed therapy has been tested in several pilot programs either in the administration of ART alone or in combination with methadone maintenance. These published observational accounts suggest that DOT may be effective (Teplin, 1990; Searight and Pound, 1994; Witbeck et al., 2000; Clarke et al., 2002; McCance-Katz et al., 2002; Mitty et al., 2002; Centers for Disease Control and Prevention [CDC], 2003; Conway et al., 2004; Kagay et al., 2004; Lucas et al., 2004; Macalino et al., 2004; Scheft and Fontanette, 2005), but a more definitive answer awaits the publication of randomized, controlled trials. As far as prisons are concerned, long-term studies will need to assess the long-term outcome following release from prison and the ability to keep these individuals connected with the health system. The correctional setting may provide an opportunity to safely treat patients with comorbid HCV and HIV (Reindollar, 2005). Potentially, DOT could be combined with pharmacotherapy for psychiatric and addictive disorders in addition to methadone, greatly improving adherence to medications in this population (Willenbring, 2005).

Psychiatric inpatient units

Persons with HIV can be admitted to a psychiatric hospital for many reasons, including psychiatric complications of the virus, psychological distress associated with the HIV diagnosis, or psychiatric symptoms related to an underlying psychiatric disorder such as substance dependence. Many persons with HIV and AIDS have multimorbid medical and psychiatric disorders. AIDS-phobic, HIV-bereaved, and factitious HIV-positive admissions are also HIV-related admissions encountered in psychiatric units. The crisis that leads to psychiatric admission can be used to help a person with a risk behavior to get HIV tested. The safe and secure setting of an inpatient unit is ideal for assisting the newly diagnosed person with coping with the news, developing a support network, and engaging in medical care. From education to testing to beginning antiretroviral therapy, the supportive setting of an inpatient psychiatric unit can be lifesaving and help a person with HIV or an established AIDS diagnosis to better cope with the illness. The public health implications of such care are significant, as is the value of care in preventing HIV illness progression. Availability of education, testing, and condoms can decrease anxiety and suffering, prevent morbidity and mortality, and protect others from HIV transmission.

NURSING HOMES AND LONG-TERM CARE FACILITIES

During the beginning of the AIDS epidemic, most persons with AIDS did not survive long enough to require long-term care. Just as medical advances have enabled more people in the general population to survive to older ages, persons with AIDS are surviving and living longer with their illnesses (Cohen, 1998). Admission of HIV-infected patients to nursing homes in the initial phase of the HIV epidemic was difficult because of prejudice and lack of knowledge (Gentry et al., 1994). During the first decade of the HIV epidemic, these nursing homes provided end-of-life and palliative care for patients whose life expectancy was very limited. With the advent of ART, life expectancy greatly increased and many patients were able to return to a functioning and overall healthy life in the community. Most of the medical and psychiatric care shifted from the general hospital and nursing home to the community.

In the last decade, the role of nursing homes in the treatment of HIV patients has changed, to meet the needs of a different reality. Many HIV nursing homes closed, while others started to integrate HIV treatment with non-HIV treatment. The number of nursing homes specifically treating HIV patients is nonetheless limited worldwide. The vast majority of nursing homes in the United States do not provide any specialty areas for HIV/ AIDS care. As our population ages and the life span of those diagnosed with HIV/AIDS continues to increase, nursing homes will see more and more patients diagnosed with HIV/AIDS among those seeking care (Pearson and Heuston, 2004).

The average person with HIV admitted to a nursing home in the United States is between age 40 and 60, male, and more likely to be African American or Latino American. Comorbid psychiatric diagnoses (especially dementia) as well as substance dependence and poor social support are prevalent among nursing home patients who are HIV infected (Cohen, 1998; Shin et al., 2002). HIV residents with dementia are significantly more likely to have other diseases, infections, and other health care conditions then other residents with HIV (Buchanan et al., 2001). Despite the multiple complications secondary to psychiatric comorbidities, patients with AIDS who have a psychiatric condition have more favorable admission characteristics and have a better prognosis. Persons with HIV and psychiatric disorders are likely to be admitted earlier in their disease course for reasons not due to HIV infection, may have fewer discharge options in the community, and, therefore, are more likely to stay in the nursing home until they die (Gentry et al., 1994; Goulet et al., 2000).

During their stay in the nursing home, patients' physical and psychological state greatly improves if specialized care is provided. The physical status of the residents improves as evidenced by an increase in body weight, increased CD4 count, and lowered viral loads. Furthermore, there is evidence of improved self-acceptance and self-confidence coupled with diminished levels of psychopathology (Carroll et al., 2000; McGovern et al., 2002). A comprehensive psychiatric program should include individual, couple, family, and group psychotherapy; bereavement interventions; pain management; and support for staff. An educational program can prevent violence and create innovative ways to maximize residual cognitive function and coping strategies. By creating a supportive and accepting environment and addressing pain and psychological distress, individuals with late-stage AIDS can live more comfortable lives, die in a more dignified and peaceful manner, and have fewer requests for hastened death (Cohen, 1998, 1999).

Despite the great improvement in treatment for HIV and AIDS, long-term nursing home care for people with AIDS has a significant role in the care of patients with advanced disease, acute convalescence, long-term care, and terminal care (Blustein et al., 1992; Dore et al., 1999). The need for long-term care may continue to grow for patients who do not respond fully to current antiretroviral therapies or have significant neuropsychiatric comorbidities (Selwyn et al., 2000). By creating a bridge between acute hospital care and the community, these facilities can provide a cost-effective alternative when people with HIV can no longer receive appropriate care using home and community-based services (McGovern et al., 2002). The prospect of increasing prevalence of HIV-associated dementia in people with advanced HIV disease similarly increases the role for the nursing home in the treatment of HIV (Cohen, 1999; Carroll et al., 2000). Finally, nursing homes may be the best and last option for the nonadherent patient with late-stage AIDS to have DOT with antiretrovirals; such treatment may prove to be a lifesaving and life-changing experience.

SUBSTANCE ABUSE TREATMENT

Methadone maintenance treatment programs

Substance abuse programs address physical and psychological treatment of individuals who are abusing alcohol, cocaine, opioids, or other substances. While treatment of most addictions includes short-term physical detoxification followed by long-term psychiatric and psychological care, treatment of opioid addiction most frequently consists of therapy with opioid or mu-receptor agonists such as methadone administered in methadone maintenance treatment programs.

There is a high prevalence of infection with blood-borne organisms in individuals who are injection drug users, and many clients are monoinfected or coinfected with HIV and hepatitis C virus. HIV infection is frequently transmitted by the sharing of contaminated needles, syringes, and other drug paraphernalia. HIV infection is also transmitted through unprotected sexual activity that may have occurred as a result of disinhibition during intoxication or the exchange of sex for drugs. More than 35% of new HIV cases are among injection drug users, their sexual partners, and their offspring (CDC, 2006a).

Methadone maintenance treatment programs provide a significant opportunity for both preventing and diagnosing HIV infection. Clients come on a regular basis and are usually required to have a counselor and to attend groups as well as 12-step programs. Staff members at these programs are in an ideal position to educate about reduction of risky behaviors and provide access to barrier contraception by making free condoms available.

Methadone maintenance programs are ideal settings for providing DOT with ART and treatment for hepatitis C. From education to testing and diagnosis to direct-observation ART treatment, methadone maintenance programs can be lifesaving to persons with HIV and AIDS.

Integrated opioid agonist maintenance treatment

In the United States, policies that would allow physicians and private group practices to provide opioid agonist treatment have been under consideration. This would entail prescribing opioid agonist treatment outside the traditional setting of methadone maintenance treatment programs.

Needle exchange programs

Syringe exchange programs (SEPs) in the United States and elsewhere were developed in response to the spread of hepatitis B virus, hepatitis C virus, and HIV among injection drug users. These programs limit one of the main vectors of blood-borne infectious diseases: the sharing of contaminated needles and syringes. Through these programs clean needles and syringes are exchanged for used ones free of charge. This practice also promotes harm reduction (Kaplan and Heimer, 1994; Normand et al., 1995). While there is scientific and individual consensus that SEPs are an important part of infectious disease prevention, there is political controversy about providing injections drug users access to clean needles at no cost.

Grau and colleagues (2005) compared psychosocial and behavioral differences among intravenous drug users who used or did not use syringe exchange programs and found no demographic or psychosocial differences between the two groups. The most significant factor distinguishing the two groups was self-efficacy.

Supervised injecting centers

Medically supervised injecting centers (SICs) are "legally sanctioned and supervised facilities designated to reduce the health and public order problems associated with illegal injection drug use" (Wright and Tompkins, 2004). The primary objectives of the these centers are reduction of fatal and nonfatal overdose, reduction of risk of infectious disease, and increased access to medical, addiction, and psychiatric care (Wright and Tompkins, 2004).

Injection drug users attending SICs are provided with a safe and clean environment, medical care, and referral resources. Supervised injecting centers are also referred to as health rooms, supervised injecting rooms, drug consumption rooms, and safer injecting rooms. They operate in over 26 European cities, Australia, and Canada. In the only comprehensive evaluation of SICs (conducted in Sydney, Australia) a reduction of injecting-related problems was reported (Dolan et al., 2000). Recent reports confirm a decrease in drug-related death rates as well as of drug users in countries with a comprehensive policy addressing harm reduction through use of SICs, such as Switzerland (Kerr et al., 2005) and the Netherlands (Wood et al., 2004). The UN International Narcotics Control Board, however, views the SIC as violating international drug conventions, and public opinion remains divided about these centers.

COMMUNITY TREATMENT

Many factors are involved in nonadherence to medical and psychiatric care of patients affected by HIV, including drug use, cognitive disorders associated with HIV, history of PTSD (Cohen et al., 2001; Kerr et al., 2004), poor financial and social support, psychiatric diagnoses, and poor access to care. Health-care plans focusing solely on the delivery of medical and psychiatric care within hospital settings are unable to provide services to the most vulnerable patients affected by HIV, mental illness, and substance abuse at the same time. Community-based services with intensive case management that provide a wide array of services and are tailored to each patient's needs have a significant impact on providing access to care as well as on retention in care. These ancillary services include case management; mental health and substance abuse treatment and counseling; advocacy; respite and buddy or companion services; food, housing, and emergency financial assistance; and transportation.

Assertive community treatment and intensive case management

Community-based treatment can be delivered through an assertive community treatment (ACT) or intensive case management. Both modalities are patient focused and attempt to create a link between the patient and medical services by addressing the specific additional needs of each patient. Assertive community treatment has a special emphasis on a team approach. These multidisciplinary teams share caseloads and meet frequently. Intensive case management, by contrast, encompasses a variety of community-based programs involving individual caseloads and a less defined structure. Assertive community treatment teams mirror the medical model of care in which psychiatrists and nurses have critical roles, and its goal is the provision of comprehensive treatment and rehabilitation that do not broker services. In contrast, the principal function of intensive case management is to link and coordinate services as well as increase community integration (Schaedle et al., 2002).

In recent years, ACT services have expanded to target the homeless population (Burnam et al., 1995; Rosenheck and Dennis, 2001). Studies examining the impact of these services on medical care show improved adherence and retention in primary care of the patients receiving multiple services. The number of services provided seems to be significantly associated with improved adherence, improved retention, and a decreased number of hospitalizations and emergency visits. These findings suggest that receipt of case management and ancillary services is associated with improvement in multiple outcomes for HIV-infected patients (Braucht et al., 1995; Rahav et al., 1995; Lin et al., 1998; Thompson et al., 1998; Magnus et al., 2001; Ashman et al., 2002; Sherer et al., 2002; Harris et al., 2003; Woods et al., 2003).

Homeless adolescents

Studies examining the impact of community services on homeless adolescents infected with and affected by HIV suggest that outreach is not only important in initially connecting hard-to-reach young persons to services but also necessary for retention in care (Woods et al., 2000, 2002). The impact of these services seems to be significantly related to the number of contacts with the community team. This higher threshold level suggests that establishing a relationship between the service provider and the client may be critical to client retention in care (Baldwin et al., 1996; Woods et al., 1998). Regardless of the way these supportive services are provided, they represent an extraordinary link between vulnerable adolescents and medical and psychiatric care.

CORRECTIONAL FACILITIES

HIV in prison

The incarcerated population in the United States has increased dramatically over the past two decades and is currently over two million individuals (Rich et al., 2005). The United States now has the highest per-capita incarceration rate in the world. This phenomenon has been fueled in large part by the "war on drugs," which has led to an increase in drug-related arrests coupled with strict mandatory sentencing requirements. Over the past 20 years, the number of people incarcerated annually for drug-related offenses has grown from 40,000 to 450,000, resulting in an incarcerated population with high rates of reported drug use. An estimated 80% of incarcerated individuals have a history of substance abuse, whereas as many as 20% of state prisoners report a history of injection drug use (Rich et al., 2005).

While injection drug use in correctional facilities is documented to be a problem, qualitative research into the HIV risks faced by inmates is lacking. The harm normally associated with drug addiction and injection drug use is exacerbated in prison. Studies examining the prevalence of medical illnesses in prison show that infectious diseases constitute the most prevalent major disease category among inmates (Baillargeon et al., 2000). Prevalence rates of HIV among male inmates have been recorded at between 6% and 8.5%, and one study of incarcerated women in New York found an 18.8% rate of HIV infection (Weisfuse et al., 1991).

The absence of adequate methadone maintenance programs, the difficult living conditions, the lack of personal space, the lack of social and inter-personal support, the violence and abuse, and the availability of drugs often increase the perceived need to use substances within the prison (Hughes, 2001), thus facilitating the spread of HIV and hepatitis C in the community (Laurence, 2005). The absence of needle exchange programs in prisons has resulted in patterns of needle sharing among large numbers of persons. Continual reuse of syringes poses serious health hazards; bleach distribution is an inadequate solution (Small et al., 2005). Depriving prisoners of the means to protect themselves from HIV infection and failing to provide prisoners living with HIV with care, treatment, and support equivalent to that available in the community at-large offend international human rights norms (Dubler et al., 1990; Betteridge, 2004; Jurgens, 2004).

It is estimated that 3%–11% of prison inmates have co-occurring mental health disorders and substance abuse disorders (Teplin, 1990; Edens et al., 1997). Patients with psychiatric disorders are more likely to engage in behaviors that increase their risk of HIV infection because of their limited impulse control, difficulties in establishing stable social and sexual relation-ships, limited knowledge about HIV-related risk factors, increased susceptibility to coercion, and comorbid alcohol and drug use. These same characteristics often lead to incarceration, making the prevalence of psychiatric disorders among inmates particularly high. Studies evaluating psychiatric disorders in prisons indicate that HIV-infected inmates exhibit consistently higher rates of psychiatric disorders than those for their uninfected counterparts. These associations persist across all psychiatric disorders and across demographic factors (Baillargeon et al., 2003).

Dual-diagnosis treatment programs have been developed in state and federal prisons. Many of these have evolved from existing substance abuse treatment programs and approaches. Dual-diagnosis treatment in prisons includes an extended assessment period, orientation and motivational activities, psychoeducational groups, cognitive-behavioral interventions such as restructuring of "criminal thinking errors," self-help groups, medication monitoring, relapse prevention, and transition into institution or community-based aftercare facilities (Edens et al., 1997).

Drug treatment in prison

The current policy for the management and treatment of addictions in prisons is highly controversial. The first needle exchange program within a prison was started in 1992 in Switzerland. All European evaluations of these programs have been favorable. Drug use decreased or remained stable over time, and syringe sharing declined dramatically. No new cases of HIV, hepatitis B, or hepatitis C were reported. The evaluations found no reports of serious unintended negative events, such as initiation of injection or use of needles as weapons (Dolan et al., 2003a).

Methadone has been widely used for over 35 years to treat opiate-dependent individuals. Short-term detoxification with methadone is rarely successful and often is followed by a rapid relapse to heroin use. The aim of methadone maintenance treatment is to stabilize opiate-dependent individuals in the long term; it has been shown to significantly reduce opiate use and its associated risks (Bellin et al., 1999). This long-term stabilization and continuous contact with medical providers greatly improve the individual's quality of life and have significant social advantages (Rich et al., 2005). In U.S. prisons, methadone treatment is currently confined to treatment of pregnant individuals, treatment of methadone withdrawal (for those in community methadone maintenance treatment), and detoxification of opiate-dependent inmates. Despite the high risk of relapse to drug use and overdose in the period immediately following release from correctional facilities, only occasionally are opiate-dependent inmates referred to methadone programs upon release (Dolan and Wodak, 1996; Dolan et al., 2003b; Rich et al., 2005). Programs enhancing the linkage between prison and community treatment have been developed in recent years. These programs show that transitional linkage to methadone maintenance treatment is feasible and extremely important in combating the cycle of drug relapse, related risk behavior, and criminality among the incarcerated, opiate-dependent population (Rich et al., 2005).

Sexual behavior in prison

Risk of HIV infection in prison is mainly from needle sharing. Unprotected sexual intercourse is another high-risk behavior that is common practice in prisons. Unprotected sexual activity can be secondary to sexual deprivation or disinhibition related to drug use, or result from exchange of sex for drugs among inmates. In addition, in the U.S. federal penitentiary system, conjugal visits are prohibited, leading to further sexual deprivation among inmates who would otherwise have a source of sexual satisfaction in a monogamous relationship.

Although there is evidence of condom use among inmates, most research has tended to focus on adolescent populations (Kingree et al., 2000; Castrucci and Martin, 2002; Nagamune and Bellis, 2002). Most studies focus on issues related to inmates' access to condoms while incarcerated. Very few studies target sexual behaviors of adult male inmates in the United States. In recent studies, both marijuana and cocaine were found to be significant predictors of not using a condom during sex prior to incarceration. Education level appears to be another predictor of the reported frequency of sexual intercourse (Braithwaite and Stephens, 2005). These data can be extremely helpful for the development of health education curricula for inmate populations.

Maltreatment, discrimination, and quarantine of HIV-seropositive individuals in correctional facilities

The correctional facility setting tends to magnify the stigma and discrimination that persons with HIV and AIDS may experience in the community at large. In the 29 years since the onset of the AIDS epidemic, some of the most overt stigma and discrimination have diminished as a result of campaigns targeting the general public and educating about risk behaviors. While obvious evidence of stigma may be lower than in the past, recent surveys have uncovered persisting attitudes of fear, judgment, and mistrust toward individuals living with HIV (Herek et al., 2002). It is understandable, therefore, that many individuals with HIV fear the consequences of stigma when their diagnosis becomes known to others.

Patients with HIV and AIDS report discrimination not only from the community but also from treatment providers. Many individuals report experiencing coerced testing; others were refused treatment after disclosing their HIV status; others reported delays in the provision of health-care services (Gruskin, 2004); Schuster et al., 2005). Such fears are likely to have detrimental effects on these individuals and persons at risk for HIV (Bird et al., 2004). They will also affect the success of programs and policies intended to prevent HIV transmission. Thus, eradicating AIDS stigma remains an important public health goal for effectively combating HIV (Cohen, 1990; Searight and Pound, 1994; Alonzo and Reynolds, 1995; Annas, 1998; Gostin and Webber, 1998; Gostin et al., 1999; Herek et al., 2002; Schuster et al., 2005).

In the correctional system, individuals living with HIV and individuals living with psychiatric conditions are forced to endure great discrimination. Mentally ill inmates are often denied reductions in sentences, parole opportunities, placement in less restrictive facilities, and opportunities to participate in sentence-reducing programs because of their status as psychiatric patients or their need for psychotropic medications (Miller and Metzner, 1994). HIV-positive inmates are often isolated and denied appropriate specialized medical treatment. The effect of this kind of discrimination is very severe, since adherence to a strict medication schedule is necessary for antiretroviral therapy to be effective. These two vulnerable populations face even more discrimination in other countries where education about psychiatric conditions and HIV is limited. In some countries patients with HIV have been quarantined or sanctioned to mandatory sanatoriums (Baldwin et al., 1996; Hansen and Groce, 2003). Both under-developed and developed countries continue to need educational policies addressing discrimination against both psychiatric and HIV-positive populations, which remain vulnerable in our societies (Merati and Supriyati, 2005).

AIDSISM AND THE MULTIPLE DISPARITIES OF HIV AND AIDS

AIDSism results from a multiplicity of prejudicial and discriminatory factors and is built on a foundation of racism, homophobia, ageism, addictophobia, misogyny, and discomfort with mental and medical illness, poverty, sexuality, infection, and death in many communities throughout the world as well as in the United States. AIDSism has contributed to disparities in the care of persons with HIV and AIDS.

Racial, ethnic, and socioeconomic disparities

Racial, ethnic, and socioeconomic disparities have been observed and documented in all aspects of the U.S. health-care system (Agency for Health Care Research and Quality, 2005a). The overall HIV death rate of African

Americans was found to be 10.95 times higher than that of whites (Agency for Health Care Research and Quality, 2005b), and racial disparities have been shown to contribute to increased HIV incidence and inadequate access to medical and psychiatric care (CDC, 2006c). U.S. correctional facilities and urban drug epicenters may be seen as microcosms of discrimination. Correctional facilities may also be instrumental in perpetuating the HIV epidemic both inside and outside of prison walls (Hammett et al., 2002; Blankenship et al., 2005; Golembeski and Fullilove, 2005; CDC, 2006b; Fullilove, 2008).

It would be difficult to estimate the true impact of these disparities on persons with HIV and AIDS. In addition to the incalculable distress, suffering, and anguish experienced (Cohen et al., 2002), many persons with AIDS have multimorbid medical illnesses and psychiatric illnesses in the setting of disparities in health care (Cohen et al., 1991; Cohen, 1996; Kolb et al., 2006).

Psychiatric disparities

Psychiatric factors take on new relevance and meaning as we approach the end of the third decade of the AIDS pandemic. Persons with AIDS are living longer and healthier lives as a result of appropriate medical care and advances in antiretroviral therapy. However, in the United States and throughout the world, some men, women, and children with AIDS are unable to benefit from medical progress. Inadequate access to care results from a multiplicity of barriers, including economic, social, political, and psychiatric obstacles. Psychiatric disorders and distress play a significant role in the transmission of, exposure to, and infection with HIV (Cohen and Alfonso, 1994, 1998; Blank et al., 2002). They are relevant to prevention, clinical care, and adherence throughout every aspect of illness from the initial risk behavior to death. They result in considerable suffering from diagnosis to end-stage illness (Cohen and Alfonso, 2004). Untreated psychiatric disorders can be exacerbated by HIV stigma to make persons with HIV and AIDS especially vulnerable to suicide (Marzuk et al., 1988; Perry et al., 1990; McKegney and O'Dowd, 1992; Alfonso and Cohen, 1997). Psychiatric treatment with individual (Cohen and Weisman, 1986; Cohen, 1987; Cohen and Alfonso, 1998, 2004), group (Alfonso and Cohen, 1997), and family therapy can help alleviate suffering, improve adherence, and prevent suicide.

CONCLUSION

Having a clear understanding of both the problems and the potentials for intervention in special settings may lead to decreased HIV transmission and to improvement in the quality of the lives of persons with HIV and AIDS.

References

Aberg JA, Kaplan JE, Libman H, Emmanuel P, Anderson JR, Stone VE, Oleske JM, Currier JS, Gallant JE (2009). Primary care guidelines for the management of persons infected with human immunodeficiency virus: 2009 Update by the HIV Medicine Association of the Infectious Diseases Society of America. *Clin Infect Dis* 49:651–681. Retrieved August 23, 2009, from http://www.journals.uchicago.edu/doi/pdf/10.1086/605292 and http://www.journals.uchicago.edu/page/cid/IDSAguidelines.html

Agency for Health Care Research and Quality (2005a). *National healthcare disparities report, 2005*. Retrieved March 20, 2007, from http://www.ahrq.gov/qual/nhdr05/nhdr05.htm.

Agency for Healthcare Research and Quality, Rockville, MD (2005b). *National healthcare disparities report, 2005. Appendix D: data tables*. Retrieved March 20, 2007, from http://www.ahrq.gov/qual/nhdr05/nhdr05.htm.

Alfonso CA, Cohen MAA (1997). The role of group psychotherapy in the care of persons with AIDS. *J Am Acad Psychoanal* 25:623–638.

Alonzo AA, Reynolds NR (1995). Stigma, HIV and AIDS: an exploration and elaboration of a stigma trajectory. *Soc Sci Med* 41:303–315.

American Psychiatric Association (2000). Practice guideline for the treatment of patients with HIV/AIDS. Work Group on HIV/AIDS. *Am J Psychiatry* 157:1–62.

Annas GJ (1998). Protecting patients from discrimination—the Americans with Disabilities Act and HIV infection. *N Engl J Med* 339:1255–1259.

Ashman JJ, Conviser R, Pounds MB (2002). Associations between HIV-positive individuals' receipt of ancillary services and medical care receipt and retention. *AIDS Care* 14:109–118.

Baillargeon J, Black SA, Pulvino J, Dunn K (2000). The disease profile of Texas prison inmates. *Ann Epidemiol* 10:74–80.

Baillargeon J, Ducate S, Pulvino J, Bradshaw P, Murray O, Olvera R (2003). The association of psychiatric disorders and HIV infection in the correctional setting. *Ann Epidemiol* 13:606–612.

Baldwin JA, Bowen AM, Trotter RR (1996). Factors contributing to retention of not-in-treatment drug users in an HIV/AIDS outreach prevention project. *Drugs Soc* 9:19–35.

Batki SL (1990). Drug abuse, psychiatric disorders, and AIDS: dual and triple diagnosis. *West J Med* 152:547–552.

Bellin E, Wesson J, Tomasino V, Nolan J, Glick AJ, Oquendo S (1999). High-dose methadone reduces criminal recidivism in opiate addicts. *Addict Res* 7:19–29.

Betteridge G (2004). Prisoners' health and human rights in the HIV/AIDS epidemic. *HIV AIDS Policy Law Rev* 9:96–99.

Bird ST, Bogart LM, Delahanty DL (2004). Health-related correlates of perceived discrimination in HIV care. *AIDS Patient Care STDS* 18:19–26.

Blank MB, Mandell DS, Aiken L, Hadley TR. (2002). Co-occurrence of HIV and serious mental illness among Medicaid recipients. *Psychiatr Serv* 53:868–873.

Blankenship KM, Smoyer AB, Bray SJ, Mattocks K (2005). Black–white disparities in HIV/AIDS: the role of drug policy in the corrections system. *J Health Care Poor Underserved* 16:140–156.

Blustein J, Schultz B, Knickman J, Kator M, Richardson H, McBride L (1992). AIDS and long-term care: the use of services in an institutional setting. *AIDS Public Policy J* 7:32–41.

Braithwaite R, Stephens T (2005). Use of protective barriers and unprotected sex among adult male prison inmates prior to incarceration. *Int J STD AIDS* 16:224–226.

Braucht GN, Reichardt CS, Geissler LJ, Bormann CA, Kwiatkowski CF, Kirby MW (1995). Effective services for homeless substance abusers. *J Addict Dis* 14:87–109.

Brunette MF, Drake RE, Marsh BJ, Torrey WC, Rosenberg SD (2003). Responding to blood-borne infections among persons with severe mental illness. *Psychiatr Serv* 54:860–865.

Buchanan RJ, Wang S, Huang C (2001). Analyses of nursing home residents with HIV and dementia using the minimum data set. *J Acquir Immune Defic Syndr* 26:246–255.

Budin J, Boslaugh S, Beckett E, Winiarski MG (2004). Utilization of psychiatric services integrated with primary care by persons of color with HIV in the inner city. *Commun Ment Health J* 40:365–378.

Burnam MA, Morton SC, McGlynn EA, Petersen LP, Stecher BM, Hayes C, Vaccaro JV (1995). An experimental evaluation of residential and nonresidential treatment for dually diagnosed homeless adults. *J Addict Dis* 14:111–134.

Carroll JF, McGovern JJ, McGinley JJ, Torres JC, Walker JR, Pagan ES, Biafora FA (2000). A program evaluation study of a nursing home operated as a modified therapeutic community for chemically dependent persons with AIDS. *J Subst Abuse Treat* 18:373–386.

Castrucci BC, Martin SL (2002). The association between substance use and risky sexual behaviors among incarcerated adolescents. *Maternal Child Health J* 6:43–47.

[CDC] Centers for Disease Control and Prevention (2003). Prevention and control of infections with hepatitis viruses in correctional settings. *MMWR Recomm Rep* 52: 1–36.

[CDC] Centers for Disease Control and Prevention (2006a) Epidemiology of HIV/AIDS—United States, 1981–2005. *MMWR Morb Mortal Wkly Rep* 55 (21):589–592.

[CDC] Centers for Disease Control and Prevention (2006b). HIV transmission among male inmates in a state prison system—Georgia, 1992–2005. *MMWR Morb Mortal Wkly Rep* 55: 421–426.

[CDC] Centers for Disease Control and Prevention (2006c). Racial/ethnic disparities in diagnoses of HIV/AIDS—33 states, 2001–2004. *MMWR Morb Mortal Wkly Rep* 55:121–125.

Clarke S, Keenan E, Ryan M, Barry M, Mulcahy F (2002). Directly observed antiretroviral therapy for injection drug users with HIV infection. *AIDS Read* 12:305–316.

Cohen MA (1987). Psychiatric aspects of AIDS: A biopsychosocial approach. In GP Wormser, RE Stahl, and EJ Bottone (eds.), *AIDS Acquired Immune Deficiency Syndrome and Other Manifestations of HIV Infection*. Park Ridge, NJ: Noyes Publishers.

Cohen MA (1989). AIDSism, a new form of discrimination. *Am Med News*, January 20, 32:43.

Cohen MA (1990). Biopsychosocial approach to the human immunodeficiency virus epidemic. A clinician's primer. *Gen Hosp Psychiatry* 12:98–123.

Cohen MA (1992). Biopsychosocial aspects of the HIV epidemic. In GP Wormser (ed.), *AIDS and Other Manifestations of HIV Infection*, second ed. (pp. 349–371). New York: Raven Press.

Cohen MAA (1996). Creating health care environments to meet patients' needs. *Curr Issues Public Health* 2:232–240.

Cohen MA (1998). Psychiatric care in an AIDS nursing home. *Psychosomatics* 39:154–161.

Cohen MA (1999). Psychodynamic psychotherapy in an AIDS nursing home. *J Am Acad Psychoanal* 27:121–133.

Cohen MAA, Aladjem AD, Horton A, Lima J, Palacios A, Hernandez L, Mehta P (1991). How can we combat excess mortality in Harlem? A one-day survey of adult general care. *Int J Psychiatry Med* 21:369–378.

Cohen MAA, Alfonso CA (1994). Dissemination of HIV: how serious is it for women, medically and psychologically? *Ann N Y Acad Sci* 736:114–121.

Cohen MA, Alfonso CA (1998). Psychiatric care and pain management in persons with HIV infection. In GP Wormser (ed.), *AIDS and Other Manifestations of HIV Infection*, third ed. Philadelphia: Lippincott-Raven.

Cohen MA, Alfonso CA (2004). AIDS psychiatry: psychiatric and palliative care, and pain management. In GP Wormser (ed.), *AIDS and Other Manifestations of HIV Infection*, fourth ed. (pp. 537–576). San Diego: Elsevier Academic Press.

Cohen MA, Alfonso CA, Hoffman RG, Milau V, Carrera G (2001). The impact of PTSD on treatment adherence in persons with HIV infection. *Gen Hosp Psychiatry* 23:294–296.

Cohen MA, Hoffman RG, Cromwell C, Schmeidler J, Ebrahim F, Carrera G, Endorf F, Alfonso CA, Jacobson JM (2002). The prevalence of distress in persons with human immunodeficiency virus infection. *Psychosomatics* 43:10–15.

Cohen MA, Weisman H (1986). A biopsychosocial approach to AIDS. *Psychosomatics* 27:245–249.

Conway B, Prasad J, Reynolds R, Farley J, Jones M, Jutha S, Smith N, Mead A, DeVlaming S (2004). Directly observed therapy for the management of HIV-infected patients in a methadone program. *Clin Infect Dis* 38:S402–S408.

Cunningham CO, Sohler NL, McCoy K, Heller D, Selwyn PA (2005). Health care access and utilization patterns in unstably housed HIV-infected individuals in New York City. *AIDS Patient Care STDS* 19:690–695.

Dolan K, Kimber J, Fry C, Fitzgerald J, McDonald D, Frautmann F (2000). Drug consumption facilities in Europe and the establishment of supervised injecting centres in Australia. *Drug Alcohol Rev* 19:337–346.

Dolan K, Rutter S, Wodak AD (2003a). Prison-based syringe exchange programmes: a review of international research and development. *Addiction*
98:153–158.

Dolan KA, Shearer JD, MacDonald M, Mattick RP, Hall W, Wodak AD
(2003b). A randomized controlled trial of methadone maintenance treatment
versus wait list control in an Australian prison. *Drug Alcohol Depend*
72:59–65.

Dolan KA, Wodak A (1996). An international review of methadone provision in
prisons. *Addict Res* 4:85–97.

Dore GJ, Correll PK, Li Y, Kaldor JM, Cooper DA, Brew BJ (1999). Changes to
AIDS dementia complex in the era of highly active antiretroviral therapy.
AIDS 13:1249–1253.

Dubler NN, Bergmann CM, Frankel ME (1990). New York State AIDS Advisory
Council. Ad Hoc Committee on AIDS in correctional facilities management
of HIV infection in New York State prisons. *Columbia Human Rights Law
Rev* 21:363–400.

Edens JF, Peters RH, Hiulls HA (1997). Treating prison inmates with co-
occuring disorders: an integrative review of existing programs. *Behav Sci
Law* 15:439–457.

Friedmann PD, Alexander JA, Jin L, D'Aunno TA (1999). On-site primary care
and mental health services in outpatient drug abuse treatment units. *J Behav
Health Serv Res* 26:80–94.

Fullilove MT (1989). Anxiety and stigmatizing aspects of HIV infection. *J Clin
Psychiatry* 50(Suppl.):5–8.

Gentry D, Fogarty TE, Lehrman S (1994). Providing long-term care for persons
with AIDS: results from a survey of nursing homes in the United States. *AIDS
Patient Care* 8:130–137.

Goldberg RW (2005). Supported medical care: a multi-faceted approach to
helping HIV/hepatitis C virus co-infected adults with serious mental illness.
AIDS 19:S215–S220.

Golembeski C, Fullilove RE (2005). Criminal (in)justice in the city and its
associated health consequences. *Am J Public Health* 95:1701–1706.

Gomez MF, Klein DA, Sand S, Marconi M, O'Dowd MA (1999). Delivering
mental health care to HIV-positive individuals: a comparison of two models.
Psychosomatics 40:321–324.

Gostin LO, Feldblum C, Webber DW (1999). Disability discrimination in
America: HIV/AIDS and other health conditions. *JAMA* 281:745–752.

Gostin LO, Webber DW (1998). HIV infection and AIDS in the public health and
health care systems. *JAMA* 279:1108–1113.

Goulet JL, Molde S, Constantino J, Gaughan D, Selwyn PA (2000). Psychiatric
comorbidity and the long-term care of people with AIDS. *J Urban Health*
77:213–221.

Gourevitch MN, Alcabes P, Wasserman WC, Arno PS (1998). Cost-
effectiveness of directly observed chemoprophylaxis of tuberculosis
among drug users at high risk for tuberculosis. *Int J Tuberc Lung Dis*
2:531–540.

Grau LE, Bluthenthal RN, Marshall P, Singer M, Heimer R (2005). Psychosocial and behavioral differences among drug injectors who use and do not use syringe exchange programs. *AIDS Behav* 9(4):495–505.

Gruskin S (2004). Bangkok 2004. Current issues and concerns in HIV testing: a health and human rights approach. *HIV AIDS Policy Law Rev* 9:99–103.

Hammett TM, Harmon MP, Rhodes W (2002). The burden of infectious disease among inmates of and releasees from US correctional facilities 1997. *Am J Public Health* 92:1789–1794.

Hansagi H, Allebeck P, Edhag O, Magnusson G (1990). Frequency of emergency department attendances as a predictor of mortality: nine-year follow-up of a population-based cohort. *J Public Health Med* 12:39–44.

Hansen H, Groce N (2003). Human immunodeficiency virus and quarantine in Cuba. *JAMA* 290:2875.

Harris SK, Samples CL, Keenan PM, Fox DJ, Melchiono MW, Woods ER; Boston HAPPENS program (2003). Outreach, mental health, and case management services: can they help to retain HIV-positive and at-risk youth and young adults in care? *Matern Child Health J* 7:205–218.

Herek GM, Capitanio JP, Widaman KF (2002). HIV-related stigma and knowledge in the United States: prevalence and trends, 1991–1999. *Am J Public Health* 92:371–377.

Hughes RA (2001). Assessing the influence of need to inject and drug withdrawal on drug injectors' perceptions of HIV risk behavior. *J Psychoact Drugs* 33:185–189.

Joyce GF, Chan KS, Orlando M, Burnam MA (2005). Mental health status and use of general medical services for persons with human immunodeficiency virus. *Med Care* 43:834–839.

Jurgens R (2004). Dublin Declaration on HIV/AIDS in prisons launched. *Can HIV/AIDS Policy Law Rev* 9:40.

Kagay CR, Porco TC, Liechty CA, Charlebois E, Clark R, Guzman D, Moss AR, Bangsberg DR (2004). Modeling the impact of modified directly observed antiretroviral therapy on HIV suppression and resistance, disease progression, and death. *Clin Infect Dis* 38:S414–S420.

Kaplan EH, Heimer R (1994). A circulation theory of needle exchange. *AIDS* 8:567–574.

Kerr T, Palepu A, Barness G, Walsh J, Hogg R, Montaner J, Tyndall M, Wood E (2004). Psychosocial determinants of adherence to highly active antiretroviral therapy among injection drug users in Vancouver. *Antivir Ther* 9:407–414.

Kerr T, Tyndall M, Li K, Montaner J, Wood E (2005). Safer injection facility use and syringe sharing in injection drug users. *Lancet* 366:316–318.

Kingree JB, Braithwaite R, Woodring T (2000). Unprotected sex as a function of alcohol and marijuana use among adolescent detainees. *J Adolesc Health* 27:179–185.

Klinkenberg WD, Sacks S (2004). HIV/AIDS treatment adherence, health outcomes and cost study group: mental disorders and drug abuse in persons living with HIV/AIDS. *AIDS Care* 16:S22–S42.

Knowlton AR, Hua W, Latkin C (2005). Social support networks and medical service use among HIV-positive injection drug users: implication to intervention. *AIDS Care* 17:479–492.

Kolb B, Wallace AM, Hill D, Royce M (2006). Disparities in cancer care among racial and ethnic minorities. *Oncology* 20:1256–1261.

Laurence J (2005). The role of prisons in dissemination of HIV and hepatitis. *AIDS Read* 15:54–55.

Leserman J, Whetten K, Lowe K, Stangl D, Swartz MS, Thielman NM (2005). How trauma, recent stressful events, and PTSD affect functional health status and health utilization in HIV-infected patients in the south. *Psychosom Med* 67:500–507.

Lin YG, Melchiono MW, Huba GJ, Woods ER (1998). Evaluation of a linked service model of care for HIV-positive, homeless and at-risk youths. *AIDS Patient Care STDS* 12:787–796.

Lucas GM, Weidle PJ, Hader S, Moore RD (2004). Directly administered antiretroviral therapy in an urban methadone maintenance clinic: a nonrandomized comparative study. *Clin Infect Dis* 38:S409–S413.

Lundgren L, Chassler D, Ben-Ami L, Purington T, Schilling R (2005). Factors associated with emergency room use among injection drug users of African-American, Hispanic and White-European background. *Am J Addict* 14:268–280.

Lyketsos CG, Fishman M, Treisman G (1995). Psychiatric issues and emergencies in HIV infection. *Emerg Med Clin North Am* 13:163–177.

Macalino GE, Mitty JA, Bazerman LB, Singh K, McKenzie M, Flanigan T (2004). Modified directly observed therapy for the treatment of HIV-seropositive substance users: lessons learned from a pilot study. *Clin Infect Dis* 38:S393–S397.

Magnus M, Schmidt N, Kirkhart K, Schieffelin C, Fuchs N, Brown B, Kissinger PJ (2001). Association between ancillary services and clinical and behavioral outcomes among HIV-infected women. *AIDS Patient Care STDS* 15:137–145.

Marzuk PM, Tierney H, Tardiff K, Gross EM, Morgan EB, Hsu MA, Mann JJ (1988). Increased risk of suicide in persons with AIDS. *JAMA* 259:1333–1337.

McCance-Katz EF, Gourevitch MN, Arnsten J, Sarlo J, Rainey P, Jatlow P (2002). Modified directly observed therapy (MDOT) for injection drug users with HIV disease. *Am J Addict* 11:271–278.

McGovern JJ, Guida F, Corey P (2002). Improved health and self-esteem among patients with AIDS in a therapeutic community nursing program. *J Subst Abuse Treat* 23:437–440.

McKegney FP, O'Dowd MA (1982). Suicidality and HIV status. *Am J Psychiatry* 149:396–398.

Merati T, Supriyati YF (2005). The disjunction between policy and practice: HIV discrimination in health care and employment in Indonesia. *AIDS Care* 17 (Suppl. 2); S175–S179.

Miller RD, Metzner JL (1994). Psychiatric stigma in correctional facilities. *Bull Am Acad Psychiatry Law* 22:621–628.

Mitty J, Stone V, Sands M, Macalino G, Flanigan T (2002). Directly observed therapy for the treatment of people with human immunodeficiency virus infection: a work in progress. *Clin Infect Dis* 34:984–990.

Nagamune N, Bellis JM (2002). Decisional balance of condom use and depressed mood among incarcerated male adolescents. *Acta Med Okayama* 56:287–294.

Normand J, Vlahov D, Moses LE (eds.) (1995). *Preventing HIV Transmission: The Role of Sterile Needles and Bleach*. Washington, DC: National Academy Press.

Okin RL, Boccellari A, Azocar F, Shumway M, O'Brien K, Gelb A, Kohn M, Harding P, Wachsmuth C (2000). The effects of clinical case management on hospital service use among ER frequent users. *Am J Emerg Med* 18:603–608.

Palepu A, Strathdee SA, Hogg RS, Anis AH, Rae S, Cornelisse PG, Patrick DM, O'Shaughnessy MV, Schechter MT (1999). The social determinants of emergency department and hospital use by injection drug users in Canada. *J Urban Health* 76:409–418.

Pearson WS, Hueston WJ (2004). Treatment of HIV/AIDS in the nursing home: variations in rural and urban long-term care settings. *South Med J* 97:338–341.

Perry S, Jacobsberg L, Fishman B (1990). Suicidal ideation and HIV testing. *JAMA* 263:679–682.

Rahav M, Rivera JJ, Nuttbrock L, Nuttbrock L, Ng-Mak D, Sturz EL, Link BG, Struening EL, Pepper B, Gross B (1995). Characteristics and treatment of homeless, mentally ill, chemical-abusing men. *J Psychoactive Drugs* 27:93–103.

Reindollar RW (1999). Hepatitis C and the correctional population. *Am J Med* 107:100S–103S.

Rich JD, Boutwell AE, Shield DC, Key RG, McKenzie M, Clarke JG, Friedmann PD (2005). Attitudes and practices regarding the use of methadone in US state and federal prisons. *J Urban Health* 82:411–419.

Rosenheck RA, Dennis D (2001). Time-limited assertive community treatment for homeless persons with severe mental illness. *Arch Gen Psychiatry* 58:1073–1080.

Rosenheck R, Lam JA (1997). Homeless mentally ill clients' and providers' perceptions of service needs and clients' use of services. *Psychiatr Serv* 48:381–386.

Schaedle R, McGrew JH, Bond GR, Epstein I (2002). A comparison of experts' perspectives on assertive community treatment and intensive case management. *Psychiatr Serv* 53:207–210.

Scheft H, Fontenette DC (2005). Psychiatric barriers to readiness for treatment for hepatitis C virus (HCV) infection among injection drug users: clinical experience of an addiction psychiatrist in the HIV-HCV coinfection clinic of a public health hospital. *Clin Infect Dis* 40:S292–S296.

Schuster MA, Collins R, Cunningham WE, Morton SC, Zierler S, Wong M, Tu W, Kanouse DE (2005). Perceived discrimination in clinical care in a nationally representative sample of HIV-infected adults receiving health care. *J Gen Intern Med* 20:807–813.

Searight HR, Pound P (1994) The HIV-positive psychiatric patient and the duty to protect: ethical and legal issues. *Psychiatry Med* 24:259–270.

Selwyn PA, Goulet JL, Molde S, Constantino J, Fennie KP, Wetherill P, Gaughan DM, Brett-Smith H, Kennedy C (2000). HIV as a chronic disease: implications for long-term care at an AIDS-dedicated skilled nursing facility. *J Urban Health* 77:187–203.

Sherer R, Stieglitz K, Narra J, Jasek J, Green L, Moore B, Shott S, Cohen M (2002). HIV multidisciplinary teams work: support services improve access to and retention in HIV primary care. *AIDS Care* 14:S31–S44.

Shin JK, Newman LS, Gebbie KM, Fillmore HH (2002). Quality of care measurement in nursing home AIDS care: a pilot study. *J Assoc Nurses AIDS Care* 13:70–76.

Small W, Kain S, Laliberte N, Schechter MT, O'Shaughnessy MV, Spittal PM (2005). Incarceration, addiction and harm reduction: inmates experience injecting drugs in prison. *Subst Use Misuse* 40:831–843.

Swartz MS, Swanson JW, Hannon MJ, Bosworth HS, Osher FC, Essock SM, Rosenberg SD (2003). Five-site health and risk study research committee: regular sources of medical care among persons with severe mental illness at risk of hepatitis C infection. *Psychiatr Serv* 54:854–859.

Taylor LE (2005). Delivering care to injection drug users coinfected with HIV and hepatitis C virus. *Clin Infect Dis* 40:S355–S361.

Teplin L (1990). The prevalence of severe mental disorders among male urban jail detainees: comparison with the Epidemiologic Catchment Area program. *Am J Public Health* 80:663–669.

Thompson AS, Blankenship KM, Selwyn PA, Khoshnood K, Lopez M, Balacos K, Altice FL (1998). Evaluation of an innovative program to address the health and social service needs of drug-using women with or at risk for HIV infection. *J Community Health* 23:419–440.

Weisfuse IB, Greenberg BL, Makki HA, Thomas P. Rooney WC, Rautenberg EL (1991). HIV-1 infection among New York City inmates. *AIDS* 5 (9):1133–1138.

Willenbring ML (2005). Integrating care for patients with infectious, psychiatric and substance use disorders: concepts and approaches. *AIDS* 19:S227–S237.

Witbeck G, Hornfield S, Dalack GW (2000). Emergency room outreach to chronically addicted individuals. a pilot study. *J Subst Abuse Treat* 19:39–43.

Wood E, Kerr T, Montaner JS, Strathdee SA, Wodak A, Hankins CA, Schechter MT, Tyndall MW (2004). Rationale for evaluating North America's first medically supervised safer injecting facility. *Lancet Infect Dis* 4:301–306.

Woods ER, Samples CL, Melchiono MW, Harris SK (2003). Boston HAPPENS program: HIV-positive, homeless and at-risk youth can access care through youth oriented HIV services. *Semin Pediatr Infect Dis* 14:43–53.

Woods ER, Samples CL, Melchiono MW, Keenan PM, Fox DJ, Chase LH, Burns MA, Price VA, Paradise J, O'Brien R, Claytor RA, Brooke R, Goodman E (2000). Needs and use of services by HIV-positive compared to at-risk youth, including gender differences. *Eval Program Plan* 23:187–198.

Woods ER, Samples CL, Melchiono MW, Keenan PM, Fox DJ, Chase LH, Tierney S, Price VA, Paradise JE, O'Brien RF, Mansfield CJ, Brooke RA, Allen D, Goodman E (1998). Boston HAPPENS program: a model of health care for HIV-positive, homeless, and at-risk youth. *J Adolesc Health* 23:37–48.

Woods ER, Samples CL, Melchiono MW, Keenan PM, Fox DJ, Harris SK (2002). Boston HAPPENS Program Collaborators: Initiation of services in the Boston HAPPENS program: human immunodeficiency virus–positive, homeless, and at-risk youth can access services. *AIDS Patient Care STDS* 16:497–510.

Wright NM, Tompkins CN (2004). Supervised injecting centres. *BMJ* 328:100–102.

Additional Resources

Aberg JA (2006). The changing face of HIV care: common things really are common. *Ann Intern Med* 145:463–465.

Brown L, Macintyre K, Trujillo L (2003). Interventions to reduce HIV/AIDS stigma: what have we learned? *AIDS Educ Prev* 15:49–69.

Chesney MA, Smith AW (1992). Critical delays in HIV testing and care: the potential role of stigma. *Am Behav Sci* 42:1162–1174.

Cochran SD, Mays VM (1990). Sex, lies and HIV. *N Engl J Med* 22:774–775.

Cohen MA (2008). History of AIDS psychiatry: a biopsychosocial approach—paradigm and paradox. In MA Cohen and JM Gorman (eds), *Comprehensive Textbook of AIDS Psychiatry* (pp. 3–14). New York: Oxford University Press.

Cohen MA, Aladjem AD, Brenin D, Ghazi M (1990). Firesetting by patients with the acquired immunodeficiency syndrome (AIDS). *Ann Intern Med* 112:386–387.

Cohen MA, Gorman JM (2008). *Comprehensive Textbook of AIDS Psychiatry*. New York: Oxford University Press.

Cohn SE, Berk ML, Berry SH, Duan N, Frankel MR, Klein JD, McKinney MM, Rastegar A, Smith S, Shapiro MF, Bozzette SA (2001). The care of HIV-infected adults in rural areas of the United States. *J Acquir Immune Defic Syndr* 28:385–392.

Cooper JR (1989). Methadone treatment and acquired immunodeficiency syndrome. *JAMA* 262:1664–1668.

Cournos F, McKinnon K, Sullivan G (2005). Schizophrenia and comorbid human immunodeficiency virus or hepatitis C virus. *J Clin Psychiatry* 66:27–33.

De Buono BA, Zinner SH, Daamen M, McCormack WM (1990). Sexual behavior of college women in 1975, 1986, and 1989. *N Engl J Med* 322:821–825.

Deuchar N (1984). AIDS in New York City with particular reference to the psychosocial aspects. *Br J Psychiatry* 145:612–619.

Fernandez F, Ruiz P (2006). *Psychiatric Aspects of HIV/AIDS* (pp. 39–47). Philadelphia: Lippincott Williams & Wilkins.

Gaughan DM, Hughes MD, Oleske JM, Malee K, Gore CA, Nachman S (2004). Psychiatric hospitalizations among children and youths with human immunodeficiency virus infection. *Pediatrics* 113:e544–e551.

Goodkin K, Heckman T, Siegel K, Linsk N, Khamis I, Lee D, Lecusay R, Poindexter CC, Mason SJ, Suarez P, Eisdorfer C (2003). "Putting a face" on HIV infection/AIDS in older adults: a psychosocial context. *J Aquir Immune Defic Syndr* 33(Suppl. 2):S171–S184.

Gottlieb MS (2001). AIDS—past and future. *N Engl J Med* 344:1788–1791.

Gottlieb MS, Schroff R, Schanker HM, Weisman JD, Fan PT, Wolf RA, Saxon A (1981). *Pneumocystis carinii* pneumonia and mucosal candidiasis in previously healthy homosexual men: evidence of a new acquired cellular immunodeficiency. *N Engl J Med* 305:1425–1431.

Hartel DM, Schoenbaum EE (1998). Methadone treatment protects against HIV infection: two decades of experience in the Bronx, New York City. *Public Health Rep* 113:107–115.

Holtz H, Dobro J, Kapila R, Palinkas R, Oleske J (1983). Psychosocial impact of acquired immunodeficiency syndrome. *JAMA* 250:167.

Hoover DR, Sambamoorthi U, Walkup JT, Crystal S (2004). Mental illness and length of inpatient stay for Medicaid recipients with AIDS. *Health Serv Res* 39:1319–1339.

Huang L, Quartin A, Jones D, Havlir DV (2006). Intensive care of patients with HIV infection. *N Engl J Med* 355:173–181.

Hunter ND (1990). Epidemic of fear: a survey of AIDS discrimination in the 1980s and policy recommendations for the 1990s. American Civil Liberties Union AIDS Project 1990. New York: ACLU.

Kaplan AH, Scheyett A, Golin CE (2005). HIV and stigma: analysis and research program. *Curr HIV/AIDS Rep* 2:184–188.

Karpiak SE, Shippy RA, Cantor MH (2006). *Research on Older Adults with HIV*. New York: AIDS Community Research Initiative of America.

Kelly JA, St. Lawrence JS, Smith S Jr, Hood HV, Cook DJ (1987). Stigmatization of AIDS patients by physicians. *Am J Public Health* 77:789–791.

MacDonald NE, Wells GA, Fisher WA, Warren WK, King MA, Doherty JA, Bowie WR (1990). High-risk STD/HIV behavior among college students. *JAMA* 263:3155–3159.

Manfredi R (2004a). HIV infection and advanced age: emerging epidemiological, clinical and management issues. *Ageing Res Rev* 3:31–54.

Manfredi R (2004b). Impact of HIV infection and antiretroviral therapy in the older patient. *Expert Rev Anti Infect Ther* 2:821–824.

Miller NS, Sheppard LM, Colenda CC, Magen J (2001). Why physicians are unprepared to treat patients who have alcohol- and drug-related disorders. *Acad Med* 76:410–418.

Mustanski B, Donenberg G, Emerson E (2006). I can use a condom, I just don't: the importance of motivation to prevent HIV in adolescents seeking psychiatric care. *AIDS Behav* 10:753–762.

National Institutes of Health (1998). NIH Consensus Development Panel on Effective Medical Treatment of Opiate Addiction: effective medical treatment of opiate addiction. *JAMA* 280:1936–1943.

Parker R, Aggleton P (2003). HIV and AIDS-related stigma and discrimination: a conceptual framework and implications for action. *Soc Sci Med* 57:13–24.

Pathela P, Hajat A, Schillinger J, Blank S, Sell R, Mostashari F (2006). Discordance between sexual behavior and self-reported sexual identity: a population-based survey of New York City men. *Ann Intern Med* 145:416–425.

Paxton S, Gonzales G, Uppakaew K, Abraham KK, Okta S, Green C, Nair KS, Merati TP, Thephthien B, Marin M, Quesada A (2005). AIDS-related discrimination in Asia. *AIDS Care* 17:413–424.

Reinisch JM, Beasley R (1990). America fails sex information test. In *The Kinsey Institute New Report on Sex: What You Must Know to Be Sexually Literate* (pp. 1–26). New York: St. Martin's Press.

Rothbard AB, Metraux S, Blank MB (2003). Cost of care for Medicaid recipients with serious mental illness and HIV infection or AIDS. *Psychiatr Serv* 54:1240–1246.

Ruiz P (2000). Living and dying with HIV/AIDS: a psychosocial perspective. *Am J Psychiatry* 157:110–113.

Sackoff JE, Hanna DB, Pfeiffer MR, Torian LV (2006). Causes of death among persons with AIDS in the era of highly active antiretroviral therapy: New York City. *Ann Intern Med* 145:397–406.

Sacks M, Burton W, Dermatis H, Looser-Ott S, Perry S (1995). HIV-related cases among 2,094 admissions to a psychiatric hospital. *Psychiatr Serv* 46:131–135.

Selwyn PA, Forstein M (2003). Overcoming the false dichotomy of curative vs. palliative care for late-stage AIDS. "Let me live the way I want to live until I can't." *JAMA* 290:806–814.

Stoff DM (2004). Mental health research in HIV/AIDS and aging: problems and prospects. *AIDS* 18(Suppl. 1): S3–S10.

Thompson LM (1987). Dealing with AIDS and fear: would you accept cookies from an AIDS patient? *South Med J* 80:228–232.

Turner BJ, Laine C, Lin YT, Lynch K (2005). Barriers and facilitators to primary care or human immunodeficiency virus clinics providing methadone or buprenorphine for the management of opioid dependence. *Arch Intern Med* 165:1769–1776.

U.S. Department of Health and Human Services (2005). *An evaluation of innovation methods for integrating buprenophrine opioid abuse treatment in HIV primary care.* Retrieved April 13, 2007, from http://hab.hrsa.gov/special/bup_index.htm

Weinrich M, Stuart M (2000). Provision of methadone treatment in primary care medical practices. *JAMA* 283:1343–1348.

Wormser GP, Joline C (1989). Would you eat cookies prepared by an AIDS patient? Survey reveals harmful attitudes among professionals. *Postgrad Med* 86:174–175, 178.

Young AS, Sullivan G, Bogart LM, Koegel P, Kanouse DE (2005). Needs for services reported by adults with severe mental illness and HIV. *Psychiatr Serv* 56:99–101.

Zaric GS, Barnett PG, Brandeau ML (2000). HIV transmission and the cost-effectiveness of methadone maintenance. *Am J Public Health* 90:1100–1111.

2

A BIOPSYCHOSOCIAL APPROACH TO PSYCHIATRIC CONSULTATION IN PERSONS WITH HIV AND AIDS

Mary Ann Cohen, Sharon M. Batista, and Joseph Z. Lux

For persons with HIV and AIDS, a thorough and comprehensive assessment has far-reaching implications not only for compassionate, competent, and coordinated care but also for adherence to medical treatment and risk reduction, as well as public health. Primary physicians, HIV specialists, as well as psychiatrists and other mental health professionals can play an important role in preventing the spread of HIV infection. Psychiatric disorders are associated with inadequate adherence to risk reduction, medical care, and antiretroviral therapy. While adherence to medical care for most medical illnesses has major meaning to patients, loved ones, and families, adherence to medical care for HIV and AIDS has major implications for reduction of HIV transmission and prevention of emergence of drug-resistant HIV viral strains (Cohen and Chao, 2008). Many persons with HIV and AIDS have psychiatric disorders (Stoff et al., 2004) and can benefit from psychiatric consultation and care. The rates of HIV infection are also higher among persons with serious mental illness (Blank et al., 2002), indicating a bidirectional relationship.

Some persons with HIV and AIDS have no psychiatric disorder, while others have a multiplicity of complex psychiatric disorders that are responses to illness or treatments or are associated with HIV/AIDS (such as HIV-associated dementia) or multimorbid medical illnesses and treatments (such as hepatitis C, cirrhosis, end-stage liver disease, HIV nephropathy, end-stage renal disease, anemia, coronary artery disease, and cancer). Persons with HIV and AIDS may also have multimorbid psychiatric disorders that are co-occurring and may be unrelated to HIV (such as posttraumatic stress disorder, or PTSD, schizophrenia, and bipolar disorder). The complexity of AIDS psychiatric consultation is illustrated in an article (Freedman et al., 1994) with the title "Depression, HIV Dementia, Delirium, Posttraumatic Stress Disorder (or All of the Above)."

Comprehensive psychiatric evaluations can provide diagnoses, inform treatment, and mitigate anguish, distress, depression, anxiety, and substance use in persons with HIV and AIDS. Furthermore, thorough and comprehensive assessment is crucial because HIV has an affinity for brain and neural tissue and can cause central nervous system (CNS) complications even in healthy seropositive individuals. Because of potential CNS complications as well as the multiplicity of other severe and complex medical illnesses in persons with HIV and AIDS (Huang et al., 2006), every person who is referred for a psychiatric consultation needs a full biopsychosocial evaluation.

This chapter will introduce the reader to some important aspects of HIV prevention; a more comprehensive approach to prevention will be presented in Chapter 5. In this chapter, we provide a basic approach to persons with HIV and AIDS who are referred to an AIDS psychiatrist and a template for a comprehensive psychiatric evaluation.

SETTINGS FOR AIDS PSYCHIATRIC CONSULTATIONS

Psychiatric consultations are requested in inpatient and ambulatory divisions of acute care facilities and in chronic or long-term care facilities. Consultations may also be requested in other settings, including nursing homes, the home care setting, marginal housing (such as shelters and single-room occupancy transitional housing), and correctional facilities, and in homeless outreach contexts. The complexities of the many special settings where persons with AIDS may be evaluated are covered in Chapter 1 of this book. Since AIDS is now regarded as a chronic severe illness in areas of the world where antiretroviral treatments are available, most persons with HIV and AIDS are seen in outpatient settings, clinics, private offices, and other ambulatory care facilities.

As medical care of persons with HIV and AIDS shifted to the ambulatory setting, psychiatric care for persons with HIV and AIDS shifted as well, particularly at academic medical centers in urban areas of nations where mental health professionals are readily available. Many models of mental health care delivery are used in the ambulatory setting. There is no clear evidence base to determine the best practice model, but many patients and clinicians are most satisfied with a colocated model of care that is based in the ambulatory HIV setting and provides comprehensive medical and mental health services in the same place. In this chapter, we will provide an integrated approach to assessing persons with HIV and AIDS in ambulatory and inpatient settings.

Comprehensive Psychosocial and Psychiatric Consultations

Outpatient consultations

A colocated AIDS psychiatry team can provide on-site psychiatric evaluations and consultations as well as follow-up psychiatric care. Since attending a psychiatric clinic and an AIDS clinic may be perceived by some patients as doubly stigmatizing, persons with HIV and AIDS are sometimes relieved to learn that psychiatric care is a routine part of their comprehensive HIV care or HIV prenatal care and may find it more acceptable than having to be seen in a psychiatric outpatient setting. In the setting of the HIV clinic, a consultation may be requested by the primary HIV clinician directly through personal contact, by telephone contact, or by written request. The HIV clinician may indirectly request a consultation through another member of the team, often a social worker or other clinician.

Process of psychiatric outpatient consultation

The consultation begins with a discussion between the HIV clinician and AIDS psychiatrist to determine the reason for the psychiatric referral, the expectations of the consultee, the urgency of the referral (manifest content of the consultation), and some of the feelings that the patient has engendered in the consultee (latent content of the consultation). During this discussion, the HIV clinician can provide a summary of the patient's medical history and current condition as well as what medications are being prescribed for the patient. The psychiatrist can review the medical record in further detail. Ideally, if the patient is in the clinic for a scheduled visit with the HIV clinician when the AIDS psychiatrist is available, an introduction by the HIV clinician may prove invaluable and demonstrate the level of coordination of care being offered to the patient. The AIDS psychiatrist can be introduced as an integral member of the multidisciplinary team providing ongoing patient care.

The HIV clinician can then discuss his or her concerns about the patient and the reasons for the psychiatric consultation. This open discussion by a sensitive and caring clinician with the psychiatric consultant in the presence of the patient can lead to better acceptance of the referral and set the stage for a continued collaborative relationship. It also serves to diminish anxiety in the patient and perhaps even serves to dispel or at least mitigate frightening myths about psychiatrists and mental health care. It is especially encouraging if the primary provider can discuss the need for the consultation as a means of providing him or her with help in better understanding and caring for the patient. The consultation is scheduled and the consulting AIDS psychiatrist reviews the chart to familiarize himself or herself with the patient's history and medical condition.

Comprehensive outpatient psychiatric consultation

When the patient arrives for the first visit, the AIDS psychiatrist can set the tone for a nonjudgmental evaluation by starting with an introduction that is sensitive to the patient's potential anxiety surrounding the encounter. Suggestions for such an introduction include greeting and shaking hands. Shaking hands is especially important since persons with HIV and AIDS are exquisitely sensitive to others' fears of contagion and may find a warm handshake reassuring. The introduction includes the AIDS psychiatrist addressing the patient by his or her title and last name (Mr. A), stating his or her title and last name (Dr. P), and accompanying the patient from the waiting area into the psychiatric consulting room. After closing the door to establish privacy and providing for appropriate seating and comfort, the psychiatrist asks the patient "How are you feeling today?" After listening to the response and following leads if applicable, the psychiatrist then describes the reason for the consultation. "Dr. M asked me to evaluate you for depression. Did she tell you that she was asking me to see you? How do you feel about seeing a psychiatrist?" This question may provide an opportunity to ask Mr. A if he has ever seen a psychiatrist or had contact with the mental health system in the past and to address the stigma that the patient may associate with mental illness.

During the process of the introduction, the psychiatrist can begin to assess the patient through careful observation. Specific observations, described in detail below, under the section on general appearance, manner, and attitude, should begin at the first moment of the encounter.

Chief complaint and history of present illness

The psychiatrist elicits the patient's chief complaint in his or her own words and follows with the history of the present illness, including the onset, course, progression, and medications if any, along with the current medical and psychiatric symptoms and illness chronology. It is important for establishment of rapport to allow the patient to tell the story of the illness in his or her words with minimal interruption or intrusion except for occasional redirection. Although the psychiatrist may wish to have a thorough review of the history in chronological order, it is better to allow the patient to provide the story and for the psychiatrist to reconstruct the chronology by asking questions if the history is unclear. Allowing the patient to tell his or her story enables the psychiatrist to observe for cognitive impairment and to determine whether the patient is an accurate historian. Hearing the history of present illness recounted as a story often provides more information about remote and recent memory than does routine questioning. Following leads is more useful than proceeding on a set course of history-taking that may serve to derail an anxious patient.

Special attention is needed when discussing how the patient learned of the diagnosis of HIV or AIDS, since this is often fraught with significant distress. A comprehensive psychiatric assessment of a person with HIV or AIDS would not be complete without a determination of the patient's understanding of his or her illness and its treatments (Cohen, 1987, 1992; Cohen and Weisman, 1986, 1988; Cohen and Alfonso, 1998, 2004; Cohen and Chao, 2008).

Past history

Although there is no special set order, the rest of the history-taking process should follow leads, if possible, and should proceed from less anxiety-provoking to more anxiety-provoking issues. The demographic information and current life situation may be easy for some individuals to start with and may enable the patient to become comfortable and used to the new setting and start to develop a connection while discussing these somewhat less charged issues. It is especially important to learn early on about the patient's occupation or former occupation (if any) and about the patient's family structure and whether or not the patient has a partner, children, or grandchildren. Expression of interest in the patient's occupational and family history can help the patient feel a sense of the psychiatrist's personal interest and perceive that the psychiatrist is thinking about him or her as not just a patient, symptom, or illness, but as a person in the context of family, society, and community.

Medical history

The general health and medical history should include information about medical illnesses and symptoms, hospitalizations, surgery, and traumatic injuries as well as medications and other treatments. It is also helpful to determine whether the patient is consulting clinicians other than the primary HIV referring clinician and, if so, whether other medications are being prescribed. Complementary and alternative healing modalities should be explored in a nonjudgmental manner. Additionally, information about nutrition and exercise can be addressed.

Specifics about HIV medical history include how and when the patient first learned about his or her serostatus, current and nadir CD4 counts if known, viral load, course and responses to illness, and treatments and responses to treatments. If the patient is known to have hepatitis C, history of course, treatments, and results are also relevant. Review of laboratory data, X-rays and other imaging studies, and other ancillary data through discussion with the primary physician and/or by a review of the medical record is a necessary part of the psychiatric consultation.

Early childhood, developmental, social, and family history

Once again, it is helpful to begin with the less affect-laden material, such as age, date of birth, and place of birth. Open-ended questions such as "What was it like for you growing up?" and "Who was in your family when you were growing up?" may be ways to begin. Exploration of relationships with parents, siblings, and other family members as well as discussions about parental drug and alcohol use can follow. Family history also includes information about illness patterns, particularly psychiatric illnesses such as bipolar disorder or schizophrenia. History and chronology of early child-hood losses are highly significant and deserve careful interest and documen-tation. Educational history includes the following questions and is relevant in determination of current level of intellectual and occupational function: (1) "How far did you go in school?" (2) "How did you do in school?" (3) "What was school like for you?" (4) "Were there any problems with learning?"

A thorough housing history includes questions about where the patient lives, whether the patient lives alone or with others, and whether the patient is homeless or marginally housed. Specific information about housing includes whether the patient is in his or her own apartment or home, if the patient is comfortable and has space, privacy, an elevator if mobility is compromised, heat, and hot water, and if the home is free of rodents or other pests. Persons who live in marginal housing, in shelters, or on the street may feel embarrassed to discuss these issues and may not disclose this information as a result.

Family history includes information about family of origin as well as relational history with partners. Since it is hard to suffer an illness in silence, it is important to ask whether the patient has disclosed his or her serostatus to anyone in the family or to any partners. Disclosure may be easier for some patients and difficult to near impossible for other patients. The multidimensional determinants in considerations of disclosure include relational, psychological, social, cultural, spiritual, and political factors. Fear of disclosure to aged parents is often used as a reason for not telling any family member about serostatus. Ages and health status of parents or dates and causes of death along with number, ages, and health of siblings are relevant. History of medical or mental illnesses and impact on the patient are also significant.

Relational history includes information about past and current partners and whether the patient is in a relationship. Allowing the patient to discuss the relationship is important. Such discussions should include questions about disclosure of serostatus to his or her intimate partner and how the partner responded. Some patients are unable to disclose serostatus because of fear of rejection, abandonment, or even violence. Since disclosure may be associated with intimate partner violence, it is important to talk about this sensitive issue as well.

It is important to ask for the number, names, ages, health, and where-abouts of children, if any, along with the status of the parent–child relationship. The complex issues of whether and when to disclose to children are relevant. The topic of disclosure to intimate partners and family is extremely anxiety provoking. In order to preserve the patient's sense of control over the process, exquisite sensitivity to the patient's feelings is critical so as not to derail the interview or to make the patient feel threatened by the clinician.

Occupational history

Occupational history is an important determinant of level of function. An individual who never worked may or may not feel distressed by being too ill to work. However, for individuals who have worked and who took pride in their career, the inability to work can be devastating and may be a significant contributor to a sense of loss or distress. It is important to ask questions about occupation in a way that is sensitive to the individual's current condition. If someone is bed-bound and near the end of life, it is helpful to acknowledge clearly that you recognize that the patient is no longer able to work but may have worked in the past. Similarly, in the ambulatory setting it is best not to make assumptions and to elicit information about occupation in a sensitive and compassionate manner. It is also important to be able to use the information in subsequent visits and to record it clearly in the medical record so that the information is available to other members of the team. A former home attendant, professional musician, foreman, teacher, nurse, or superintendent may take considerable pride in his or her hard work. For those individuals who are still able to work, this can be a source of validation and meaning for some and a source of stress and fatigue for others.

Trauma history and response to trauma history

History of early childhood and other trauma is not easy to obtain. Trauma may be accompanied by amnesia, regardless of whether traumatic brain injury was involved. Trauma may also be followed by intense repression of horrific events. Some patients may refuse to talk about painful experiences whether distant or recent, particularly on a first encounter with the psychiatrist. Furthermore, if there is a history of trauma and such trauma was perpetrated by a parent or other close relative, this absolute violation and betrayal leads to loss of the most significant paradigm and basis for future development of trusting relationships. Hence, the patient may find it difficult to trust physicians and other health professionals who may represent those very figures of parental authority. A brief, supportive statement validating the difficulty of talking about early trauma may serve to mitigate discomfort. Additional reassurance that it is normal for persons who have experienced early-childhood abuse or neglect to have problems with trust can also be comforting.

If the patient is willing to discuss the painful experiences, it is helpful to ask direct and closed-ended questions unless the patient proceeds to tell the story in his or her own words. The patient may, in fact, feel relieved to be able to talk about these secrets after many decades. Questions may include those about physical and emotional abuse as well as neglect. Asking about being a witness to physical or threatened violence on a repeated basis or to seeing one parent trying to hurt or kill the other parent may be relieving to the patient who has not been able to tell anyone about it because of threats or fear of reprisals.

Specific questions about sexual abuse should elicit information about unwanted touching, molesting, or fondling as well as penetration, intercourse, and rape. It is also important to determine the dates of the traumatic events whenever possible. Later trauma such as rape, life-threatening robbery, kidnapping, or the witnessing of trauma, including combat-related trauma, can be explored in detail as well. Finally, head trauma, often accompanied by amnesia, should be specifically addressed.

A history of trauma is significant in evaluating for trauma sequelae, including dissociative phenomena, hyperarousal, depression, eating disorders, substance use disorders, psychiatric disorders (especially posttraumatic stress disorder), intimate-partner violence, and commercial sex work. Specific questions about posttraumatic stress disorder include those about dissociation, intrusive thoughts, flashbacks, nightmares, easy startle, hypervigilance, insomnia, and a sense of a foreshortened future.

Sexual history

Persons with HIV and AIDS have sexual needs as well as needs for companionship, tenderness, love, and romance. Many individuals are extremely uncomfortable discussing sexual feelings and may suffer in silence with problems of arousal, pain, or excitement. Some persons find it difficult to ask a partner to use a condom. Men and women with HIV and AIDS have a high prevalence of alcohol and other drug use and some may continue substance use and associated HIV risk behaviors such as sharing of needles and exchange of sex for drugs or money. The AIDS psychiatrist needs to be comfortable with taking a sexual history and as well as drug and alcohol histories. Suggestions for taking a sexual history are summarized in Table 2.1.

TABLE 2.1 Sexual History-Taking

Setting the Tone

1. Often people with chronic medical illness experience problems with their sexual function. What is your sexual function like since you have been ill?
2. How does your sexual function since you have been physically ill compare with that when you were healthy?
3. Often people with psychiatric illness such as depression experience problems with their sexual function. What is your sexual function like since you have been ill?
4. How is your sexual function since you have been depressed (or had another psychiatric illness) compared with that when you were healthy?
5. Often people who need to take medications experience problems with their sexual function. What is your sexual function like since you have been on (the medication)?
6. How does your sexual function since you have been on (the medication) compare with that before starting on (the medication)?

Sexual Experience

7. When did you have your first period?
8. What was the experience of having your first period like for you?
9. When did you have your first ejaculation?
10. What was the experience of having your first ejaculation like for you?
11. How has your period changed over the years?
12. How have the changes in your hormones affected your sexual function?
13. How enjoyable is sex for you?
14. How enjoyable is masturbation for you?
15. Do you have (a) sexual partner(s)?
16. Are you sexually active?
17. What is the frequency of your sexual activity?
18. Have you noticed a change in the frequency of your sexual activity?
19. How do your religious beliefs affect your sexuality?
20. How do your cultural beliefs affect your sexuality?
21. Which of your sexual practices do you associate with feelings of shame?
22. Which of your sexual practices do you associate with feelings of anxiety?
23. Which of your sexual practices do you associate with feelings of unhappiness?

Safe and Unsafe Sex

24. What methods are you using to prevent yourself from getting sexually transmitted infections (herpes, gonorrhea, chlamydia, syphilis, HPV) or HIV infection? How many sexual partners do you have?
25. How many sexual partners have you had?
26. How has your number of sexual partners changed over time?
27. What kind of barrier contraception are you using?
28. What kind of spermicidal preparation are you using?
29. What lubricants do you use during sexual intercourse?
30. Are you aware that petroleum-based lubricants (Vaseline and others) can cause leakage of condoms?

(continued)

TABLE 2.1 (Continued)

---

31. How do you put on a condom?
32. At what point during intercourse do you put on a condom?
33. How do you ensure that there is no air bubble trapped inside the condom?
34. While wearing a condom, how do you ensure that there is no leakage during intercourse?
35. How do you ensure that there is no leakage upon condom removal?

Talking about sexuality

Sexuality is so much more than sex. It is integral to a person's identity because it encompasses much more than a person's sexual behaviors. This is also a specific area where lesbian, gay, bisexual, and transgender (LGBT) individuals may identify anxieties, trauma, or alternatively, a rich developmental history and concept of self. LGBT patients deserve, desire, and benefit from understanding and supportive clinicians. Being clear and open regarding issues related to sexual identity and gender role will not only help gain a patient's confidence and trust but also demonstrate respect on the part of the clinician. The questions asked and language used will determine whether patients perceive clinicians as nonjudgmental, accepting, and open or as judgmental, discriminatory, or biased.

A common frustration on the part of clinicians and LGBT persons alike is the "misreading" of sexuality, namely making assumptions about gender, sexual orientation, and sexual behaviors (Greenfield, 2007) based on cultural stereotypes. One way to avoid reflexively resorting to stereotypes is to be respectful of the terminology that patients use in reference to themselves or to describe their experiences and to mirror that terminology as a form of respect. There is never any shame in asking a patient for further elaboration regarding what they mean to describe—it may even be gratifying to them that a clinician is paying attention to their sexuality, as this aspect of a person's intimate life is often overlooked. Gaining an understanding of the patient's experiences and perspective regarding their sexuality is beneficial for the clinician beyond being a means of establishing rapport with the patient—it also enhances the psychosocial formulation. While some of these questions may seem irrelevant, they can open the door to taking a full sexual history, which is essential to assess for behavior-specific risks of infection or transmission.

Characteristics to assess when talking about sexuality (Greenfield, 2007)

1. *Gender identity:* refers to biological and psychological aspects of a person's experience of their gender, i.e., how one thinks of one's own gender.
   Examples: man, woman, transsexual, transgender, intersex

2. *Gender role:* refers to the role the person acts or appears as and often connotes differing degrees and combinations of both masculinity and femininity.

Examples: masculine, feminine, effeminate

Slang terms (can be used both as pejorative or with humor or pride): butch, fem, tomboy, sissy, top or bottom, dyke, lesbo

3. Sexual orientation: refers to gender to which the person is attracted.

Examples: heterosexual, homosexual, bisexual, gay, lesbian, straight

Questions to assist in sexuality history-taking for LGBT persons

1. What is your sexual orientation?
2. With which gender do you identify?
3. When and how did you discover your gender identity?
4. What words do you prefer to use to describe your sexual identity?
5. Do feelings about your sexual identity play a role in your current level of distress?
6. Have you come out as LGBT to your family? To your friends? To your coworkers or classmates?
7. Do you currently experience any conflicts regarding religion or spirituality and your sexuality?
8. Do you experience any conflicts in your daily life regarding your sexuality?
9. Have you been in significant love or romantic relationships in your life?
10. Have you ever been a victim of a hate crime?

Follow-up questions to assist to assess sexual orientation and behavior

10. What is your sexual orientation?
11. What is your sexual activity like?
12. Do you have sex with men? With women? With both?
13. What types of sex do you engage in?
14. Do you engage in any form of sexual behavior that worries you or your partner?
15. Have you ever had a sexually transmitted disease?

Psychiatric history

Persons with HIV and AIDS are at especially high risk for cognitive disorders, affective disorders, substance use disorders, and posttraumatic stress disorder. There is also an association between serious mental illness and HIV-related illness, documented in a large study of treated Medicaid recipients. In this study, Blank and colleagues (2002) found a high HIV seroprevalence rate among treated Medicaid recipients with serious mental illness. They found that the HIV seroprevalence rate was four times higher among persons with schizophrenia and five times higher among persons with mood disorder than for persons without serious mental illness. They estimate that the untreated rates may be 10 to 20 times higher for persons with serious mental illness than those for persons without serious mental illness.

A comprehensive assessment of prior psychiatric symptoms, a history of psychiatric disorders, and a history of treatment for psychiatric illness include a history of inpatient and outpatient treatment, types of treatment, course of illness, history of illness as it relates to seroconversion (for example, whether there were symptoms preceding or following HIV infection), and current involvement in psychiatric care. It is important to ascertain whether the patient is still in the care of other mental health clinicians and to obtain permission to contact the treating mental health clinician, if appropriate.

A full review of both current psychotropic medications and those previously prescribed is important. Since there is a high prevalence of mood disorders in persons with HIV and AIDS, a history of episodes of depression and mania should be elicited. Because there is a high prevalence of substance use disorders and suicidal ideation among persons with HIV and AIDS, these histories will be delineated separately. Both of these topics are explored in depth in Chapter 6 of this book.

Suicide history-taking

There is no treatment for suicide, only prevention and education. To evaluate for suicide risk in vulnerable persons with HIV and AIDS, AIDS psychiatrists and other clinicians need to be able to take a suicide history, recognize and ensure that depression and other psychiatric disorders are treated, determine risk factors and etiologies, and ultimately help to resolve the suicidal crisis. Psychiatrists need to feel comfortable with taking a suicide history and discussing suicide in depth with a person with HIV and AIDS. This discussion entails the establishment of a trusting relationship, discussion of suicide and death in relation to both the illness and the individual's philosophies and religious beliefs, and awareness of the value of continuity of care and reassurance that the patient will not be abandoned (Cohen, 1992). No suicidal patient ever gets the idea for suicide from talking openly about suicide. Persons who are suicidal are able to admit to suicidal ideation and even to plans for suicide. They are also able to discuss prior attempts as well as precipitants. From these discussions, risk factors for the patient can be determined and crisis intervention initiated. Risk factors for suicide are summarized in Table 2.2 and suicide history-taking is summarized in Table 2.3.

TABLE 2.2 Risk Factors for Suicide

1. Hopelessness
2. Impulsivity
3. Substance use disorder
4. Previous suicide attempts
5. Recent illness
6. Recent hospitalization
7. Living alone
8. Inexpressible grief
9. Depression

TABLE 2.3 Suicide History-Taking

1. Have you ever thought about killing yourself?
2. What specifically made you think of suicide?
3. Have you ever tried to commit suicide?
4. What precipitated your previous attempt or attempts?
5. How did you try to kill yourself?
6. When did you try to kill yourself?
7. Do you know anyone in your family or outside your family who committed suicide?
8. Do you feel like killing yourself now?
9. What would you accomplish?
10. Do you plan to rejoin someone you lost?
11. Who would miss you?
12. Do you have any reasons for living, such as spiritual beliefs?
13. What would you miss?
14. Do you have any specific plans?
15. What are they?
16. Have you obtained the means necessary to go through with the plan?

Far from harming the suicidal individual with HIV and AIDS, being able to speak openly about suicidal thoughts and feelings is highly cathartic. Thoughts of suicide while providing some measure of consolation and control may also be frightening, distressing, and painful. Sharing suicidal feelings with an empathic listener is not only relieving but may also provide the patient with a new perspective. To resolve a suicidal crisis, it is important to reestablish bonds, provide the patient with a supportive network of family, loved ones, friends, and caregivers, and identify and treat psychiatric disorders. Crisis intervention, networking, and ongoing psychiatric care may help prevent suicide.

When is "intent to die" not really a suicide? Traditional suicide assessments have numerous limitations, particularly that they tend to pathologize almost all decisions that are not life prolonging, including deferring potentially futile or aggressive treatments. In the context of terminal or end-stage illness, patients often desire control over the manner in which they die. In the face of chronic incurable illness and progressive decline, it can be appropriate for a patient and their loved one to welcome an end to their suffering, such as by withdrawing care or deferring aggressive life-prolonging measures that are futile. Such decisions should be put into context and compared with those that are more idiosyncratic, such as overt suicidal feelings or behavior. Bostwick and Cohen (2009) explain that it is important to verify that the patient is not making such choices because of psychiatric illness but rather that the medical and psycho-social contexts are in agreement, that the patient has made his or her wishes known to others, and that the decision is consistent with the patient's pre-viously held values. Bostwick and Cohen propose that the concept of colla-boration is a key factor in such assessments: while social supports and doctors may not be in support of a particular choice, they are aware of the patient's reasoning behind that choice and are able to contextualize this reasoning as being in agreement with other values that the patient has previously held.

Key factors of a nonsuicidal decision by a patient with intent to die include the following:

1. Has the patient discussed their wishes with their physician? With their family or friends?
2. Are their social supports (family, friends, etc.) aware of their reasoning for their decision?
3. Is there evidence of collaboration on the part of others? Lack of collaboration with others, e.g., "taking matters into one's own hands" or planning death in secret, can be a warning sign of psychiatric illness as an underlying factor.

Violence History-Taking

Often health-care practitioners are called into a medical setting to help assess and manage the risk of harm to others in addition to the more obvious risk of self-harm that can present in the acutely ill patient. Whenever possible, it is also important to take a history related to the potential for violence toward others. Some patients with history of impulsive behavior or who have anti-social personality disorder or psychotic-spectrum disorders can act out in the acute setting, especially in times of medical instability or crisis. Risk factors for violence include prior violence, substance use, severity of mental illness, psychopathy, personality disorder, young age at first violence, impulsivity, and stress (McNiel et al., 2008). Patients are most at risk of violence in the medical setting when they feel they lack control over their care and are acutely ill. Questions for violence history-taking are listed in Table 2.4.

TABLE 2.4 Violence History-Taking

1. Have you ever become so physically out of control that you hurt another person?
2. Would you consider yourself an impulsive person? In what way?
3. Have you ever encountered problems with the law?
4. Were you violent at a young age?
5. What situations make you feel out of control?

Drug History-Taking

It is important to be able to take a complete history of substance use for each individual with HIV or AIDS who is referred for psychiatric consultation. Patients are often reluctant to discuss drug addiction and may see their addiction as so much a part of their everyday lives that it is not even given a second thought. This can be as true for a business executive who has a three-martini lunch and continues to drink during and after dinner on a daily basis as it is for a chronic heroin-, cocaine-, or sedative-hypnotic-addicted individual. Furthermore, defensiveness and denial may need to be understood as concomitants of addictive disorders. For each individual, it is important to obtain a history of the chronology of the substance use from the first use to the last, as well as to identify any periods when substance use coincided with or was independent of other symptoms.

An extremely benevolent and nonjudgmental approach is essential to help diminish defensiveness. An important part of the history-taking is to be able to ask questions that are ego supportive. Addiction history can be obtained after learning about crises, traumas, and losses and later determining if substances may have been used to console or self-medicate at the times of crisis, loss, or trauma. Using "how," "when," and "what" questions generally is useful and can facilitate history-taking and help to avoid the potential blaming aspects of "why" questions. Specific questions for substance use history-taking are summarized in Table 2.5.

The comprehensive and thorough history-taking of substance use can provide information of significance to all members of the treatment team. It is essential to assess for withdrawal or intoxication, especially in the acute setting (discussed below). It is also vital to understand what drugs will be induced or inhibited by such substances as heroin or methadone. Drugs that induce isoenzyme cytochrome P4503A4 may lead to lowering opioid levels, resulting in a need for increased heroin use or an increase in the dose of methadone to obtain the same serum levels as before enzyme induction. If the patient is on an antiretroviral, the patient may stop taking the medication because he or she is feeling uncomfortable symptoms of opioid withdrawal.

TABLE 2.5 Substance Use History-Taking

1. Many people who are ill may use drugs or alcohol to get through difficult times. What have you used to get through these times?
2. Specifically ask about all drugs by name and street name:
   Alcohol
   Heroin—dope, smack, horse
   Cocaine—crack, freebase
   Cannabis—marijuana, weed, dope, pot, joints
   Sedative-hypnotics—primarily benzodiazepines such as alprazolam, Xanax, or sticks
   Inhalants—printer cartridges, rubber cement and other glues, aerosolized chemicals
   Hallucinogens
       Lysergic acid dethylamide, LSD, or acid
       Psilocybin or mushrooms
       Methamphetamine or speed, ice, crystal meth, crank
       Dimethoxymethylamphetamine or DOM, STP
       Methylenedioxymethamphetamine or MDMA, Ecstasy, X, XTC
       Ketamine or K, special K, Ket, super K, vitamin K
       Gamma-hydroxybutyric acid or GHB, liquid E, Georgia Home Boy
       Phencyclidine or angel dust, PCP
3. Precipitants
   a. What led to your first trying (the specific substance or substances) _____?
   b. What was your reaction to it?
   c. How were you able to get it?
   d. What effect did it have on the problem, crisis, or trauma in your life?
4. Chronology
   a. When did you first use _____?
   b. What happened after that?
   c. What other drugs or alcohol did you use?
   d. How did using _____ affect your school, work, and relationships?
   e. What kind of trouble did you get into?
   f. When did you last use?
5. Amounts, routes, and access
   a. What is the most you can hold or use in a day?
   b. How do you take it?
       Intravenous—with or without sharing of needles or works
       Insufflation or snorting
       Smoking
       Subcutaneous or skin-popping
       Oral
   c. What illegal means did you resort to in order to get it?
       Exchange of sex for drugs
       Selling drugs
       Selling belongings
       Selling family belongings
       Robbery, violent crime
6. Course, stage of change, and treatments
   Have you been in substance abuse treatment programs?
   Have you ever wanted to or tried to stop using? If so, when?
   Does substance use pose a risk or harm to you at this time?

Other drug–drug interactions, including those with psychotropic medication, are also significant. A patient with comorbid HIV and hepatitis C who stops all alcohol use during interferon treatment and eagerly resumes daily use after successful treatment and eradication of hepatitis C virus puts his or her hepatic function in jeopardy once again. For individuals who have unprotected sexual encounters in the context of alcohol or drug use, history-taking has public health implications. For individuals exposed to drug- or alcohol-related intimate partner violence, the implications are both tragic and obvious. Hence, for medical, psychological, and social reasons, a comprehensive drug history is essential in assessing persons with HIV and AIDS.

Inpatient general care consultations

For patients who are not known to the facility, it is important to obtain as much information as possible from members of the medical, surgical, obstetric, or other team providing care for the patient. A review of the chart, laboratory data, and current medications should be assessed. Clinicians should ascertain the correct name and room number, and check to be certain that the patient fits the description and that his or her identification bracelet matches the name of the patient referred. This is especially important because of the confidential nature of HIV illness. Specific recommendations for history-taking in the inpatient general care setting are summarized in Table 2.6.

PSYCHIATRIC EXAMINATION

The complete psychiatric assessment of a person with HIV and AIDS includes an evaluation of all the aspects of psychological functioning listed below. Every patient deserves the full baseline cognitive assessment suggested here, since early cognitive changes may be very subtle.

A patient may have no evidence of disorientation to person, place, or time, may be able to register and recall, and may not have a subjective awareness of any cognitive difficulty even though executive dysfunction may be evident through a clock drawing and preclinical findings may be indicated in constructional apraxia on three-dimensional cube or Bender-Gestalt drawings. Early-stage dementia may be indicated on formal testing in the comprehensive assessment described. In addition to cognitive disorders, a comprehensive psychiatric examination will provide evidence of any other psychiatric disorders. It will also help inform decisions on the patient's ability to adhere to care and help determine psychiatric treatment to alleviate

TABLE 2.6 Recommendations for History-Taking on Inpatient General Care

1. Knock on the door of the room even if it is open, and await a response.
2. Ascertain the patient's identity verbally and with identification bracelet while beginning introductions.
3. Introduction by name and title: "Good morning, Ms. B, I am Dr. P and I am a psychiatrist (while shaking hands).
4. Establish privacy by using the privacy curtains or door of the room.
5. Sit down near the bedside, preferably at the same level as the patient, if possible.
6. Attend to distractions with the patient's permission.
7. If the television is on at high volume, ask to turn it down.
8. If visitors are present, determine whether to proceed with the interview, request time alone, or reschedule after the visitors leave. Visits by partners, family members, or friends are especially important to persons with HIV and AIDS who, in addition to feeling isolated and alone as with any severe illness, are extremely sensitive to rejection and discrimination and may place a higher value on the presence of visitors.
9. Attend to comfort and address pain or other urgent issues.
10. Obstacles to communication
    a. The sleeping patient
       Since sleep disturbances are prevalent in persons with HIV and AIDS, consider allowing the patient to rest, and come back later.
          One may attempt to arouse the patient and obtain permission to proceed with the introduction and interview, with appropriate apology for disturbing his or her sleep.
    b. Pain
       Address pain issues with the primary nurse or physician.
    c. Nausea or vomiting
       Provide an emesis basin and report to the primary nurse.
    d. Need for bedpan or assistance to the bedside commode
       Provide a bedpan if available or contact a nursing assistant.
    e. Sensory deficits
       i. Visual impairment
          Describe what you are doing and what is happening and be certain not to touch the patient before fully explaining that you would like to shake hands in greeting and who and where you are.
       ii. Hearing impairment
          Ascertain that hearing aids are in place or obtain amplifiers. Ask if it is all right to turn off the television or radio to eliminate as much background noise as possible.
             Use lip reading if possible.
             Speak slowly, loudly, and clearly and on the side of the ear with the better hearing.
    f. Obtain interpreters if there is a language barrier.
    g. Communication barriers: endotracheal tube, tracheostomy, or ventilator
          Use a clipboard, paper, and pen to enable the patient to write responses to simple questions, if possible.
          Make use of a communication board if writing is not feasible because of paralysis or paresis.
          If these measures are not possible, use closed-ended questions with a code, such as head-nodding, blinking (1 blink designates "yes" and 2 blinks designates "no"), or finger squeezing (1 squeeze means "yes" and 2 squeezes means "no").

distress and suffering and decrease potential morbidity and mortality associated with nonadherence to care.

As with history-taking, there is no set order for the psychiatric examination. The least challenging and affect-laden areas should be addressed first and the more complex and difficult ones last. Many of the functions being evaluated will have been observed during the process of meeting the patient and taking the history. However, time has to be set aside to complete a full evaluation of the patient's current presentation, including assessment for depression, anxiety, psychosis, suicidality, danger to others, and cognition. The setting of the consultation is meaningful—a higher prevalence of delirium can be anticipated in acute general-care units and especially intensive care units, and a higher prevalence of HIV-associated dementia can be expected in the nursing home or long-term care facility settings.

General appearance, manner, attitude, and relevant physical signs and symptoms

The psychiatrist can observe for signs of medical or psychiatric illnesses: mobility, gait, abnormal movements, general appearance, grooming, appropriateness and neatness of attire, responsiveness, cooperation, and ability to maintain eye contact.

Observation for psychomotor retardation (slowing) or agitation can be helpful. The psychiatrist can listen carefully for rate, quality, tone, audibility, modulation, and form of speech, including evidence of prosody, aphasias, or dysphasias.

Additionally, observation of skin for icterus, pallor, cyanosis, edema, rashes, or other lesions can be useful. The psychiatrist should also evaluate whether the patient appears healthy or ill, robust or cachectic, with signs of wasting and protein energy undernutrition.

Obvious signs of specific medical illness or organ impairment include seizures, involuntary movements, tremors, paresis, paralysis, facial droop or asymmetry, exophthalmos, neck fullness, spider angiomata, ascites, anascarca, dyspnea, clubbing, and pedal edema.

The psychiatrist can look for signs of delirium such as fluctuating levels of consciousness or attention (as evidenced by ability to change mental set during the interview, ability to follow the content and meaning, and ability to follow complex commands), mood, and behavior, and falling asleep during the evaluation. Similarly, delirium related to intoxication or withdrawal can be observed with signs of slurred speech, "nodding out," or flattening of the nasal cartilage (due to cocaine insufflation). Also note the presence of tremulousness (especially if there is postural tremor, which indicates alcohol or benziodiazepine withdrawal), pinpoint pupils (from use of opioids), dilated pupils (from opioid withdrawal or PCP), diaphoresis (from opiate withdrawal or stimulant intoxication), tracks and abscesses from injection drug use, and skin lesions indicative of subcutaneous drug use.

Attention to vital signs can show elevated systolic or diastolic blood pressure as well as tachycardia in either intoxication with stimulants or withdrawal from alcohol, benzodiazepines, or stimulants.

Finally, the psychiatrist can look for signs of side effects of medications, such as lipodystrophy from antiretroviral medications or orobuccolingual movements (tardive dyskinesia) from psychotropic medications.

It is also important to determine whether the patient appears his or her stated age and, if the patient is working, whether he or she is appropriately attired for the occupation. Observing for relational ability, eye contact, handshake, and ability to engage is also significant. The patient's cooperativeness, hostility, depression, anxiety, and fear should be noted.

Affectivity and mood

Observation of affect includes attention to euthymia, depression, anxiety, elation, irritability, hostility, expansiveness, appropriateness of affect in relation to reported mood and thought content, and constriction or fullness of range. Affectivity is a somewhat objective assessment by the clinician, whereas mood is more subjective and reflects the patient's assessment of how he or she feels. Moods can be sad, tearful, anxious, angry, or suspicious. Often, before physical signs are apparent, the first hallmark of withdrawal from any substance of abuse is irritability or emotional lability. Suicidal ideas or intentions as well as plans or thoughts should be explored. Violent or homicidal ideas or plans need to be discussed.

Thought content and mental trend

Delusions, ideas of reference, flight of ideas, tangentiality, preoccupation, paranoid ideation, and expansiveness are important to assess. Specific well-formed and systematic delusions or grandiose ideas as well as general suspiciousness and guarding are indicative of underlying psychotic processes.

Perception

The patient should be asked about perceptions in a supportive manner that does not create defensiveness. Asking whether the patient "ever sees shadows" or feels that his or her "mind may be playing tricks" may be helpful.

Specific questions to determine the presence of auditory, visual, olfactory, or tactile (coenesthetic) hallucinations and formication are necessary. Visual hallucinations include those of colorful, frightening, Lilliputian, and specific people, alive or deceased. Observation for signs that the patient is responding to internal stimuli should be documented.

Cognition

This is a crucial part of the evaluation and needs to be done in a systematic and comprehensive and nonthreatening manner. The initial aspects have to do with observation as described above in the section on general appearance, manner, and attitude, observing for level of alertness, consciousness, confusion, fluctuation, somnolence, or stupor. Careful observation may reveal perseveration on words, numbers, or actions. Perseveration may be evident in the absence of hearing impairment when the patient responds to a prior question more than one time as if he or she had not heard the subsequent question.

Specific questions regarding orientation can be approached in an ego-supportive manner and can be asked as part of the routine. Memory is best tested by observing the patient's ability to provide his or her medical history in an organized manner and asking direct and specific questions about onset, course, and treatments. If a patient spontaneously reveals that memory is a problem, this lead can be followed with a statement such as "Let's see how your memory is working now." This can provide a smooth transition into a formal assessment of cognitive abilities. Memory is tested with evaluation of remote, recent, registration, and recall (the four Rs of memory). Asking the patient to repeat the four words "hat," "car," "tree," and "twenty-six" from a cognitive screening device (Jacobs et al., 1977) and then recall them again 5 minutes later provides a test for registration and 5-minute recall. However, given that HIV affects primarily subcortical processes, standard memory tests alone can often underestimate cognitive difficulties in these patients. Other tests that involve aspects of executive functioning and processing speed can often be quite helpful.

While a complete neuropsychological battery is often beyond the reach of many practitioners and clinics, referral for neuropsychological testing can be helpful in clinically unclear areas, especially when dealing with areas related to patient safety. Also, the clinician can perform basic testing within the consultation model by including such tasks as Trails A/B or the Digit Symbol Substitution Test, which reflect aspects of executive function and processing speed. Frontal-executive function testing by means of the Frontal Assessment Battery is a useful bedside test that can also be quite sensitive in picking up subcortical deficits and processing delays.

Drawings can help in the assessment of visuospatial function as well as for perseveration and fine hand tremor that may be present as part of the motor syndrome of HIV. The copying of Bender-Gestalt drawings and a three-dimensional cube assesses for constructional apraxia, as does a clock drawing (Bender, 1938; Lyketsos et al., 2004). Clock drawing is especially helpful in assessing executive function and planning as well as for constructional apraxia and hemineglect. Irregular spacing of clock numbers with some too close together or too far apart indicates executive dysfunction with difficulty in planning. Left hemineglect may be associated with a lesion in the right parietal lobe. Repetition of the clock numbers is indicative of perseveration.

Repetition of numbers indicates perseveration, as does repetitive movements when performing Luria maneuvers (repeated and mimicked patterns of fist, edge, and palm to palm gestures) or copying repetitive figures. The patient should be asked to draw the face of a clock, starting with a circle and placing the numbers on the face. The patient should then be asked to draw the hands to represent a time of 10 after 11 on the clock drawing to assess ability to change mental sets.

Further testing for abstract thinking with similarities and proverb interpretation as well as interpretation of current events is helpful. Intellectual function should be assessed in relation to educational and occupational levels and can be tested by observing vocabulary usage, comprehension level, and reasoning.

To assess for concentration, calculation, and spelling, the patient can be asked to subtract serial 7's or 3's and spell the word "world" both forward and backward. Performance on this task may vary between individuals according to their level of education and what native language they speak. Another task that can assess performance in this domain is to have the patient repeat the months of the year or the days of the week forward and backward. Asking the patient about their understanding of their illness can provide an assessment of insight and judgment as well as abstract thinking.

Screening Tools and Instruments

In the authors' view, a comprehensive biopsychosocial assessment by an AIDS psychiatrist is the gold standard for the assessment and management of HIV-positive patients with substance abuse or mental illness. However, resources are limited, and it is not feasible for an AIDS psychiatrist to perform a detailed psychiatric assessment on every HIV-infected patient.

In these circumstances, there is a risk that psychiatric issues may remain unrecognized and untreated, and for this reason brief psychiatric screening instruments may be useful for HIV staff and clinicians. However, the use of screening scales has important caveats and limitations. In order to remain brief, screening scales often focus on just one or a limited number of psychiatric disorders, and to avoid missing cases, they are prone to sacrificing diagnostic specificity for sensitivity. Referral and treatment algorithms also need to be in place for those HIV-infected patients who are identified by screening instruments as requiring further psychiatric assessment.

This section is not intended to provide a comprehensive review of screening instruments but instead will focus on a limited number of scales that have been validated or are commonly used in the HIV-infected population. For a description of other psychiatric screening instruments developed for use in medically ill patients, the reader is directed to reference sources such the *Textbook of Psychosomatic Medicine* (Levenson, 2005).

The 16-item substance abuse (SA)/mental illness (MI) Symptoms Screener (SAMISS), which can be administered in less than 10 minutes, was developed to screen for substance abuse, manic and depressive episodes, generalized anxiety disorder, panic disorder, post-traumatic stress disorder, and adjustment disorder in a HIV clinic population (Pence et al., 2005; Whetten et al., 2005). The authors chose to focus on these psychiatric disorders because of the increased prevalence of these disorders in the HIV population and their association with worsened medication adherence and treatment outcomes. A validation study of the SAMISS conducted in an HIV-positive clinic population had 86% sensitivity and 75% specificity for substance abuse, and 95% sensitivity and 49% specificity for mental illness as compared to the Structured Clinical Interview for DSM-IV (Pence et al., 2005).

The Client Diagnostic Questionnaire (CDQ), with an administration time of 15–20 minutes and based on the Primary Care Evaluation of Mental Disorders (PRIME-MD), was designed to screen for depression, PTSD, panic and other anxiety-spectrum disorders, substance abuse, and psychosis in a diversity of HIV service settings (Aidala, et al., 2004). For the diagnosis of any disorder, the sensitivity of the CDQ was 91% and specificity 78% as compared to clinician assessment.

Although the Mini-International Neuropsychiatric Interview (M.I.N.I) was not specifically designed for a HIV service setting, a number of HIV providers have reported its usefulness in this population. The M.I.N.I, a structured diagnostic interview with an administration time of approximately 15–20 minutes, screens for a broad range of anxiety, mood, substance abuse, eating and psychotic disorders, antisocial personality disorder, and suicidality (Sheehan et al., 1998). The instrument may be individualized, and modules such as eating disorders, which are less important for the HIV-infected population, may be excluded.

Depression is common among HIV-infected individuals and is associated with worsened medication adherence (Starace et al., 2002; Ammassari et al.,

2004). Although not specifically developed for the HIV-infected patient, a number of brief screening scales, including the Hamilton Rating Scale for Depression (Hamilton, 1968), Hospital Anxiety and Depression Scale (Zigmond and Snaith, 1983), Beck Depression Inventory-II, Center for Epidemiologic Studies Depression Scale, Zung Self-Rating Depression Scale (Coulehan et al., 1989), and nine-question Patient Health Questionnaire (Spitzer et al., 1999) may be used to screen for depression in the HIV-infected patient.

As previously described, neuropsychological deficits are prevalent in HIV-infected patients. Commonly used cognitive assessments such as the Folstein Mini Mental State Exam (MMSE) (Folstein et al., 1975) are inaccurate for detecting HIV-associated subcortical dementia. Assessments designed for the HIV-infected population such as the HIV Dementia Scale (Power et al., 1995; Berghuis et al., 1999), modified HIV Dementia Scale (Davis et al., 2002), and Mental Alternation Test (Jones et al., 1993) are superior to the MMSE for detecting HIV-associated dementia but are not sensitive for identifying patients with less severe HIV-associated minor cognitive or motor disorder.

CONCLUSIONS

A biopsychosocial approach to psychiatric evaluation of a person with HIV and AIDS can provide a way to get to know the individual in the context of family, society, and community. This approach to psychiatric assessment is a significant part of the comprehensive care of a person with HIV and AIDS. It can help prevent the spread of HIV infection, improve adherence to medical care, reduce stigma associated with HIV and AIDS, and alleviate distress in persons with HIV and AIDS, their loved ones, and their caregivers.

REFERENCES

Aidala A, Havens J, Mellins CA, Dodds S, Whetten K, Martin D, Gillis L (2004). Development and validation of the Client Diagnostic Questionnaire (CDQ): a mental health screening tool for use in HIV/AIDS service settings. *Psychol Health Med* 9:362–380.

Ammassari A, Antinori A, Aloisi MS, Trotta MP, Murri R, Bartoli L, Monforte AD, Wu AW, Starace F (2004). Depressive symptoms, neurocognitive impairment, and adherence to highly active antiretroviral therapy among HIV-infected persons. *Psychosomatics* 45:394–402.

Bender L (1938). *A Visual Motor Gestalt Test and Its Clinical Use*. New York: American Orthopsychiatry Association.

Berghuis JP, Uldall KK, Lalonde B (1999). Validity of two scales in identifying HIV-associated dementia. *J Acquir Immune Defic Syndr* 21:134–140.

Blank MB, Mandell DS, Aiken L, Hadley TR (2002). Co-occurrence of HIV and serious mental illness among Medicaid recipients. *Psychiatr Serv* 53:868–873.

Bostwick JM, Cohen LM (2009). Differentiating suicide from life-ending acts and end-of-life decisions: a model based on chronic kidney disease and dialysis. *Psychosomatics* 50(1):1–7.

Cohen MA (1987). Psychiatric aspects of AIDS: a biopsychosocial approach. In GP Wormser, RE Stahl, and EJ Bottone (eds.), *AIDS and Other Manifestations of HIV Infection*. Park Ridge, NJ: Noyes Publishers.

Cohen MA (1992). Biopsychosocial aspects of the HIV epidemic. In GP Wormser (ed.), *AIDS and Other Manifestations of HIV Infection*, second ed. (pp. 349–371). New York: Raven Press.

Cohen MA, Alfonso CA (1998). Psychiatric care and pain management in persons with HIV infection. In GP Wormser (ed.), *AIDS and Other Manifestations of HIV Infection*, third edition. Philadelphia: Lippincott-Raven Publishers.

Cohen MA, Alfonso CA (2004). AIDS psychiatry: psychiatric and palliative care, and pain management. In GP Wormser (ed.), *AIDS and Other Manifestations of HIV Infection*, fourth ed. (pp. 537–576). San Diego: Elsevier Academic Press.

Cohen MA, Chao D (2008). Comprehensive psychosocial and psychiatric diagnostic consultation in persons with HIV and AIDS. In MA Cohen and JM Gorman (eds.), *Comprehensive Textbook of AIDS Psychiatry* (pp. 61–73). New York: Oxford University Press.

Cohen MA, Weisman H (1986). A biopsychosocial approach to AIDS. *Psychosomatics* 27:245–249.

Cohen MA, Weisman HW (1988). A biopsychosocial approach to AIDS. In RP Galea, BF Lewis, and LA Baker (eds.), *AIDS and IV Drug Abusers*. Owings Mills, MD: National Health Publishing.

Coulehan JL, Schulber HC, Block MR (1989). The efficiency of depression questionnaires for case finding in primary medical care. *J Gen Intern Med* 4:541–547.

Davis HF, Skolasky RL Jr, Selnes OA, Burgess DM, McArthur JC (2002). Assessing HIV-associated dementia: modified HIV Dementia Scale versus the grooved pegboard. *AIDS Read* 12:29–38.

Folstein MF, Folstein SE, McHugh PR (1975). "Mini-Mental State." A practical method for grading the cognitive state of patients for the clinician. *J Psychiatr Res* 12:189–198.

Freedman JB, O'Dowd MA, Wyszynsk B, Torres JR, McKegney FP (1994). Depression, HIV dementia, delirium, posttraumatic stress disorder (or all of the above). *Gen Hosp Psychiatry* 16:426–434.

Greenfield J (2007). Coming out: the process of forming a positive identity. In HJ Makadon, KH Mayer, J Potter, and H Goldhammer (eds.), *The Fenway Guide to Lesbian, Gay, Bisexual, and Transgender Health*. Philadelphia: American College of Physicians.

Hamilton M (1968). Development of a rating scale for primary depressive illness. *Br J Soc Clin Psychol* 6:278–296.

Huang L, Quartin A, Jones D, Havlir DV (2006). Intensive care of patients with HIV infection. *N Engl J Med* 355:173–181.

Jacobs JN, Bernhard MR, Delgado A, Strain JJ (1977). Screening for organic mental syndromes in the medically ill. *Ann Intern Med* 86:40–46.

Jones BN, Teng EL, Folstein MF, Harrison KS (1993). A new bedside test of cognition for patients with HIV infection. *Ann Intern Med* 119:1001–1004.

Levenson JL (2005). *The American Psychiatric Publishing Textbook of Psychosomatic Medicine*. Washington, DC: American Psychiatric Publishing.

Lyketsos CG, Rosenblatt A, Rabins P (2004). Forgotten frontal lobe syndrome or "executive dysfunction syndrome." *Psychosomatics* 43(3):345–355.

McNiel DE, Chamberlain JR, Weaver CM, Hall SE, Fordwood SR, Binder RL (2008). Impact of clinical training on violence risk assessment. *Am J Psychiatry* 165:195–200.

Pence BW, Gaynes BN, Whetten K, Eron JJ Jr, Ryder RW, Miller WC (2005). Validation of a brief screening instrument for substance abuse and mental illness in HIV-positive patients. *J Acquir Immune Defic Syndr* 40:434–444.

Power C, Selnes OA, Grim JA, McArthur JC (1995). HIV Dementia Scale: a rapid screening test. *J Acquir Immune Defic Syndr Hum Retrovirol* 8:273–278.

Sheehan DV, Lecrubier Y, Sheehan KH, Amorim P, Janavs J, Weiller E, Hergueta T, Baker R, Dunbar GC (1998). The Mini-International Neuropsychiatric Interview (M.I.N.I.): the development and validation of a structured diagnostic psychiatric interview for DSM-IV and ICD-10. *J Clin Psychiatry* 59 (Suppl 20):22–33.

Spitzer RL, Kroenke K, Williams JB (1999). Validation and utility of a self-report version of PRIME-MD: the PHQ primary care study. Primary Care Evaluation of Mental Disorders. Patient Health Questionnaire. *JAMA* 282:1737–1744.

Starace F, Ammassari A, Trotta MP, Murri R, de Longis P, Izzo C, Scalzini A, d'Arminio Monforte A, Wu AW, Antinori A, AdICoNA and the Neuro IcoNA Study Groups (2002). Depression is a risk factor for suboptimal adherence to highly active antiretroviral therapy. *J Acquir Immune Defic Syndr* 31:S136–S139.

Stoff DM, Mitnick L, Kalichman S (2004). Research issues in the multiple diagnoses of HIV/AIDS, mental illness and substance abuse. *AIDS Care* 16 (Suppl 1):S1–S5.

Whetten K, Reif S, Swartz M, Stevens R, Ostermann J, Hanisch L, Eron JJ Jr (2005). A brief mental health and substance abuse screener for persons with HIV. *AIDS Patient Care STDs* 19:89–99.

Zigmond AS, Snaith RP (1983) The Hospital Anxiety and Depression Scale. *Acta Psychiatr Scand* 67:361–370.

Appendix A

Initial Consultation or Evaluation

TABLE 2.A   Initial Consultaion or Evaluation

Consult requested by:

Reason for Consultation: (include pertinent observations and questions by
  health-care professional requesting consult)

Chief Complaint:

History of Present Illness:

Past Psychiatric History: (especially note history of psychiatric admission or
  outpatient care, suicide attempts and suicide risk factors, and history of
  violence or impulsive behavior)

Substance Abuse History: (besides specific substances of abuse and time course
  also include history of substance abuse treatment such as rehabilitation and
  detoxification)

Social and Occupational History:

Sexual History:

Trauma History:

Developmental History:

Family History:

Past Medical History:

Allergies:

Current Medications: (also indicate if any recent changes to regimen)

Laboratory Results:

Imaging Results and Other Tests:

Vital Signs: (especially note any abnormalities over last 24–48 hours)

Neurological Exam: (for patients being evaluated for alcohol or benzodiazepine
  withdrawal include presence of postural tremor or hyperreflexia; include pupil

(continued)

TABLE 2.A (Continued)

size and light reflex in assessing patients with possible history of opiate abuse or withdrawal; also note presence and nature of any involuntary movements for patients with neuroleptic treatment experience)

Mental Status Exam:

Appearance/Behavior:

Speech:

Affect:

Mood:

Thought Process:

Thought Content:

Cognitive: (also include clock and Bender-Gestalt drawings)

Insight:

Judgment:

Diagnostic Impression: (comment on both suspected acute and chronic processes)

Psychic Strengths and Weaknesses: (Is this patient very resilient in a particular way? Do they have a specific point of weakness that can obstruct treatment such as denial of their illness or inability to relate to others?)

Recommendations: (This is an opportunity for the consultant to make recommendations to facilitate the global medical and psychiatric care, i.e., the total well-being of the patient, and reinforce their strengths. There may be comfort factors of other physical complaints that the patient would like to have addressed or pain control may be inadequate. In situations where there are multiple dimensions to address, e.g., in a patient requiring multimodal treatment for addiction, anxiety disorder, and insomnia, it would be beneficial for the primary team to have a clear understanding of how to prioritize these complaints and in which order to treat them, if applicable.)

3

HIV through the Life Cycle

Mary Ann Cohen, Sharon M. Batista, and Jocelyn Soffer

HIV infection can occur at any time in the life cycle from the newborn period, through childhood and adolescence to adulthood, older age. The unique issues and special vulnerabilities involved with each aspect of the life cycle, from family planning to pregnancy and the newborn to older aged person with HIV, are addressed from the biopsychosocial standpoint. While some features of HIV illness are common to any age group, specific challenges arise at various stages of the life cycle, as well as different patterns of transmission, clinical course, and service needs. This chapter will consider such differences at various stages of the life cycle.

HIV in Infants and Toddlers

At the beginning of the AIDS epidemic almost 30 years ago, infected blood products represented a common mode of transmission, with many children diagnosed with HIV infection after receiving transfusions for hemophilia and blood disorders. Because of current practices of screening blood products prior to transfusion, the face of neonatal and early-childhood HIV has changed considerably, to one of children who are infected mostly perinatally through vertical transmission, rather than through exposure to blood products.

While the incidence of perinatally acquired infections is decreasing in areas of the world where there is access to HIV care and antiretroviral medication, some transmission of HIV from mother to child remains, both in the United States and throughout the world. In 2007, approximately 79 infants were born with HIV in the United States, compared with 330 in

1994 (CDC, 2007). The primary means of HIV infection of a newborn is vertical transmission during gestation, birth, or breastfeeding of an infant by an HIV-positive mother. It is strongly recommended that all pregnant women be screened for HIV infection as part of routine prenatal care. Such screening is not legally mandatory, however, and may not be performed without the mother's consent.

It is advantageous to obtain HIV testing as early as possible in the course of a pregnancy so that preparation can be made to reduce the risk of transmission to the infant. Without preventive care during gestation or delivery, the risk of transmission from mother to child is 15%–35% (Newell, 1991; Gabiano et al., 1992). This risk is reduced to less than 1% risk with antiviral therapy, elective cesarean section, and exclusive bottle-feeding (European Collaborative Study, 2005). Presently, recommendations for treatment of HIV infection in pregnant women are the same as those for non-pregnant women. As of 2007, guidelines during pregnancy are as follows: "For HIV-infected pregnant women who do not require therapy for their own health, antiretroviral drugs are recommended for prevention of mother-to-child transmission. HAART [highly active antiretroviral therapy] is recommended for all women with HIV RNA levels of ≥ 1000 copies/mL, along with consideration of elective cesarean section. For women with HIV RNA levels <1000 copies/mL, a 3-parts zidovudine regimen (prenatal, intrapartum, and neonatal) should be used alone or in combination with antiretroviral drugs" (Jamieson et al., 2007).

Even with treatment of the mother during gestation and delivery, it is important that the infant be tested for HIV at the time of birth, as well as periodically thereafter as indicated. Many states allow or even mandate testing of the infant without consent by the mother at the time of delivery if the HIV status of the mother is unknown. These states include New York, Connecticut, and Indiana (Kaiser Family Foundation, 2008). This surveillance is performed so that appropriate treatment can be initiated immediately. It is also important in such situations to counsel the mother so that she can anticipate both her and her infant's needs for HIV-related primary care.

HIV antibody detection is not useful for neonatal diagnosis of HIV infection. If vertical HIV transmission is suspected, virological tests to identify antibody to the virus or components, including DNA polymerase chain reaction (PCR) and RNA PCR, are made within 48 hours of birth, at 1 to 2 months, and at 3 to 6 months to distinguish decreasing maternal antibody from infant antibody. Other tests include enzyme-linked immunosorbent assay (ELISA) or enzyme immunoassay, Western blot, p24 antigen capture assay, and culture. CD4 count and HIV RNA provide additional complementary and independent information about prognosis and may later help determine when to start or change antiretroviral therapy.

At times, a mother learns of her own infection during routine HIV testing during pregnancy or mandatory testing of her newborn. Any unexpected positive test result represents a crisis point and a critical time for psychosocial intervention and education. Common immediate questions include how and when the mother became infected, with whom the diagnosis can be shared, and how the infant's life and her caregiver role will be affected. For mothers who are HIV positive, it is recommended that they abstain from all breast-feeding following delivery, as this carries risk of transmission of the virus. The lack of breastfeeding can also lead to concerns regarding nutrition for the growing infant as well as for the development of maternal infant attachment.

When assessing the emotional health and development of infants and toddlers, one must remember that toddlers younger than 2 years of age are themselves unable to grasp the concept of a life-threatening illness. Infants are nonetheless certainly affected by the behaviors and emotional states of their caregivers; delays in development, failure to thrive, and other behavioral changes can reflect the distress of an infant.

HIV in Children and Adolescents

Emotional and physical reactions to illness

Upon diagnosis with HIV, many reactions are possible, spanning from denial to the activation of anticipatory grief. The latter reaction may be especially prominent and compounded in families with the loss of multiple relatives from HIV infection. The parents and family of a child with HIV may feel that their child has a foreshortened future; such reactions must be addressed and education provided about realistic expectations (Pao and Wiener, 2008).

Despite tremendous advances in social awareness about HIV as well as advances in treatment of the illness, stigmatization persists. Massive public education campaigns to increase knowledge that HIV cannot be acquired through casual contact such as hugging, kissing, using a toilet, or sharing utensils have not fully eradicated continuing AIDSism (Cohen, 1989; Cohen, 2008), fear of AIDS, and AIDS discrimination. (Please refer to Chapter 4 for further general discussion regarding stigma in HIV.) AIDSism can particularly affect children. Others may respond anxiously and with unnecessary caution toward, or even avoidance of, a child with HIV. Families and children may find themselves adapting their behavior in anticipation of or in reaction to the fears of others.

Often, children with HIV live with the illness as a secret, sharing the diagnosis with only very close and trusted family and friends. In some cases, the parent may hide the illness from everyone but the child, going to great

TABLE 3.1 Stresses Associated with Illness in Children and Adolescents

1. Medical factors (complex medical regimens, side effects of therapy)
2. Psychological stressors (secrecy, guilt, fear of ostracism and death, uncertainties about future, sexual activity)
3. Social stressors (concerns surrounding disclosure, dating, insurance, academic and vocational success)

lengths to do so. Such efforts to maintain a cohesive cover story about the child's illness are not only exhausting for the family but also result in an elaborate network of lies and deception that is disruptive to the child's psychological development (Havens et al., 2005). If the child is not allowed to discuss the illness with anyone, he or she learns at an early age that there is something to feel ashamed and fearful about. This leads to social isolation and increased difficulty adjusting to illness-related challenges.

Children infected with HIV can experience delays in growth and the delayed onset of puberty. Cognitive deficits have also been noted. Although the mechanisms for these developmental changes are likely multi-factorial and not yet well understood, it is known that close pediatric care is essential for the child with HIV. As shown in Table 3.1, the stress associated with HIV infection in children and adolescents can be divided into three categories (Belman et al., 1992). Approaching a child through the lens of these categories can help the clinician to decipher changes in a child's behavior and affect, with the resulting understanding of the child incorporated into comprehensive psychosocial assessment and treatment planning.

CDC definition in children and adolescents

The Centers for Disease Control and Prevention (CDC) AIDS case definition for children is used for surveillance and reporting and is similar to the one used for adults, with several exceptions. Lymphoid interstitial pneumonia/pulmonary lymphoid hyperplasia (LIP/PLH) and multiple or recurrent serious bacterial infections are AIDS defining for children, but not for adults. Additionally, certain types of cytomegalovirus (CMV), herpes simplex virus infections, and toxoplasmosis of the brain are AIDS defining only for adults and for children older than 1 month of age. An expanded definition for AIDS in adolescents and adults, amended in 1993, does not apply to children younger than 13 years old. A separate classification system has been developed to describe the spectrum of HIV disease to include HIV-exposed infants with undetermined infection status. Degree of immunosuppression is defined on the basis of age-adjusted CD4+ lymphocyte counts and percentages (Kline, 2007).

In vertically acquired HIV infection, clinical manifestations do not usually appear in the neonatal period and in infants and children are varied and often nonspecific. Lymphadenopathy, often in association with hepatosplenomegaly, can be an early sign of infection. During the first year of life, oral candidiasis, failure to thrive, and developmental delay are other common presenting features of HIV infection. Table 3.2 lists the most common AIDS-defining conditions observed among children in the United States with vertically acquired HIV infection.

Coping with stigma and the school setting

Children must also cope with stigma as it arises in school settings. It is illegal to discriminate against children with HIV in the public school system, but parents continue to report concerns as well as troubling experiences with disclosing serostatus to a child's school. Disclosure, even to trusted teachers and school staff, should be made with great consideration and support. HIV medication regimens present one major barrier to not disclosing a child's diagnosis to the school, as young children cannot take medications independently. This is particularly challenging with medications that need to be dosed multiple times a day or taken with food. Children often need assistance with explaining the need to take medications, any obvious illness, or school absences to both their peers and teachers.

If the family decides it is in the child's best interest to share the diagnosis with the school, the health-care team can assist families with the school process. Possible interventions include those indicated in Table 3.3 (Armstrong et al., 1993; Cohen et al., 1997; Wiener et al., 1998). Balancing academic expectations for the child and flexibility in assignments according to what the child can keep up with (e.g., in light of frequent clinic visits or cognitive deficits) is a challenge for parents and teachers. Nevertheless, this balance is of great importance in preparing the child for the responsibilities of adolescence and young adulthood (Wiener et al., 2003).

Other barriers to care

There are other issues that may affect children as they cope with illness and treatment and subsequently lead to nonadherence with medication. Children often complain that pill sizes are large and difficult to swallow. Some medications require refrigeration or must be taken with particular food requirements (e.g., on an empty stomach or with a high-fat meal) (Koenig and Bachanas, 2007). Although it may sound trivial, forgetfulness is cited as a major reason for young people missing doses of medication. To increase adherence in this population, technology can be very helpful, including the use of pagers, PDAs with password-protected reminders, and cell phones, which are especially popular with teens. Pharmacies have developed special blister packs in which all doses for a particular time of day are sealed in a

TABLE 3.2 1994 Revised HIV Pediatric Classification System: Clinical Categories

Category N: Not Symptomatic

Children who have no signs or symptoms considered to be the result of HIV infection or who have only one of the conditions listed in category A

Category A: Mildly Symptomatic

Children with two or more of the following conditions but none of the conditions listed in categories B and C:

- Dermatitis
- Hepatomegaly
- Lymphadenopathy (>0.5 cm at more than two sites; bilateral—one site)
- Parotitis
- Recurrent or persistent upper respiratory infection, sinusitis, or otitis media
- Splenomegaly

Category B: Moderately Symptomatic

Children who have symptomatic conditions other than those listed for category A or category C that are attributed to HIV infection. Examples of conditions in clinical category B include but are not limited to the following:

- Anemia (<8 g/dL), neutropenia (<1000/mm^3), or thrombocytopenia (<100,000/mm^3) persisting >30 days
- Bacterial meningitis, pneumonia, or sepsis (single episode)
- Candidiasis, oropharyngeal (i.e., thrush) persisting for >2 months
- Cardiomyopathy
- Cytomegalovirus (CMV) infection with onset before age 1 month
- Diarrhea, recurrent or chronic
- Fever lasting >1 month
- Hepatitis
- Herpes simplex virus (HSV) stomatitis, recurrent (i.e., more than two episodes within 1 year)
- HSV bronchitis, pneumonitis, or esophagitis with onset before age 1 month
- Herpes zoster (i.e., shingles) involving at least two distinct episodes or more than one dermatome
- Leiomyosarcoma
- Lymphoid interstitial pneumonia (LIP) or pulmonary lymphoid hyperplasia (PLH) complex
- Nephropathy
- Nocardiosis
- Toxoplasmosis with onset before age 1 month
- Varicella, disseminated (i.e., complicated chickenpox)

Category C: Severely Symptomatic

Children who have any condition listed in the 1987 surveillance case definition for acquired immunodeficiency syndrome, with the exception of LIP (which is a category B condition)

Source: Centers for Disease Control and Prevention (1994). *Morbidity and Mortality Weekly Report,* 43 (no. RR-12): 1–10. Accessed from Kline (2007).

TABLE 3.3 How the Health-Care Team Can Assist with School Issues

a. Inform parents of a child's right to an education
b. Meet with school officials and school personnel to educate them about HIV infection and apprise them of the individual needs of a specific child
c. Accompany parents to a school board meeting when they feel this would be of support
d. Provide consultation to teachers and principals in talking to the other classmates about HIV and AIDS
e. Provide up-to-date information to the school about the child's progress if the child has been out ill for a period of time

TABLE 3.4 Treatment Nonadherence and Strategies to Improve Adherence in Children

Barrier	Strategies to Overcome Barrier
Pill sizes are large and difficult to swallow	Training children to swallow pills with more comfort
Forgetfulness	Use of technology: pagers, PDAs with password-protected reminders, cell phones
Complex pill regimens	Special blister packs and/or pillboxes

packet together, which represents an alternative to using the traditional pillbox. Combinations of these approaches can be helpful; Lyon and colleagues (2003) demonstrated that a group method was effective in educating adolescents and young adults about how to use a pillbox, combined with a calendar or alarm watch, to appropriately remember dosage times. In this study, they noted decreased viral loads in some participants and increased health-related behaviors overall. Workshops and videos have also been studied (Sampaio-Sa et al., 2008).

Table 3.4 summarizes some of the barriers to treatment adherence and strategies to address them.

Gaining access to care may provide additional challenges for families. Medications and office visits are expensive and many providers require insurance. Patients must travel to various providers' offices, which can be logistically challenging for families. Additionally, business hours may coincide with school hours, causing absences at school.

The teenage years

A developmental task of teenagers is negotiating a balance between becoming more independent and maintaining ties with the family of origin. Risk reduction in adolescents is thus particularly challenging given that many adolescents, as part of this stage of life, question or even act against the very limitations and rules that are initiated to protect them. They may be unreceptive to education efforts regarding safe and healthy sex practices, HIV and other sexually transmitted diseases, pregnancy prevention and planning, and substance abuse prevention or treatment.

In addition to this predilection for challenging protective guidelines, other factors have been identified as risk factors in teenagers. Lesbian, gay, bisexual, or transgender (LGBT) youth may be particularly at risk for unhealthy behaviors associated with transmission of HIV and poor self-care. A recent study found that young men who have sex with men and who seek partners on the Internet also identified other behaviors that place them at risk for contracting sexually transmitted infections. These behaviors include risky sexual intercourse, sexual activity at a club or bathhouse, and multiple anal intercourse partners during the past 3 months (Garofalo et al., 2007). Another study of bisexual and lesbian adolescents found an increased likelihood of engaging in prostitution, having frequent intercourse, and using ineffective contraception (Saewyc et al., 1999). Housing instability is another risk factor for HIV infection in adolescents. In a study by Marshall and colleagues (2009), homelessness was inversely associated with condom use, and unstable housing was associated with increased numbers of sex partners.

HIV testing and treatment are more complicated in the care of minors, who by definition are not of legal age to consent to treatment without the consent of a legal guardian. Laws regarding parental consent in such cases vary from state to state. Public health campaigns have demonstrated that there is an overwhelming advantage in establishing rapport and offering treatment to an adolescent who presents requesting care without the knowledge or presence of a parent, specifically in the case of sexual health or pregnancy. In most states, these two areas are exempt from laws requiring parental consent for treatment. But this is not the case in all states, so it is important for providers to know the law as it applies to their specific state.

Psychotherapy for children and adolescents

Psychotherapy is an important part of the care of a child coping with HIV infection. Interventions are diverse and often include the entire family or support network. As treatment of HIV has improved with antiretroviral therapy (ART), psychosocial and psychiatric management of HIV-infected children and adolescents has evolved from primarily bereavement and family stabilization models to those promoting quality of life in chronic illness. Preparing for long-term survival, achieving academic success, living independently, and preventing secondary infection have become important goals in the care of HIV-infected youth. Frequently, youths with HIV have complex social and psychiatric needs, with histories of disrupted home life, family history of mental illness and substance abuse, and exposure to trauma and urban violence. Social, psychological, and treatment issues are age specific and usually involve difficulties with peers, self-image, sexuality, and planning for life as an adult.

The way in which the school-age child copes with illness depends on many factors, including age and developmental stage, parental adaptation, social skills, and psychological makeup (Wiener et al., 2003). Children tend to ask many questions, including "why," "what," "when," "how," and "what if" questions. Psychosocial treatment should be guided by the child's developmental stage, cognitive abilities, stage of illness, and disclosure status (see Table 3.5). These factors determine the meaning that the illness carries for the child and the kind of psychological and intellectual resources available.

The efficacy of group treatment modalities in children affected by HIV was assessed by Funck-Brentano and colleagues (2005). In this pilot study, a peer support group intervention was associated with an improvement in children's emotional well-being, which can have a positive influence on medical outcomes.

Children are also affected by the illness of parents and siblings; it is common for some of these youngsters to become "parentified," prematurely taking on adult responsibilities and roles before they are emotionally or developmentally ready (Bekir et al., 1993; Valleau et al., 1995). The greater the severity of their parents' illness, the more children tend to assume inappropriate adult role behaviors. Psychotherapeutic interventions for children in HIV-affected households should be sensitive to such issues. They should also assist with permanency and legacy planning and promote social-support networks (Wiener et al., 2003). Special attention must be given to the rivalry and envy that might arise in the well child when the HIV-infected child receives special medical care and parental attention (Fanos and Wiener, 1994).

The teenage years represent a time of developmental transitions, with the usual stresses compounded in those also dealing with HIV, whether in themselves or in family members. Many teens are reluctant to seek mental health services or attend traditional support groups, although such interventions can offer tremendous benefit. Providers can help teens to believe that their life has

TABLE 3.5 Factors Guiding Treatment in Children Affected by and Infected with HIV/AIDS

- Child's developmental stage, which affects his or her ability to trust, tolerate pain or frustration, engage in relationships, and cope with change and separation
- Child's cognitive abilities and ability to understand illness and death
- Disclosure status
- Stage of illness

purpose, keep themselves mentally active, adapt to loss and change, and create a backup plan in case they become ill (Wiener et al., 2003).

Support groups can offer a sense of belonging for these teens, a place where they can openly share fears about their illness and traumatic experiences. Overnight camping or summer-camp specialty programs for infected teens can also offer such benefits and represent an alternative to mental health services explicitly designated as such. Such programs may provide opportunities to obtain counselor training and find summer employment. Peer empowerment programs provide HIV-positive youths the opportunity to deliver prevention messages to other young people (Luna and Rotheram-Borus, 1999), and community-based service providers may hire HIV-positive youth to serve as peer leaders, with close supervision and guidance. Please see Chapter 14 for a list of relevant summer camps.

Disclosure in the pediatric population

One of the greatest sources of psychological stress for children and adolescents, as well as for their caregivers, is the tension generated by questions surrounding disclosure, including when, how, and to whom (Wiener and Battles, 2006; Wiener et al., 2007). Such issues may lead to disclosure of other family secrets, including paternity, history of parental sexual behavior, and substance abuse (Havens et al., 2005). Parental guilt about transmission may complicate decisions about disclosure and should be addressed in psychotherapeutic interventions. Parents and other caretakers may have the sense that nondisclosure will protect children from unnecessary psychological pain and even mental illness, that children may not understand what the illness means, or that the knowledge will cause children to feel that they have a foreshortened future. The parent of a child with HIV may anticipate rejection by both their child and their community at large. In addition to these stressors, disclosure to children leads to forced disclosure of parental illness and concerns about keeping the illnesses secret from others, as discussed earlier (Havens et al., 2005). Finally, inevitable disclosure of parental illness feeds into the child's anxiety about potential abandonment and additional loss.

In addressing these concerns, most current guidelines and opinions support the benefits and importance of disclosure (Wiener and Battles, 2006; Wiener et al., 2007). In 1999, the American Academy of Pediatrics published guidelines that endorse disclosure of HIV to older children and adolescents as beneficial and ethically appropriate (American Academy of Pediatrics Committee on Pediatric AIDS, 1999). Many studies have suggested positive outcomes associated with disclosure, including the promotion of trust, improved adherence, enhanced support services, open family communication, and better long-term health and emotional well-being. In today's era of technology, a caretaker must also take into account the vast amount of readily available information in libraries and on the Internet. For most children, the trauma of discovering their diagnosis through piecing together information retrieved on the Internet, for instance, by researching their medications, would be far worse than learning about it in the presence of their doctor and family. It is therefore important that disclosure take place in as supportive an atmosphere as possible, with cooperation between health professionals and parents. It can be helpful to conceive of disclosure as a process, rather than as a single event, occurring over several visits.

Despite these recommendations and the clear benefits to disclosure, there is also evidence that knowledge of serostatus may in some cases contribute to depression, anxiety, and behavioral problems in children. Caregivers should be prepared for the possible emotional reactions of children following disclosure, ranging from no reaction to acute panic to delayed reactions, including the onset of new psychosomatic complaints, nightmares, emotional lability, and regressive behavior. While some children present with an adult-like acceptance, parents and therapists should be sensitive to the underlying sense of shame and personal defectiveness often associated with the diagnosis. Artwork following disclosure often reveals confusion, guilt, or a sense of damage that the child may have internalized.

For all these reasons, post-disclosure counseling is recommended. With time and support, most children demonstrate reduction of guilt, a sense of pride with mastery of information, and increased comfort with medical procedures such as blood draws and pill swallowing (Wiener and Battles, 2002; Wiener et al., 2003).

The mental health practitioner should also assess for unresolved and complicated grief reactions, which can manifest with difficulty making decisions, oppositional behavior, or symptoms of depression and anxiety. Inquiring into the inner world of children and helping them make sense of their struggles facilitates psychological growth and healing (Wiener and Figueroa, 1998).

A summary of steps involved in preparing for and carrying out disclosure of HIV status is provided in Table 3.6.

In addition to the feelings that the child may have about their HIV status, the parents and caretakers also develop strong emotional reactions during the process of disclosure. These can range from anxiety about the outcome of the disclosure, fear of stigma as they anticipate that their child may become labeled as ill or contaminated, to shame and guilt as they anticipate questions from their child about the means of transmission, particularly for parents who have used intravenous drugs or have a history of sexually transmitted HIV. Parents may be uncomfortable explaining related issues of sexuality, such as homosexuality, bisexuality, prostitution, and promiscuity. Caregiver

TABLE 3.6 HIV Disclosure Process Involving Children

Step 1. Preparation

- Have a meeting with the parent or caregivers involved in the decision-making process.
- Address the importance of disclosure and ascertain whether the family has a plan in mind. Respect the intensity of feelings about this issue. Obtain feedback on the child's anticipated response. Explore the child's level of knowledge and his or her emotional stability and maturity.
- If the family is ready to disclose, guide them in various ways of approaching disclosure (Step 2).
- If the family is not ready, encourage them to begin using words that they can build on later, such as *immune problems, virus,* or *infection.* Provide books on viruses for the family to read with the child. Strengthen the family through education and support and schedule a follow-up meeting.
- Respect the family's timing, but strongly encourage the family not to lie to the child if he or she asks directly about having HIV, unless significant, identifiable safety concerns render the decision to disclose inadvisable. Also remind the family to avoid disclosure during an argument or in anger.

Step 2. Disclosure

- In advance, have the family think through or write out how they want the conversation to go.
- Choose a place where the child will be most comfortable to talk openly.
- Provide the family with questions the child may ask so that they are prepared with answers. Such questions include the following: "How long have you known this?" "Who else has the virus?" "Will I die?" "Can I ever have children?" "Who can I tell?" "Why me?" "Who else knows?"
- Keep medical facts to a minimum (immunology, virology, the effectiveness of therapy) and reinforce hope.
- The child should be told that nothing has changed, except that a name is now being given to what they have been living with.
- The child needs to hear that he or she didn't do or say anything to cause the disease and that the family will always remain by their side.

Step 3. After Disclosure

- Schedule appropriately spaced and regular follow-up meetings.
- Provide the child with a journal or diary to record their questions, thoughts, and feelings. If appropriate, provide books about children living with HIV.
- Ask the child to tell you what they have learned about their virus. This question may provide an opportunity to clarify misconceptions. Writing and art may be useful techniques.
- Asses changes in emotional well-being and provide the family with information about symptoms that could indicate the need for more intensive intervention.
- Support parents for having disclosed the diagnosis and, if interested and available, refer them to a parents support group. Encourage them to think about the emotional needs of the other children in the family in the disclosure process.

- Remind parents that disclosure is not a one-time event. Ongoing communication will be needed. Ask parents what other supports they feel would be helpful to them and their child. Provide information about HIV camp programs for HIV-infected and HIV-affected children and families.

Source: Adapted from Pao and Weiner (2008, Table 24.3), based on Wiener LS, Battles HB (2006). Untangling the web: a close look at diagnosis disclosure among HIV-infected adolescents. *J Adolesc Health* 38(3):307–309. Copyright (2006), with permission from Elsevier.

support groups and individual therapy can help parents to confront and work through these discomforts and challenges.

In rare instances, the medical team may find itself in conflict with the parents of a child with HIV who is not aware of the diagnosis. When does the medical team have the right or obligation to disclose the diagnosis to the child? Current guidelines indicate that the medical team has the authority to disclose to the child their serostatus against the wishes of the parent if there is a significant risk that the child will pass on the virus, for example, if the child is a teenager who has begun to share injection drugs or has become sexually active. (Please also refer to Chapter 13: Ethical and Legal Aspects.)

Transition to young adulthood and long-term survivors

A significant number of children with HIV live into their late adolescent years and are now graduating from high school, attending trade schools or colleges, and holding down part-time or full-time jobs. The goal for these young adults with HIV/AIDS is to increase self-care behaviors, such as medical adherence and health-related interactions, reduce secondary transmission, and enhance their quality of life (Rotheram-Borus and Miller, 1998). The psychological transition from anticipating an early death to planning for one's future, however, along with uncertainty about the effectiveness of HIV drug regimens and fears of losing health insurance or disability insurance can result in significant anxiety. The cumulative effects of multiple losses can also lead to increased anxiety and depression.

Reports of multiple losses, or "loss overload," are frequently heard when describing the psychological impact of HIV/AIDS. As many HIV-positive youngsters age, they find themselves grieving for parents, siblings, and/or close friends who did not live long enough to benefit from currently available drug treatments. Others have been shuffled between care providers, households, schools, neighborhoods, and social service agencies. It is often not until late adolescence that the impact of these losses "hits home." This distress often occurs at a time when the transition from pediatric care providers to adult programs or centers is required; this move is experienced as yet another loss (Battles and Wiener, 2002). Unresolved and complicated grief reactions can mask difficulty making decisions, feeling "lost," guilt surrounding survival, oppositional behavior, or depression and anxiety, each of which can lead to disabling mental health problems. Assessing for grief reactions needs to be a part of the mental health care provided for each HIV-positive child, adolescent, and surviving young adult.

Summary

HIV-infected youth will remain at high risk for psychological distress and at greater risk for comorbid psychiatric symptoms. Therefore, providers from multiple disciplines will need to work together to enable optimal growth and development, to maximize the child's function and quality of life, and to promote mental health and resiliency.

HIV IN YOUNG ADULTHOOD AND ADULTHOOD

Risk of transmission

The most common routes of exposure in newly diagnosed younger adults are sexual contact among men who have sex with men, injection drug use, and heterosexual sex (Luther and Wilkin, 2007). One study identified specific risk factors for HIV transmission: a history of more than five casual partners or use of drugs and alcohol (Cooperman et al., 2007). The literature establishing early-childhood trauma as a risk for HIV infection is extensive (Masten et al., 2007; Pence et al., 2007; Sikkemma et al., 2009), including history of sexual assault (Gwandure, 2007).

Pregnancy, discussed later in this section, is also a risk factor for HIV infection, especially in adolescents and younger adults. This risk association is poorly understood. In a recent study, it was observed that only 52% of HIV-positive adolescent mothers knew their serostatus prior to the pregnancy, and approximately 83% of all pregnancies were unplanned (Koenig et al., 2007). This finding suggests that as many as half of pregnant HIV-positive adolescents are first learning of their HIV-positive status while also discovering that they are going to become mothers.

Challenges related to fertility and pregnancy

Issues surrounding fertility and family planning present many challenges for couples in which one or both members have HIV. Some of these difficulties may be compounded in serodiscordant couples. Despite HIV infection, many couples desire a pregnancy but may feel that their health-care providers will not support such efforts, perceiving pregnancy as unnecessarily risky. Couples may doubt that their interests and concerns will be adequately addressed (Panozzo et al., 2003). Challenges include maintaining the health of the mother before, during, and after the pregnancy, and preventing transmission of HIV to the seronegative partner and to the infant (Matthews and Mukkerjee, 2009).

Fertility counseling is an important opportunity for educating about harm reduction. The risk of HIV transmission to the uninfected partner is too great to endorse natural conception through unprotected intercourse. One study involving serodiscordant couples (HIV-positive male, HIV-negative female) showed seroconversion in 4% of women (Mandelbrot et al., 1997). For those with access to assistive reproductive technologies, pregnancy can be achieved with an extremely low risk of transmission of HIV (Matthews and Mukkerjee, 2009). For couples in which the male partner is seropositive and the female is seronegative, several technologies are available, including intrauterine insemination using washed sperm (recommended as first line), in vitro fertilization, and intracytoplasmic sperm injection (Waters et al., 2007).

Many of these technologies are expensive, however, and often not covered by insurance. This makes it difficult for couples to pursue the safest path toward a pregnancy without incurring significant financial hardship. While unprotected intercourse is not recommended within a serodiscordant couple, some data indicate that with a low or suppressed viral load, a couple may be able to conceive naturally with minimal risk of transmission (Castilla et al., 2005; Barreiro et al., 2006). An HIV-infected woman with an HIV-negative partner can attempt insemination using her partner's semen and a syringe to eliminate the risk of transmitting the virus to her partner.

Men who have sex with men

A particular subset of men who have sex with men, or men who have identified themselves as "down-low," (living in heterosexual relationships but secretly having same-sex relationships) have been the subject of much attention in the popular press, as it has been proposed that these men may pose risks within their communities as vectors of HIV transmission to multiple sexual partners, both male and female. Bond and colleagues (2009) found that down-low identification was not associated with unprotected sex. Furthermore, contrary to popular perception, down-low men were less likely to be HIV positive than were non–down-low-identifying peers, and identifying as down-low did not actually mean that the men had sex with female partners. In this study, down-low men reported lower rates of unprotected receptive anal intercourse (Bond et al., 2009). Conversely, in another study of heterosexually identified men, those men who reported having sex with both men and women were more likely to have a sexually transmitted infection, to have unprotected intercourse, and to have sex while intoxicated with drugs or alcohol (Zellner et al., 2009).

Depression in HIV-positive pregnant women

HIV-positive women are especially at risk for depression during pregnancy, which can interfere with essential prenatal and general medical care. A recent study has shown prenatal depression to be associated with substance use and CD4 counts less than 200 (Kapetanovic et al., 2009). Women with depression are more likely to have difficulty with adherence to antiretroviral medications, placing themselves at risk for complications and their fetus as risk for transmission of the virus. In one study, social isolation and perceived stress on the part of the patient were independently correlated with depression in pregnant women with HIV (Blaney et al., 2004).

Current guidelines for screening and treatment of depression in HIV-positive pregnant women can be found online at hivguidelines.org. These guidelines are summarized here (New York State Department of Health AIDS Initiative, 2009). Clinicians should screen all HIV-infected pregnant women for depression at least once each trimester, including at the first prenatal visit, and should educate patients about the risks of perinatal depression.

When treatment is indicated, the clinician and HIV-infected pregnant woman should discuss the risks and benefits of antidepressant therapy. The discussion should include the patient's history of depression, past response to medication, and assessment of risk for postpartum depression. Possible drug–drug interactions and the risks of prenatal exposure to psychotropic medication must be weighed against the benefit of stabilizing the patient's depressive symptoms in open discussion with the patient. It is common for primary care physicians to prescribe antidepressants, but in some cases it is preferable to refer patients to a psychiatrist. Primary care clinicians should consider referring the pregnant HIV-infected woman with depression to a psychiatrist in the situations listed in Table 3.7.

TABLE 3.7 When to Consider Referral of a Pregnant HIV-Infected Woman with Depression to a Psychiatrist

- Existence of co-occurring mental health disorder
- Patient's depression is a feature of an underlying mental health disorder
- History of poor response to previous antidepressant therapy
- Possible complex drug–drug interactions with other medications
- History of prior allergic reaction to antidepressant medication

Mania in HIV-positive pregnant women

While less common, the development of manic symptoms during pregnancy represents a medical and psychiatric emergency, necessitating urgent evaluation and treatment. Mania substantially increases the risk for antiretroviral nonadherence, poor general self-care, and high-risk behavior, including sexual promiscuity and substance use. Psychopharmacological treatment of mania is discussed in Chapter 7.

OLDER ADULTS AND HIV AND AIDS

Prevalence and rate of new diagnoses

There are limited data regarding the prevalence of HIV infection or rates of transmission in the population of older adults in the United States. In this chapter, the term *older adult* will be used to refer to all adults age 50 and older, and not to the stereotypical "geriatric" age of 65 and older. In 2007, it was estimated that there were more than 116,000 older adults living with HIV or AIDS in the United States (Paul et al., 2007). This accounts for 24% of those living with HIV/AIDS, with some estimates of infection rates in this population as high as 15% of all new diagnoses (CDC, 2005). It is predicted that by the year 2015, 50% of persons living with HIV/AIDS will be age 50 and older (U.S. Senate Special Committee on Aging, 2005). While the epidemiology may be changing and the statistics complicated by use of better surveillance methods in more recent years, older adults appear to be at the same or even higher level of risk compared to that of younger and middle-aged adults.

Troubleshooting: Vulnerability factors related to prevention, testing, and diagnosis

Trends in societal perceptions likely contribute to the increasing rates of HIV infection in the older adult population. Interventions focus primarily on younger persons (Lovejoy et al., 2008), with older adults frequently excluded from most public health campaigns targeting HIV transmission and prevention. Thus older adults may be receiving less education about HIV risk reduction than their younger counterparts. Maes and Louis (2003) demonstrated that older adults do not feel that AIDS is a problem in their age group, despite infection rates reflecting the contrary. It may be that older adults are not getting the message from their providers that they should be concerned about their HIV risk.

Numerous factors contribute to the delay in diagnosis of HIV infection in older adults. Older adults do not receive routine screening as frequently as younger adults, even though the current CDC guidelines contain expanded recommendations regarding HIV testing that include testing up to age 64 (Simone and Appelbaum, 2008). In order to be diagnosed, therefore, an older adult must often express concern about or interest in be tested. Physical symptoms related to HIV can also mimic age-related problems (Lee, 2006; Simone and Appelbaum, 2008); a primary care physician may treat the complaint rather than discovering the underlying HIV infection that is the cause. This bias may account for the shorter time from diagnosis to onset of AIDS in older adults (Schmid et al., 2009).

As humans, physicians are also susceptible to their own biases. Health-care practitioners perceive that sexual activity and interest decrease with age and may expect older patients to be retired not only from employment but also from sex. Common but inaccurate assumptions about older adults are that they are celibate or monogamous (Allison-Ottey et al., 1999), do not engage in sexual activity, do not abuse substances, and do not carry sexually transmitted infections. Additionally, physicians may underestimate the prevalence of gay men in this population or mistakenly assume that married people and those in long-term relationships are monogamous. Physicians may also perceive older adults to be less willing to change their behaviors and therefore might be less likely to address risk factors with their older patients when they arise. Physicians have expressed discomfort in discussing sexuality and sexual health practices with older adults; they may feel uncomfortable taking sexual histories in persons of their parents' or grandparents' age.

For all these reasons, developing rapport with the patient and facilitating comfort with this potentially sensitive area of personal history is essential. Health-care providers often omit the sexual history during their assessment in these patients (Levy-Dweck, 2005), but as with any other age group, it is important to communicate interest and concern so that patients can talk openly. This approach will also enable patients to maximally benefit from the educational opportunity that an office visit provides. Sexual history taking and psychiatric assessment are similar to that for other adults, but more attention may be paid to drug interactions, medications, or conditions that cause sexual dysfunction. For further information about sexual history taking and psychiatric assessment, please refer to Chapter 2 in this handbook.

Transmission and risk factors according to subset of the older population

Despite popular perception, older age remains a crucial time for HIV prevention efforts. This section will highlight specific areas of vulnerability for older adults and differences in HIV risk and transmission from those in the general population.

Sexual contact

While older adults do not always perceive themselves to be at risk for HIV, the same high-risk behaviors (including unprotected sex and intravenous drug use) as those practiced by younger adults are the predominant mechanisms of HIV transmission in older adults (Goodroad, 2003). Other contributors to increasing HIV transmission in older adults include physiological factors. Age-related thinning and decreased lubrication of vaginal mucosa may facilitate transmission of the virus through increased exposure to blood. Condom use is rare in older persons (Allison-Ottey et al., 1999; Schensul et al., 2003), making sexual activity a major source of transmission risk in this population, although there are limited data about the prevalence of specific modes of transmission. Generally, heterosexual sex poses the greatest risk for older women, especially when condoms are not used. Older women may consider condoms to be for birth control only (Zablotsky and Kennedy, 2003). In a study of older women, 21% of women interviewed with a current sexual partner reported that condom use was not necessary because they were no longer able to become pregnant (Tessler Lindau et al., 2006).

It may also be difficult for older women to insist on condom use because of fears of rejection or intimate-partner violence. Married women are at risk for HIV infection in situations where partners are engaging in sexual activity or injection drug use outside of their marriage, at times unbeknownst to them. Men also tend to exert more control over and resistance to condom use. It is commonly believed that insistence on using a condom implies lack of trust in the relationship. In one study, HIV-positive women in Nairobi had a two-fold higher incidence of intimate-partner violence (Fonck et al., 2005). Another study in India found that women experiencing sexual and physical intimate-partner violence had increased rates of HIV infection (Silverman et al., 2008). Such data suggest links between partner violence and HIV infection.

Substance use

There are limited data on the prevalence of substance use in HIV-positive older adults. One study on the influence of alcohol use on risk perception found that intoxication decreased insistence on condom use from the female partner and increased the likelihood of unprotected sex, but this finding was in a simulated situation and must be interpreted in this context (Stoner et al., 2008). While rates of depression and substance use decrease with age in the general population worldwide, this cannot be assumed to be the same with HIV infection (Rabkin et al., 2004). Both cognitive impairment and substance use have been shown to pose serious impediments to antiretroviral adherence in older adults (Hinkin et al., 2004).

Gender

Numerous studies have focused on the sexual risk-taking behavior of older men. Grossman (1995) has argued that denial of sexuality due to internalized homophobia and anonymous sexual encounters present risks for HIV transmission that are often undetected in older men. Older men tend to have more partners and more simultaneous partners than women (Allison-Ottey et al., 1999). Some authors have proposed that the advent of phosphodiesterase inhibitors (such as sildenafil) may have contributed to increased sexual activity in older age, by enabling older men to engage in sexual activity who would otherwise be unable to do so, but there are no current data to support this hypothesis. Older men may also feel that condoms affect sexual performance and thus avoid using them.

There may be variation in risk behavior across this age spectrum. In a study of older adults that was conducted in two U.S. cities, a younger subset of the male population (ages 50–61) was more likely to engage in high-risk sex-related and drug-related behavior (Schensul et al., 2003). In this same study, 29% of sexually active male residents reported having sex with commercial sex workers and only 31% of these men reported always using a condom.

Relationship status and HIV diagnosis

Marriage itself has not been found to impact risk behavior. "Relationship status," particularly not being in a married relationship, has been shown to be a risk for engaging in high-risk sexual behavior (Coleman and Ball, 2007). It may be perceived that unprotected intercourse enhances trust and intimacy in relationships (Davidovich et al., 2004).

HIV treatment also does not reduce risk-behavior in older adults. Crawford and colleagues (2003) conducted a study demonstrating that merely being in treatment for HIV can lessen risk-reduction techniques, which may suggest that being treated leads to a perception that one cannot acquire other sexually transmitted diseases or transmit them.

Minorities and men who have sex with men

In a study of 110 self-identified older Black and Latino men who have sex with men, it was found that the majority perceived themselves to be at minimal risk for contracting HIV, despite findings that these older men were sexually active, were often with multiple partners, and included drug use as a frequent part of their sexual encounters (Jimenez, 2003). Dolcini and colleagues (2003) found higher prevalence rates among older men who were Black, substance users, or had sex with men and were relatively less "closeted," meaning they were more likely to disclose their sexuality.

Impact of HIV/AIDS on older adults

Older adults tend to experience a poorer quality of life than that of their HIV-negative peers because symptoms of HIV-related disease can worsen with age. Health maintenance and preventive care are of crucial importance, particularly in women who have specific health maintenance needs and complaints compared to those of men (Lee, 2006). Older adults also face numerous psychosocial stressors and often live in environments where they have limited social contacts. They may feel ashamed of their illness and thus less likely to disclose the diagnosis to relatives or friends. Additionally, they may face increased financial strains from unemployment or retirement.

Older adults are susceptible to increased distress because they must simultaneously combat AIDS phobia and ageism (and at times homophobia), all while typically having more fragile support systems (Shippy and Karpiak, 2005). Violations of confidentiality were found to be common among older adults with HIV infection (Emlet, 2008). Older adults also tend to have smaller social support networks than those of younger adults. It has been well documented that social support lessens psychological distress in HIV-positive older adults, improving mood and general feeling of well-being (Chesney, 2003; Mavandadi et al., 2009).

Psychotherapy and enhanced supportive services can be helpful to prevent or mitigate the effects of social isolation and demoralization, particularly in this age group. Support from social contacts can also be very useful if the patient is comfortable disclosing their serostatus. Social services such as local community groups, senior centers, food pantries, and housing services can alleviate some of the distress experienced by those with limited family or friends. Support groups for older persons with HIV or chronic medical illness, individual supportive therapy, and other group therapies are all options for targeting illness-related symptoms and enhancing older adults' ability to cope. Adults who are socially isolated, have cognitive impairment, and are experiencing greater symptoms may particularly come to rely on such groups and social services as their source of support and socialization with others. Please refer to Chapter 8 for more information regarding psychotherapy for HIV-positive adults, and Chapter 14 for resources for older adults with HIV.

Little is known about the relationship between aging and manifestations of psychiatric disorders in HIV-positive persons. The possibility of superimposed neurocognitive deficits on pre-existing mental illness or medical illness should always be a consideration in older persons with HIV infection who have a psychiatric complaint. In a neuropsychological assessment, Becker and colleagues (2004) found that dementia was most common in older persons, whereas younger HIV-positive patients most commonly had cognitive impairment that was significant but did not meet criteria for dementia. Viral load seems to be of particular importance in the development of cognitive impairment. It was also observed that HIV viral load was higher in those who developed dementia during the 1-year follow-up period (Becker et al., 2004). Cherner and colleagues (2004) found that viral load and age were significant predictors of neuropsychological impairment; older adults with detectable cerebrospinal fluid (CSF) HIV virus had twice the prevalence of cognitive impairment compared with those with undetectable viral load. The consequences of cognitive impairment are numerous and range from nonadherence with treatment to hypersexuality.

The older population is especially vulnerable to medication side effects, a situation further compounded by the likelihood that older adults are taking multiple medications concurrently. General principles regarding psychiatric treatment in the older-adult population can be applied to treating those with HIV disease as well; the clinician should start with very low doses of psychotropic agents to minimize side effects. More consideration should be given to psychotherapy as a supplementary or initial treatment in this population. For details regarding the evaluation and treatment of psychiatric and cognitive complaints, please refer to Chapters 6 and 8 in this handbook.

End-of-life issues

End-of-life concerns arise with frequency in the older-adult age group as patients come to anticipate the course of their illness and cope with setbacks and gradual physical decline due to their HIV infection, other comorbid conditions, and the general aging process. One of the most important things a physician can do for a patient with HIV is to assist with anticipatory guidance regarding end-of-life concerns, palliative care, and advance directives. It is also crucial to involve family members or the patient's social network, if applicable, as they may have concerns about arranging end-of-life care for their loved one. Information about palliative care can be found in Chapter 12. Information about ethics and advance directives is given in Chapter 13, and resources related to advance directives for caregiving can be found in Chapter 14 of this handbook.

HIV ACROSS THE LIFE CYCLE: CONCLUSIONS AND FURTHER RECOMMENDATIONS

This chapter has highlighted the risks and challenges of HIV infection across varied life stages and as manifested differently in men and women. Primary care and mental health practitioners must keep in mind that efforts to reduce risk of transmission, education about barrier methods, psychoeducation, and improved access to care are fundamental for HIV prevention in all age groups (Rotherdam-Borus et al., 2009). In addition, all age groups benefit from good rapport with and education from their providers. General health maintenance that includes sexual health education as well as health-care providers' attention and curiosity regarding potential substance use and sexuality are also necessary.

Despite such commonalities, the age groups covered in this chapter face different vulnerabilities related to their specific population characteristics. The different developmental tasks faced by different age groups across various stages of the life cycle will shape a patient's experience of diagnosis and treatment. Providers who can be sensitive to both physiological and psychological variations, as manifested throughout the life cycle, will be able to provide a more compassionate, more effective, and higher level of care to those persons whose lives are affected by HIV.

REFERENCES

Allison-Ottey S, Weston C, Hennawi G, Nichols M, Eldred L, Ferguson RP (1999). Sexual practices of older adults in a high HIV prevalence environment. *Md Med J* 48(6):287–291.

American Academy of Pediatrics Committee on Pediatric AIDS (1999). Disclosure of illness status to children and adolescents with HIV infection. *Pediatrics* 103(1):164–166.

Armstrong FD, Seidel JF, Swales TP (1993). Pediatric HIV infection: a neuropsychological and educational challenge. *J Learn Disabil* 26:92–103.

Battles HB, Wiener LS (2002). From adolescence through young adulthood: psychosocial adjustment associated with long-term survival of HIV. *J Adolescent Health* 30(3):161–168.

Becker JT, Lopez OL, Dew MA, Aizenstein HJ (2004). Prevalence of cognitive disorders differs as a function of age in HIV virus infection. *AIDS* 18(Suppl. 1):S11–S18.

Bekir P, McLellan T, Childress AR, Gariti P (1993). Role reversals in families of substance abusers: a transgenerational phenomenon. *Int J Addict* 28:613–630.

Belman A, Brouwers P, Moss H (1992). HIV-1 and the central nervous system. In DM Kaufman, GE Solomon GE, and CR Pfeffer (eds.), *Child and Adolescent Neurology for Psychiatrists* (p. 238). Baltimore: Williams & Wilkins.

Blaney NT, Fernandez MI, Ethier KA, Wilson TE, Walter E, Koenig LJ (2004). Psychosocial and behavioral correlates of depression among HIV-infected pregnant women. *AIDS Patient Care STDS* 18(7):405–415.

Bond L, Wheeler DP, Millett GA, LaPollo AB, Carson LF, Liau A (2009). Black men who have sex with men and the association of down-low identity with HIV risk behavior. *Am J Public Health* 99(Suppl. 1):S92–S95.

Castilla J, Del Romero J, Hernando V, Marincovich B, Garcia S, Rodriguez C (2005). Effectiveness of highly active antiretroviral therapy in reducing heterosexual transmission of HIV. *J Acquir Immune Defic Syndr* 40(1):96–101.

[CDC] Centers for Disease Control and Prevention (2005). HIV/AIDS topics: Persons aged 50 and over. Retrieved April 21, 2009, from http://www.cdc.gov/hiv/topics/over50/

[CDC] Centers for Disease Control and Prevention (2007). Cases of HIV infection and AIDS in the United States and dependent areas, Table 25. Retrieved April 21, 2009, from http://www.cdc.gov/hiv/topics/surveillance/resources/reports/2007report/table25.htm

Cherner M, Ellis RJ, Lazzaretto D, Young C, Mindt MR, Atkinson JH, Grant I, Heaton RK (2004). Effects of HIV-1 infection and aging on neurobehavioral functioning: preliminary findings. *AIDS* 18(Suppl. 1):S27–S34.

Chesney M (2003). Adherence to HAART regimens. *AIDS Patient Care STDS* 17:169–177.

Cohen J, Reddington C, Jacobs D, et al. (1997). School-related issues among HIV-infected children. *Pediatrics* 100:e8.

Cohen MA (1989). AIDSism, a new form of discrimination. *Am Med News*, January 20, 32:43.

Cohen MA (2008). History of AIDS psychiatry—a biopsychosocial approach—paradigm and paradox. In MA Cohen and JM Gorman (eds.), *Comprehensive Textbook of AIDS Psychiatry* (pp. 3–14). New York: Oxford University Press.

Coleman CL, Ball K (2007). Determinants of perceived barriers to condom use among HIV-infected middle-aged and older African-American men. *J Adv Nurs* 60(4):368–376.

Cooperman NA, Arnsten JH, Klein RS (2007). Current sexual activity and risky sexual behavior in older men with or at risk for HIV infection. *AIDS Educ Prev* 19(4):321–333.

Crawford I, Hammack PL, McKirnan DJ, Ostrow D, Zamboni BD, Robinson B, Hope B (2003). Sexual sensation seeking, reduced concern about HIV and sexual risk behaviour among gay men in primary relationships. *AIDS Care* 15 (4):513–524.

Davidovich U, de Wit JB, Stroebe W (2004). Behavioral and cognitive barriers to safer sex between men in steady relationships: implications for prevention strategies. *AIDS Educ Prev* 16(4):304–314.

Dolcini MM, Catania JA, Stall RD, Pollack L (2003). The HIV epidemic among older men who have sex with men. *J Acquir Immune Defic Syndr* 33 (Suppl. 2):S115–S121.

Emlet CA (2008). Truth and consequences: a qualitative exploration of HIV disclosure in older adults. *AIDS Care* 20(6):710–717.

European Collaborative Study (2005). Mother-to-child transmission of HIV infection in the era of highly active antiretroviral therapy. *Clin Infect Dis* 40(3):458–465.

Fanos JH, Wiener L (1994). Tomorrow's survivors: siblings of HIV-infected children. *J Dev Behav Pediatr* 15:S43–S48.

Fonck K, Leye E, Kidula N, Ndinya-Achola J, Temmerman M (2005). Increased risk of HIV in women experiencing physical partner violence in Nairobi, Kenya. *AIDS Behav* 9(3):335–339.

Funck-Brentano I, Dalban C, Veber F, Quartier P, Hefez S, Costagliola D, Blanche S (2005). Evaluation of a peer support group therapy for HIV-infected adolescents. *AIDS* 19:1501–1508.

Gabiano C, Tovo PA, de Martino M, Galli L, Giaquinto C, Loy A, Schoeller MC, Giovannini M, Ferranti G, Rancilio L, et al. (1992). Mother-to-child transmission of human immunodeficiency virus type 1: risk of infection and correlates of transmission. *Pediatrics* 90(3):369–374.

Garofalo R, Herrick A, Mustanski BS, Donenberg GR (2007). Tip of the Iceberg: young men who have sex with men, the Internet, and HIV risk. *Am J Public Health* 97(6):1113–1117.

Goodroad BK (2003). HIV and AIDS in people older than 50. A continuing concern. *J Gerontol Nurs* 29(4):18–24.

Grossman AH (1995). At risk, infected, and invisible: older gay men and HIV/AIDS. *J Assoc Nurses AIDS Care* 6(6):13–19.

Gwandure C (2007). Sexual assault in childhood: risk HIV and AIDS behaviours in adulthood. *AIDS Care* 19(10):1313–1315.

Havens JF, Mellins CA, Ryan S (2005). Child psychiatry: psychiatric sequalae of HIV and AIDS. In B Sadock and V Sadock (eds.), *Kaplan & Sadock's Comprehensive Textbook of Psychiatry*, eighth ed. (p. 3434). Philadelphia: Lippincott Williams & Wilkins.

Hinkin CH, Hardy DJ, Mason KI, Castellon SA, Durvasula RS, Lam MN, Stefaniak M (2004). Medication adherence in HIV-infected adults: effect of patient age, cognitive status, and substance abuse. *AIDS* 18(Suppl. 1): S19–S25.

Jamieson DJ, Clark J, Kourtis AP, Taylor AW, Lampe MA, Fowler MG, Mofenson LM (2007). Recommendations for human immunodeficiency virus screening, prophylaxis, and treatment for pregnant women in the United States. *Am J Obstet Gynecol* 197(3 Suppl.):S26–S32.

Jimenez AD (2003). Triple jeopardy: targeting older men of color who have sex with men. *J Acquir Immune Defic Syndr* 33(Suppl. 2):S222–S225.

Kaiser Family Foundation (2009). HIV testing for mothers and newborns. Retrieved May 1, 2009, from http://www.statehealthfacts.org/compare-table.jsp?ind=563&cat=11

Kapetanovic S, Christensen S, Karim R, Lin F, Mack WJ, Operskalski E, Frederick T, Spencer L, Stek A, Kramer F, Kovacs A (2009). Correlates of perinatal depression in HIV-infected women. *S Patient Care STDS* 23(2):101–108.

Kline MW (2007). Pediatric HIV infection. Baylor International pediatric AIDS initiative. Retrieved April 3, 2007, from http://bayloraids.org/resources/ped-aids/manifestations.shtml

Koenig LJ, Bachanas PJ (2007). Adherence to medications for HIV: teens say, "Too many, too big, too often." In M Lyons and L D'Angelo (eds.), *Teenagers, HIV, and AIDS: Insights from Youths Living with the Virus*. Westport, CT: Praeger/Greenwood.

Koenig LJ, Espinoza L, Hodge K, Ruffo N (2007). Young, seropositive, and pregnant: epidemiologic and psychosocial perspectives on pregnant adolescents with human immunodeficiency virus infection. *Am J Obstet Gynecol* 197(3 Suppl.):S123–S31.

Lee S (2006). Women and HIV. Aging with HIV. *BETA* 18(2):33–35.

Lester P, Chesney M, Cooke M, et al. (2002). When the time comes to talk about HIV: factors associated with diagnostic disclosure and emotional distress in HIV-infected children. *J Acquir Immune Defic Syndr* 31:309–317.

Levy-Dweck S (2005). HIV/AIDS fifty and older: a hidden and growing population. *J Gerontol Soc Work* 46(2):37–50.

Lovejoy TI, Heckman TG, Sikkema KJ, Hansen NB, Kochman A, Suhr JA, Garske JP, Johnson CJ (2008). Patterns and correlates of sexual activity and condom use behavior in persons 50-plus years of age living with HIV/AIDS. *AIDS Behav* 12(6):943–956.

Luna GC, Rotheram-Borus MJ (1999). Youth living with HIV as peer leaders. *Am J Community Psychol* 27:1–23.

Luther V, Wilkin A (2007). HIV infection in older adults. *Clin Geriatr Med* 23 (3):567–583, vii.

Lyon ME, Trexler C, Akpan-Townsend C, Pao M, Selden K, Fletcher J, Addlestone IC, D'Angelo LJ (2003). A family group approach to increasing adherence to therapy in HIV-infected youths: results of a pilot project. *AIDS Patient Care STDS* 17(6):299–308.

Maes CA, Louis M (2003). Knowledge of AIDS, perceived risk of AIDS, and at-risk sexual behaviors among older adults. *J Am Acad Nurse Pract* 15 (11):509–516.

Mandelbrot L, Heard I, Henrion-Geant R, Henrion R (1997). Natural conception in HIV negative women with HIV infected partners. *Lancet* 349:850–851.

Marshall BD, Kerr T, Shoveller JA, Patterson TL, Buxton JA, Wood E (2009). Homelessness and unstable housing associated with an increased risk of HIV and STI transmission among street-involved youth. *Health Place* 15 (3):753–760.

Masten J, Kochman A, Hansen NB, Sikkema KJ (2007). A short-term group treatment model for gay male survivors of childhood sexual abuse living with HIV/AIDS. *Int J Group Psychother* 57(4):475–496.

Matthews LT, Mukherjee JS (2009). Strategies for harm reduction among HIV-affected couples who want to conceive. *AIDS Behav* 13(Suppl. 1):5–11.

Mavandadi S, Zanjani F, Ten Have TR, Oslin DW (2009). Psychological well-being among individuals aging with HIV: the value of social relationships. *J Acquir Immune Defic Syndr* 51(1):91–98.

Moskowitz DA, Roloff ME (2007). The existence of a bug-chasing subculture. *Cult Health Sex* 9(4):347–357.

Newell ML (1991). The natural history of vertically acquired HIV infection. The European Collaborative Study. *J Perinat Med* 19(Suppl. 1):257–262.

New York State Department of Health AIDS Initiative (2009). Guidelines for treatment of depression in pregnant women. Retrieved April 21, 2009, from http://www.hivguidelines.org/GuideLine.aspx?GuideLineID=39#E

Panozzo L, Battegay M, Friedl A, Vernazza PL; Swiss Cohort Study (2003). High risk behaviour and fertility desires among heterosexual HIV-positive patients with a serodiscordant partner—two challenging issues. *Swiss Med Wkly* 133 (7-8):124–127.

Pao M, Wiener L (2008). Childhood and adolescence. In MA Cohen and JM Gorman (eds.), *Comprehensive Textbook of AIDS Psychiatry* (pp. 307–339). New York: Oxford University Press.

Paul SM, Martin RM, Lu SE, Lin Y (2007). Changing trends in human immunodeficiency virus and acquired immunodeficiency syndrome in the population aged 50 and older. *J Am Geriatr Soc* 55(9):1393–1397.

Pence BW, Reif S, Whetten K, Leserman J, Stangl D, Swartz M, Thielman N, Mugavero MJ (2007). Minorities, the poor, and survivors of abuse: HIV-infected patients in the US Deep South. *South Med J* 100 (11):1114–1122.

Rabkin JG, McElhiney MC, Ferrando SJ (2004). Mood and substance use disorders in older adults with HIV/AIDS: methodological issues and preliminary evidence. *AIDS* 18(Suppl. 1):S43–S48.

Rotheram-Borus MJ, Miller S (1998). Secondary prevention for youths living with HIV. *AIDS Care* 10:17–34.

Rotheram-Borus MJ, Swendeman D, Chovnick G (2009). The past, present, and future of HIV prevention: integrating behavioral, biomedical, and structural intervention strategies for the next generation of HIV prevention. *Annu Rev Clin Psychol* 5:143–167.

Saewyc EM, Bearinger LH, Blum RW, Resnick MD (1999). Sexual intercourse, abuse and pregnancy among adolescent women: does sexual orientation make a difference? *Fam Plan Perspect* 31(3):127–131.

Sampaio-Sa M, Page-Shafer K, Bangsberg DR, Evans J, Dourado Mde L, Teixeira C, Netto EM, Brites C (2008). 100% adherence study: educational workshops vs. video sessions to improve adherence among ART-naïve patients in Salvador, Brazil. *AIDS Behav* 12(4 Suppl.):S54–S62.

Schensul JJ, Levy JA, Disch WB (2003). Individual, contextual, and social network factors affecting exposure to HIV/AIDS risk among older residents living in low-income senior housing complexes. *J Acquir Immune Defic Syndr* 33(Suppl. 2):S138–S152.

Schmid GP, Williams BG, Garcia-Calleja JM, Miller C, Segar E, Southworth M, Tonyan D, Wacloff J, Scott J (2009). The unexplored story of HIV and ageing. *Bull World Health Organ* 87(3):162–162A.

Schwarcz S, Scheer S, McFarland W, Katz M, Valleroy L, Chen S, Catania J (2007). Prevalence of HIV infection and predictors of high-transmission sexual risk behaviors among men who have sex with men. *Am J Public Health* 97(6):1067–1075.

Shippy RA, Karpiak SE (2005). The aging HIV/AIDS population: fragile social networks. *Aging Ment Health* 9(3):246–254.

Sikkema KJ, Hansen NB, Meade CS, Kochman A, Fox AM (2009). Psychosocial predictors of sexual HIV transmission risk behavior among HIV-positive adults with a sexual abuse history in childhood. *Arch Sex Behav* 38(1):121–134.

Silverman JG, Decker MR, Saggurti N, Balaiah D, Raj A (2008). Intimate partner violence and HIV infection among married Indian women. *JAMA* 300 (6):703–710.

Simone MJ, Appelbaum J (2008). HIV in older adults. *Geriatrics* 63(12):6–12.

Stoner SA, Norris J, George WH, Morrison DM, Zawacki T, Davis KC, Hessler DM (2008). Women's condom use assertiveness and sexual risk-taking: effects of alcohol intoxication and adult victimization. *Addict Behav* 33(9):1167–1176.

Tessler Lindau S, Leitsch SA, Lundberg KL, Jerome J (2006). Older women's attitudes, behavior, and communication about sex and HIV: a community-based study. *J Women Health* 15:747–753.

U.S. Senate Special Committee on Aging (2005). HIV over fifty: exploring the new threat [Web cast]. May 12, 2005. Retrieved April 28, 2009, from http://aging.senate.gov/hearing_detail.cfm?id=270655&

Valleau MP, Bergner RM, Horton CB (1995). Parentification and caretaker syndrome: an empirical investigation. *Fam Ther* 22:157–164.

Waters L, Gilling-Smith C, Boag F (2007). HIV infection and subfertility. *Int J STD AIDS* 18(1):1–6.

Wiener L, Battles H (2002). Mandalas as a therapeutic technique for HIV-infected children and adolescents. *J HIV/AIDS Soc Work* 1:27–39.

Wiener L, Battles H (2006). Untangling the web: a close look at diagnosis disclosure among HIV-infected adolescents. *J Adolesc Health*.38(3): 307–310.

Wiener L, Figueroa V (1998). Children speaking with children and families about HIV infection. In P Pizzo and K Wilfert (eds.), *Pediatric AIDS: The Challenge of HIV Infection in Infants, Children, and Adolescents*, third edition (p. 729). Baltimore: Williams and Wilkins.

Wiener L, Havens J, Ng W (2003). Psychosocial problems in pediatric HIV infection. In WT Shearer (ed.), *Medical Management of AIDS in Children*. Philadelphia: WB Saunders.

Wiener L, Mellins CA, Marhefka S, Battles HB (2007). Disclosure of an HIV diagnosis to children: history, current research, and future directions. *J Dev Behav Pediatr* 28(2):155–166.

Wiener LS, Septimus A, Grady C (1998). Psychosocial support and ethical issues for the child and family. In PA Pizzo and CM Wifert (eds.). *Pediatric AIDS: The Challenge of HIV Infection in Infants, Children, and Adolescents*, third ed. Baltimore: Williams & Wilkins.

Zablotsky D, Kennedy M (2003). Risk factors and HIV transmission to mid-life and older women: knowledge, options, and the initiation of safer sexual practices. *J Acquir Immune Defic Syndr* 33(Suppl. 2):S122–S130.

Zellner JA, Martínez-Donate AP, Sañudo F, Fernández-Cerdeño A, Sipan CL, Hovell MF, Carrillo H (2009). The interaction of sexual identity with sexual behavior and its influence on HIV risk among Latino men: results of a community survey in northern San Diego County, California. *Am J Public Health* 99(1):125–132.

4

Stigma of HIV and AIDS— Psychiatric Aspects

Sami Khalife, Jocelyn Soffer, and Mary Ann Cohen

Understanding HIV Stigma: A Historical Perspective

Since 1981, when previously healthy young adults were first stricken with a mysterious illness that was eventually described as "a new acquired cellular immunodeficiency" (Gottlieb et al., 1981), understanding of HIV and AIDS, both the in the medical community and general society, has come a long way. There remains, however, an unfortunate degree of stigma that persists since its development in the early days of the illness (Cohen and Weisman, 1986; Cohen, 1987, 1992; Cohen and Alfonso, 1998; Cohen, 2008). Early in the course of this epidemic, as it became evident that the immune deficiency had an infectious etiology and could lead to rapidly fatal complications, many became fearful of the possibility of contagion. An "epidemic of fear" (Hunter, 1990) thus began to develop along with the AIDS epidemic. During the first decade, even many physicians surveyed had negative attitudes toward persons with HIV and AIDS (Kelly et al., 1987; Thompson, 1987; Wormser and Joline, 1989).

At the beginning of the HIV epidemic some persons hospitalized with AIDS experienced difficulty receiving even minimally adequate care, including getting their rooms cleaned, obtaining water or food, and receiving proper medical attention. Psychiatric consultations for AIDS patients with depression, withdrawal, and treatment refusal often revealed the heightened feelings of isolation and depression experienced by the patients, in part as a result of the reactions of staff members to their illness, including the palpable fear of contagion. Holtz and coauthors (1983) were the first to describe the profound withdrawal from human contact as the "sheet sign," observed when persons with AIDS hid under their sheets and completely covered their faces.

Thus, since the beginning of the AIDS epidemic, people with AIDS have been stigmatized. They have felt shunned and ostracized by not only medical caregivers but also the general community and even by their own families and friends. In some areas of the world, persons with AIDS have been quarantined because of the irrational fears, discrimination, and stigma associated with this pandemic. In the United States, persons with AIDS have lost their homes and jobs, and some children and adolescents have been excluded from classrooms. While this level of discrimination is no longer common in the United States, children still experience subtle and not so subtle discrimination in some classrooms as well as rejections from summer camps. In the early 1980s, a diagnosis of AIDS led to rejection by homeless shelters, nursing homes, long-term care facilities, and even facilities for the terminally ill. As recently as 2009, a retired university provost and Unitarian minister was forced to leave an Arkansas assisted living facility one day following his admission when a review of his medical record revealed that he was HIV positive (Lambda Legal, 2009). The attitudes of families, houses of worship, employers, teachers, hospital staff, and funeral directors were marked by catastrophic stigma and discrimination, such that persons with AIDS had difficulty finding support, obtaining health care, keeping a job, or finding a chronic-care facility or even a place to die. Discrimination against persons with AIDS was described and labeled as "AIDSism" (Cohen, 1989). AIDSism is built on a foundation of homophobia, misogyny, addictophobia, and fears of contagion and death.

Although the medical profession has made great strides against discrimination and stigma, with most physicians now "accustomed to caring for HIV-infected patients with concern and compassion" (Gottlieb, 2001), these problems remain at the societal level, both globally and within the United States. Despite the burgeoning literature to support the benefits of addressing the psychiatric needs of persons with HIV from a biopsychosocial approach and increased understanding of the illness, there remains considerable stigma and AIDSism. Such stigma has implications not only for the mental and physical health of the individuals who experience it but also for public health. Stigma and AIDSism present barriers to getting tested for HIV, obtaining test results, disclosing serostatus to intimate partners, obtaining optimal medical care in a timely manner, and engaging in safer sex practices. HIV stigma remains a potent stressor for persons living with HIV, and is a major limiting factor in primary and secondary prevention and care. Please see Chapter 5 of this handbook for a more extensive discussion of primary and secondary prevention.

Psychosomatic medicine psychiatrists who specialize in AIDS psychiatry as well as general psychiatrists and other mental health clinicians are in a unique position to work with primary HIV clinicians, infectious-disease specialists, and other physicians and health professionals to combat

HIV and AIDS stigma, or AIDSism. The remainder of this chapter will review the epidemiology and characteristics of such stigma, factors that lead to and perpetuate the stigma, the impact of stigma on persons with HIV and AIDS, and strategies to address stigma against persons with HIV.

EPIDEMIOLOGY AND CHARACTERISTICS OF HIV STIGMA

Definition, characteristics, and forms of expression

In this chapter, we refer to stigma associated with HIV and AIDS interchangeably as AIDSism or HIV stigma. *AIDSism* refers to all unfavorable attitudes, beliefs, and policies directed toward people perceived as having HIV or AIDS, as well as toward the people with whom they are close and the communities with which they are associated. Patterns of prejudice, which include discounting, discrediting, and discriminating against groups of people, play into and strengthen existing social inequalities, especially those of gender, sexual orientation, and race, that lie at the root of HIV stigma (Herek et al., 1998). AIDSism includes a set of attitudes, behaviors, and beliefs that can be conceptualized at cultural, societal, and individual levels. Both HIV and AIDSism are global pandemics, and persons with HIV are stigmatized throughout the world to varying degrees and in different forms.

AIDSism can be manifested in laws and policies that punish persons with HIV or legitimize further discrimination against them. This includes electoral campaigns that avoid HIV-related issues or even foster negative attitudes against persons with HIV and their loved ones, associates, caregivers, or advocates. AIDSism is reflected in the institutional failures to address needs related to HIV, such as inadequate funding for research, public awareness campaigns, and free treatment for persons with limited resources, throughout the United States and globally. Policies that fail to protect the rights of persons with HIV and AIDS in the workplace and health-care system and in obtaining adequate insurance, housing, and education are also reflections of ongoing stigma.

Laws mandating compulsory HIV testing without prior consent or protection of confidentiality, such as mandatory HIV testing for immigrants or prisoners, are ethically problematic. While universal testing increases the identification of persons who did not previously know they were infected, this must be coupled with adequate resources for pre- and post-test counseling.

At the individual level, HIV stigma can be expressed by avoidance, abuse (physical, verbal, or emotional), and social rejection of persons with HIV and people associated with them (including injection drug users, gay men, and

TABLE 4.1 Questions to Ask about HIV Stigma

- Have you disclosed your serostatus to close friends or relatives?
- Have you regretted having told some people that you have HIV?
- Have you lost friends by telling them that you have HIV?
- Do you feel that you have to hide the fact that you have HIV?
- Do you worry that people who know will tell others?
- Do you worry that people may judge you if they learn that you have HIV?
- Do you feel guilty or ashamed because you have HIV?
- Do you worry about people discriminating against you because of your HIV status?
- Do you worry about losing your job if your employer knows that you have HIV?
- Do you feel that telling people about your status has negatively affected your relationship with them?

sex workers) (Swendeman et al., 2006). It is important for HIV clinicians to explore levels of stigma experienced by persons with HIV, as patients may find it very difficult to raise issues about HIV stigma and may find it relieving if clinicians encourage discussion of these painful issues. Table 4.1 provides a summary of basic questions that the clinician can ask to inquire about the level of stigma experienced.

Prevalence and Trends

Since the beginning of the AIDS epidemic, people with HIV have been stigmatized (Herek et al., 2002). Although overt expressions of HIV-related stigma have declined in the past decade, in many countries significant HIV stigma remains, serving as a limiting factor in primary and secondary prevention and care (Weiss and Ramakrishna, 2006). Although methodologically difficult to quantify, stigma has nonetheless been well described and even quantified in multiple studies.

In one study assessing the prevalence of HIV stigma and misinformation about HIV transmission in the United States during the 1990s, Herek and colleagues (2002) compared answers to telephone surveys conducted in 1991, 1996–1997, and 1998–1999 that were devised to assess such stigma. The surveys included questions about support for AIDS-coercive policies such as quarantine, publicly identifying persons with HIV, and mandatory testing (of pregnant women, immigrants, and people perceived to be at high risk). It examined attribution of responsibility and blame toward persons with HIV (e.g., the belief that persons with HIV are responsible for their disease or that they deserve it), as well as negative beliefs about persons with HIV (e.g., that they do not care about infecting others). Affective responses to persons with HIV were also surveyed, including feelings of anger, fear, and disgust. Finally, the study looked at comfort with and avoidance of persons with HIV in hypothetical situations (e.g., having one's child attend school with a classmate with HIV, or working in an office with a person with HIV).

The authors concluded that although support for punitive policies (quarantine and public identification of persons with HIV) and negative feelings toward persons with HIV and AIDS had declined over the 1990s, with fewer than 1 in 5 adults supporting coercive measures by 1999, significant stigma remained at the end of the decade. By 1999, one-fifth of those surveyed expressed fear of persons with HIV and one-sixth expressed disgust toward or supported public naming of persons with HIV. More covert forms of stigma persisted as well, with roughly one-fourth of respondents reporting discomfort with direct or symbolic contact with a person with HIV, and nearly one-third stating that they would avoid shopping at a neighborhood grocery store whose owner had AIDS. Approximately one-half of respondents perceived persons with HIV to be responsible for their illness, with the proportion overestimating the risk of infection posed by casual social contact actually increasing over the decade.

In an Internet-based survey conducted in 2000 by the Centers for Disease Control and Prevention (CDC), approximately 40% of respondents displayed misinformed beliefs, stating that HIV transmission could occur through sharing a glass or from being coughed or sneezed on by an HIV-infected person. Also, 19% of respondents endorsed the stigmatizing belief that persons who acquired AIDS through sex or drug use "have gotten what they deserve." Stigmatizing responses were relatively more common among men, whites, persons aged ≥ 55 years, those with only a high school education, those with an income $<\$30,000$, and those in poorer health. Misinformation tended to correlate with stigmatizing beliefs (Lentine et al., 2000).

Comparison to stigma associated with other illnesses

Few studies have compared HIV-related stigma to stigma related to other chronic medical conditions (Triplet and Sugarman, 1987; Crawford, 1996; Greene, 2000). Because other chronic illnesses may not conjure the attribution of blame that HIV often invokes, HIV stigma tends to be higher than that associated with other illnesses such as epilepsy, diabetes (Fernandes et al., 2007), hepatitis, tuberculosis, or severe adult respiratory syndrome (SARS) (Mak et al., 2006). Comparison of stigma associated with other sexually transmitted diseases and HIV stigma will be discussed below.

Historically, while cancer patients have also suffered from stigma, often because of the public's lack of information about the disease (Romano, 1986), there has been a counterbalancing tendency to view these patients as victims. Some studies have demonstrated increased positive social support for cancer patients compared to that for a random population sample and for non-cancer surgery patients (Bloom and Kessler, 1994) (Tempelaar et al., 1989).

Persons with mental illness form another group facing societal discrimination, with documented adverse effects on the quality of life of these patients (Crisp et al., 2000; Angermeyer et al., 2004). While few studies have directly compared the degree of stigma toward these two groups of patients, a particularly marginalized population is those with both HIV and mental illness, as associated stigma tends to be additive for the two conditions (Walkup et al., 2004; Lau and Tsui, 2007).

Origins of HIV Stigma and Perpetuating Factors

Means of transmission

The means of transmission of an illness usually relates to the development of illness-related stigma. Historically, sexually transmitted diseases (STDs) have been stigmatized because of their mode of infection. Persons with HIV carry the additional risk of association with groups already stigmatized on the basis of race, gender, sexual orientation, drug use, and lifestyle. Some means of HIV transmission represent negatively sanctioned social behaviors and thus lead to a judgmental distinction between various persons with HIV depending on how the illness was acquired. Some persons are perceived as "innocent" because they are infected with HIV through transplantation of organs, blood transfusions, or perinatally, while others are considered "guilty" and "deserving" of the illness when infection with HIV resulted from unprotected sexual contact or injection drug use (Skinner and Mfecane, 2004).

Victim blaming

People with an undesirable condition are generally subjected to even greater stigma when they are perceived to be personally responsible for that condition (Weiner, 1993). Not only is AIDS a life-threatening illness, but those affected by it are at times viewed as responsible for both getting infected with HIV and transmitting HIV to others (De Bruyn, 1999). From a list of 18 conditions, including having a criminal record, being HIV positive was assigned the highest degree of social disapproval, ranked in 14 different countries in a World Health Organization (WHO) study (Ustun et al., 2001).

Victim blaming harms HIV patients, perpetuates HIV stigma, and may in turn increase stigma of previously stigmatized behaviors or populations by contributing to vicious cycles of negative attitudes. It may also lead to further stigma subgrouping based on negative stereotypes, for example, that promiscuous sexual behaviors are more common in certain ethnic populations.

Since the first cases of AIDS were reported in communities of gay men and injection drug users, these negative reactions have continued to affect how people living with HIV and AIDS experience the illness. HIV was initially labeled GRID, or gay-related immunodeficiency. Gay men have been particularly affected by HIV stigma because they are viewed as blameworthy for having brought the illness upon themselves by engaging in sexual behaviors perceived as socially unacceptable.

In couples, victim blaming can lead to interpartner violence or exclusion from the household. Clinicians should be aware that victim blaming may be an unintended consequence of public education campaigns that stress the importance of personal decision making in HIV prevention. Health educators and clinicians face the challenge of communicating the importance of protecting oneself from HIV without blaming individuals who have become infected while not protecting themselves (Herek et al., 2002).

Religious groups may intentionally or inadvertently contribute to discrimination by making explicit or implicit judgments against persons with HIV and AIDS. Some groups have gone so far as to label the epidemic as God's punishment for sinners (including gay men, sex workers, and drug users) (Johnson, 1995).

Addictophobia and homophobia

Despite the evidence that addiction is an illness similar to other severe and complex chronic illnesses, it is often still viewed as the substance user's voluntary, deliberate, and repetitive choice and bad behavior. Moral judgments about addiction are common and elicit high degrees of social disapproval or stigma (Ustun et al., 2001). Since addiction has been perceived to be associated with HIV, persons with both conditions carry a double stigma: there is judgment against the disease itself and against associated behaviors that are viewed as deviant (Nardi, 1990).

Homophobia, or *heterosexism*, is defined as the belief that heterosexuality is or should be the only acceptable sexual orientation. It is associated with fear and hatred of persons who love and are sexually attracted to others of the same sex (Blumenfeld, 1992). There are at least 20 million gay and lesbian individuals living in the United States today, or approximately 10% of the population (Carl, 1990). Negative attitudes and feelings associated with homosexuality are common in almost all cultures. The AIDS epidemic has negatively impacted general attitudes toward homosexuals, as well as attitudes of health care professionals, leading to overt discrimination, social ostracism, and deprivation of various rights (Douglas et al., 1985). Stereotypic and stigmatizing attitudes toward homosexuality may interfere directly and indirectly with the care provided to gay and lesbian patients.

On a larger scale, negative reactions to socially unacceptable character-istics ascribed to people with HIV, such as homosexuality, promiscuity, and illicit drug use (Chenard, 2007), lie at the root of HIV/AIDS stigma. Indeed, some have argued that preexisting stigma helped to give rise to the AIDS epidemic by creating social conditions that foster HIV transmission. For example, opposition to needle exchange programs, despite their effectiveness in reducing HIV transmission rates, is based on the need to maintain the stigma associated with illegal drug use (Herek et al., 1998).

Misperceptions about HIV

An increasing number of people understand how HIV is transmitted, but many still lack understanding of how it is *not* transmitted. In the study mentioned earlier on prevalence of HIV stigma and misinformation about HIV transmission in the 1990s, almost half of the respondents believed that HIV could be contracted from sharing a drinking glass, and more than a third believed that it could be contracted from using a public toilet or through exposure to a cough or sneeze (Herek et al., 2002). At times during the epidemic, available blood supplies for transfusions have been in shortage because of decreased donations for fear of contracting HIV by donating blood. This situation emphasizes the need to continue to educate successive generations about how HIV is and is not transmitted, since stigma is more likely to thrive in an environment of ignorance.

Impact of Stigma on Persons with HIV

Measurement of stigma associated with HIV

Being able to measure the beliefs and attitudes that relate to AIDSism among community members and persons with HIV and AIDS is key to under-standing the complexity of this phenomenon. Such measurement is necessary in order to conduct research assessing the impact of AIDSism on affected individuals and to evaluate the effectiveness of interventions aimed at redu-cing AIDSism at both the individual and community levels (Visser et al., 2008). However, measuring HIV stigma is challenging, in part because stigma can be perceived and experienced in many different ways. A refined conceptualization and measurement of stigma may enable those who provide care to both develop and assess improved interventions.

Berger and her colleagues have developed an HIV-stigma scale that measures perceived stigma in persons with HIV and AIDS. This scale is used to examine the perceived consequences of other people knowing that the respondent has HIV, such as losing friends, feeling that people are avoiding him or her, and feeling regrets for having told some people. This scale has been found to be reliable and valid in a sample of persons with HIV (Berger et al., 2001). A more recent shorter version, using 32 instead of 40 items, was also validated (Bunn et al., 2007) and can be used in both research protocols and clinical settings.

Effects on the well-being of people living with HIV

Stigma affects both the physical and psychological well-being of people with HIV and AIDS. Physical conditions associated with HIV and AIDS, including cognitive impairment (such as HIV-associated dementia), lipodystrophy, skin lesions (such as Kaposi's sarcoma), weight loss, impaired vision, and limb amputation, represent major obstacles to adherence to treatment and can be psychologically damaging for the infected person. Stigmatizing beliefs can be internalized into a person's self-perception and sense of identity. Stigmatized persons often accept some of the negative social judgments that label them and disqualify them from equal participation. This adds to the stress of being diagnosed with HIV and increases the likelihood of depression and anxiety (Skinner and Mfecane, 2004; Varas-Diaz et al., 2005; Vanable et al., 2006). By increasing patients' vulnerability to depression, stigma may also affect longer-term health outcomes, as depressive symptoms may further compromise functioning of the immune system and contribute to more rapid progression to AIDS and mortality (Leonard, 2000; Ickovics et al., 2001).

It is helpful for the clinician to be aware of the potential impact of HIV stigma when caring for people with HIV. In practical terms, clinicians should inquire about existing support systems, attitudes of family members, and the patient's perception of others' reactions toward his or her HIV/AIDS diagnosis. People with HIV may not share this information with their physician if not directly asked. They may feel ashamed because of their internalized stigma or rejection by their family. Some persons with HIV may choose not to disclose their serostatus to any family members and do not expect support from them.

Discussing stigma and available support systems early in the treatment not only helps to foster the physician–patient therapeutic relationship but can also positively affect the long-term prognosis of the illness. Persons with HIV who have an intact support system are more likely to adhere to treatment recommendations and to disclose serostatus to their loved ones, including significant others (Ware et al., 2006). This support and openness can become particularly important later on in the course of the illness, if a patient loses full decision-making capacity (from HIV dementia or other CNS disease) and needs assistance with medical and other decisions.HIV stigma and fear of disclosure make it difficult to persuade people to get tested and can thus delay diagnosis as well as entry into treatment and the adoption of a healthier lifestyle (Skinner and Mfecane, 2004). As a result, many cases of HIV infection go undiagnosed and untreated, increasing further the like-lihood of HIV transmission. A person who is aware of his or her serostatus may nonetheless choose not to disclose it because of stigma-related fears, and may delay seeking care and treatment. The benefits of testing need to be considered and be part of the assessment by the clinician when caring for patients with an unknown serostatus.

Strategies for addressing stigma in the care of persons with HIV

Numerous interventions have been suggested to reduce stigma related to HIV and AIDS. These interventions can be implemented at different levels: intrapersonal, interpersonal, and organizational (including community and governmental) (McLeroy et al., 1988; Richard et al., 1996). Regardless of the level of intervention, it is important to understand that working to reduce or eliminate stigma will not be an overnight or short-term undertaking, but rather a process requiring ongoing efforts. As stigma is multifaceted and highly resistant to change, it is best targeted in multiple ways. Educating people about HIV, while important and beneficial, is not in itself sufficient to eliminate stigma. Providing information alone does not adequately change sexual behavior in relation to HIV or address racism and sexism (Skinner and Mfecane 2004). Since stigma toward people with HIV is related to other kinds of stigma, anti-stigma campaigns also need to address these related areas of prejudice—for example, those based on race, gender, sexual orienta-tion, and lifestyle.

Interventions at the intrapersonal level aim to identify and change cogni-tive distortions and unhealthy attitudes that people living with HIV and AIDS may have as a result of stigma. People with HIV often internalize guilt and blame, leading to unwillingness to seek treatment because they view them-selves as undeserving or unworthy of care. They may not disclose their HIV serostatus out of fear of rejection and mistreatment. Individual counseling, psychotherapy, cognitive-behavioral therapy, and support groups that aim to enhance knowledge, self-image, and self-esteem, as well as to change attitudes and behavior, are important components of decreasing stigma.

Interventions at the interpersonal level deal with the impact of social support and networks on health status and behavior. Even care provided by family members, community volunteers and health-care providers can be accompanied by stigma. It is important to educate those caring for and supporting HIV-affected individuals not only about the disease (including symptoms and modes of transmission) but also about the language to use in discussing the illness.

Clinicians and other health-care providers need to be aware of illness-related word choices that may have pejorative connotations. For example, practitioners should avoid use of the words "crackhead" (instead of "cocaine user"), "clean" (instead of "drug free"), "bareback" (instead of "unprotected anal sex") and "prostitute" (instead of "to have sex in exchange for money" or "commercial sex work"). Clinicians also need to be aware of their own attitudes toward sexuality and must closely examine any homophobic feelings and attitudes to be sure they do not interfere with the provision of treatment (Smith, 1993). During history taking, instead of asking how a patient got infected, it is less blaming to ask when and how a patient learned or knew about their serostatus and what provided an incentive for getting tested. This nonjudgmental approach reassures the patient and helps in building a therapeutic relationship.

Interventions at the organizational level aim to develop new policies within an organization, such as offering voluntary counseling and testing services to its employees. Such policies should define an employer's responsibility toward employees living with HIV and AIDS, to fully protect them from possible discrimination. At the community level, educational outreach is important to provide accurate information about HIV, both to the general public and community groups. Such education should aim to counter false assumptions on which stigma can be based. Advocacy programs that work toward changing policies and discriminatory laws play a major role in improving access to treatment and care for persons affected (Heijnders and Van Der Meij, 2006). At the governmental level, policies to limit discrimination and ensure access to confidential care make a significant impact on reducing the burden of stigma on affected individuals and their communities.

In summary, many types of stigma-reduction strategies can be implemented at different levels. Stigma is a social phenomenon and not an attribute of individuals. While persons living with HIV and AIDS cannot alone carry the burden of activism against stigma, they must also play an active and important part of the stigma-reduction process. Strategies should thus be multitargeted, with health-care professionals playing a significant role in their implementation (Heijnders and Van Der Meij, 2006).

CONCLUSION

We have seen how AIDSism, stigma, discrimination, and fear, in conjunction with denial and lack of awareness, complicate and perpetuate the HIV pandemic. Multidimensional approaches to reducing AIDS stigma have been described and need to be integrated into the care of persons with HIV. The creation of educational programs and supportive, nurturing, nonjudgmental health-care environments can help combat AIDSism and provide comprehensive and compassionate care. In order for persons with HIV and AIDS to live more comfortable lives, with preservation of independence and dignity, it is important to establish special nurturing, supportive, and loving health-care environments. Such environments can enable persons with HIV, their loved ones, and caregivers to meet the challenges of AIDS and AIDSism with optimism and dignity while at the same time preventing the perpetuation of the HIV pandemic (Cohen and Alfonso, 2004; Cohen, 2008).

References

Angermeyer MC, Beck M, Dietrich S, Holzinger A (2004). The stigma of mental illness: patients' anticipations and experiences. *Int J Soc Psychiatry* 50 (2):153–162.

Berger BE, Ferrans CE, Lashley FR (2001). Measuring stigma in people with HIV: psychometric assessment of the HIV stigma scale. *Res Nurs Health* 24 (6):518–529.

Bloom JR, Kessler L (1994). Emotional support following cancer: a test of the stigma and social activity hypotheses. *J Health Soc Behav* 35(2):118–133.

Blumenfeld W (1992). *Homophobia: How We All Pay the Price*. Boston: Beacon.

Bunn JY, Solomon SE, Miller C, Forehand R (2007). Measurement of stigma in people with HIV: a reexamination of the HIV Stigma Scale. *AIDS Educ Prev* 19(3):198–208.

Carl D (1990). *Counseling Same-Sex Couples*. New York: Norton.

Chenard C. (2007). The impact of stigma on the self-care behaviors of HIV-positive gay men striving for normalcy. *J Assoc Nurses AIDS Care* 18(3):23–32.

Cohen MA (1987). Psychiatric aspects of AIDS: a biopsychosocial approach. In GP Wormser, RE Stahl, and EJ Bottone (eds.), *AIDS Acquired Immune Deficiency Syndrome and Other Manifestations of HIV Infection*. Park Ridge, NJ: Noyes Publishers.

Cohen MA (1989). AIDSism, a new form of discrimination. *Am Med News*, January 20, 32:43.

Cohen MA (1992). Biopsychosocial aspects of the HIV epidemic. In GP Wormser (ed.), *AIDS and Other Manifestations of HIV Infection*, second edition (pp. 349–371). New York: Raven Press.

Cohen MA, Alfonso CA (1998). Psychiatric care and pain management in persons with HIV infection. In GP Wormser (ed.), *AIDS and Other Manifestations of HIV Infection*, third edition. Philadelphia: Lippincott-Raven.

Cohen MA, Alfonso CA (2004). AIDS psychiatry: psychiatric and palliative care, and pain management. In GP Wormser (ed.), *AIDS and Other Manifestations of HIV Infection*, fourth edition (pp. 537–576). San Diego: Elsevier Academic Press.

Cohen MA, Weisman H (1986). A biopsychosocial approach to AIDS. *Psychosomatics* 27:245–249.

Cohen MA (2008). History of AIDS psychiatry—a biopsychosocial approach—paradigm and paradox. In MA Cohen, JM Gorman (eds.), *Comprehensive Textbook of AIDS Psychiatry* (pp. 3–14). New York: Oxford University Press.

Crawford AM (1996). Stigma associated with AIDS: a meta-analysis. *J Appl Soc Psychol* 26:398–416.

Crisp AH, Gelder MG, Rix S, Meltzer HI, Rowlands OJ (2000). Stigmatisation of people with mental illnesses. *Br J Psychiatry* 177:4–7.

De Bruyn M (1999). Intersecting health risks: adolescent unwanted pregnancy, unsafe abortion and AIDS. *Initiat Reprod Health Policy* 3(1):4–5.

Douglas CJ, Kalman CM, Kalman TP (1985). Homophobia among physicians and nurses: an empirical study. *Hosp Community Psychiatry* 36(12):1309–1311.

Fernandes PT, Salgado PC, Noronha AL, et al. (2007). Prejudice towards chronic diseases: comparison among epilepsy, AIDS and diabetes. *Seizure* 16(4):320–323.

Gottlieb MS (2001). AIDS—past and future. *N Engl J Med* 344:1788–1791.

Gottlieb MS, Schroff R, Schanker HM, Weisman JD, Fan PT, Wolf RA, Saxon A (1981). *Pneumocystis carinii* pneumonia and mucosal candidiasis in previously healthy homosexual men: evidence of a new acquired cellular immunodeficiency. *N Engl J Med* 305:1425–1431.

Greene K (2000). *Disclosure of Chronic Illness Varies by Topic and Target: The Role of Stigma and Boundaries in Willingness to Disclose.* Mahwah, NJ: Lawrence Erlbaum Associates.

Heijnders M, Van Der Meij S (2006). The fight against stigma: an overview of stigma-reduction strategies and interventions. *Psychol Health Med* 11 (3):353–363.

Herek GM, Capitanio JP, Widaman KF (2002). HIV-related stigma and knowledge in the United States: prevalence and trends, 1991–1999. *Am J Public Health* 92(3):371–377.

Herek GM, Mitnick L, Burris S, et al. (1998). Workshop report: AIDS and stigma: a conceptual framework and research agenda. *AIDS Public Policy J* 13(1):36–47.

Holtz H, Dobro J, Kapila R, Palinkas R, Oleske J (1983). Psychosocial impact of acquired immunodeficiency syndrome. *JAMA* 250:167.

Hunter ND (1990). Epidemic of fear: a survey of AIDS discrimination in the 1980s and policy recommendations for the 1990s. American Civil Liberties Union AIDS Project 1990. New York: ACLU.

Ickovics JR, Hamburger ME, Vlahov D, et al. (2001). Mortality, CD4 cell count decline, and depressive symptoms among HIV-seropositive women: longitudinal analysis from the HIV Epidemiology Research Study. *JAMA* 285 (11):1466–1474.

Johnson SD (1995). Model of factors related to tendencies to discriminate against people with AIDS. *Psychol Rep* 76(2):563–572.

Kelly JA, St. Lawrence JS, Smith S, Jr, Hood HV, Cook DJ (1987). Stigmatization of AIDS patients by physicians. *Am J Public Health* 77:789–791.

Lambda Legal (2009, Aug 10). Protecting our seniors. Retrieved September 14, 2009, from http://www.lambdalegal.org/publications/articles/protecting-our-seniors.html

Lau JT, Tsui H (2007). Comparing the magnitude of discriminatory attitudes toward people living with HIV/AIDS and toward people with mental illness in the Hong Kong general population. *Health Educ Res* 22(1):139–152.

Lentine DA, Iannacchione VG, Laird GH, McClamroch K, Thalji L (2000). HIV-related knowledge and stigma: United States 2000. *MMWR Morb Mortal Wkly Rep* 49(47):1062–1064.

Leonard B (2000). Stress, depression and the activation of the immune system. *World J Biol Psychiatry* 1(1):17–25.

Mak WW, Mo PK, Cheung RW, Woo J, Cheung FM, Lee D (2006). Comparative stigma of HIV/AIDS, SARS, and tuberculosis in Hong Kong. *Soc Sci Med* 63 (7):1912–1922.

McLeroy KR, Bibeau D, Stecker A, Glanz K (1988). An ecological perspective on health promotion programs. *Health Educ Q* 15(4):351–377.

Nardi PM (1990). AIDS and obituaries: the perpetuation of stigma in the press. In DA Feldman (ed.), *Culture and AIDS* (pp. 159–168). New York: Praeger Publishers.

Richard L, Potvin L, Kishchuk N, Prlic H, Green LW (1996). Assessment of the integration of the ecological approach in health promotion programs. *Am J Health Promot* 10(4):318–328.

Romano RM (1986). *The Cancer Prevention Awareness Program: Approaching Public Understanding with Good News*. Oxford, UK: Pergamon.

Skinner D, Mfecane S (2004). Stigma, discrimination and the implications for people living with HIV/AIDS in South Africa. *SAHARA J* 1(3):157–164.

Smith GB (1993). Homophobia and attitudes toward gay men and lesbians by psychiatric nurses. *Arch Psychiatr Nurs* 7(6):377–384.

Swendeman D, Rotheram-Borus MJ, Comulada S, Weiss R, Ramos ME (2006). Predictors of HIV-related stigma among young people living with HIV. *Health Psychol* 25(4):501–509.

Tempelaar R, De Haes JC, De Ruiter JH, et al. (1989). The social experiences of cancer patients under treatment: a comparative study. *Soc Sci Med* 29 (5):635–642.

Thompson LM (1987). Dealing with AIDS and fear: would you accept cookies from an AIDS patient? *South Med J* 80:228–232.

Triplet RG, Sugarman DB (1987). Reactions to AIDS victims: ambiguity breeds contempt. *Pers Soc Psychol Bull* 13:265–274.

Ustun TB, Chatterji S, Rehm J, Saxena S, Bickenbach JE, Trotter RE, Room R (2001). *Disability and Culture: Universalism and Diversity*. Ashland, OH: Hogrefe & Huber Publishers.

Vanable PA, Carey MP, Blair DC, Littlewood RA (2006). Impact of HIV-related stigma on health behaviors and psychological adjustment among HIV-positive men and women. *AIDS Behav* 10(5):473–482.

Varas-Diaz N, Serrano-Garcia I, Toro-Alfonso J (2005). AIDS-related stigma and social interaction: Puerto Ricans living with HIV/AIDS. *Qual Health Res* 15(2):169–187.

Visser MJ, Kershaw T, Makin JD, Forsyth BW (2008). Development of parallel scales to measure HIV-related stigma. *AIDS Behav* 12(5):759–771.

Walkup J, Cramer LJ, Yeras J (2004). How is stigmatization affected by the "layering" of stigmatized conditions, such as serious mental illness and HIV? *Psychol Rep* 95(3 Pt 1):771–779.

Ware NC, Wyatt MA, Tugenberg T (2006). Social relationships, stigma and adherence to antiretroviral therapy for HIV/AIDS. *AIDS Care* 18(8):904–910.

Weiner B (1993). AIDS from an attributional perspective. In JB Pryor and GD Reeder (eds.), *The Social Psychology of HIV Infection* (pp. 287–302). Hillsdale, NJ: Lawrence Erlbaum Associates.

Weiss MG, Ramakrishna J (2006). Stigma interventions and research for international health. *Lancet* 367(9509):536–568.

Wormser GP, Joline C (1989). Would you eat cookies prepared by an AIDS patient? Survey reveals harmful attitudes among professionals. *Postgrad Med* 86:174–184.

Wright K, Naar-King S, Lam P, Templin T, Frey M (2007). Stigma scale revised: reliability and validity of a brief measure of stigma for HIV+ youth. *J Adolesc Health* 40(1):96–98.

5

STRATEGIES FOR PRIMARY AND SECONDARY PREVENTION OF HIV TRANSMISSION

Sami Khalife, Mary Ann Cohen, and Harold W. Goforth

Since HIV disease was first recognized three decades ago, numerous efforts have been made to prevent its continued transmission. The Centers for Disease Control and Prevention (CDC) estimates that more than 56,000 Americans become infected each year—one person every 9 1/2 minutes—and that more than one million people in this country are now living with HIV (CDC, 2008, 2009; Hall et al., 2008). The CDC estimates that roughly 1 in 5 people infected with HIV in the United States is unaware of his or her infection and may be unknowingly transmitting the virus to others (CDC, 2008).

Over the past 15 years, many behavioral HIV risk reduction interventions have been developed, with prevention efforts targeting mostly HIV-negative individuals and focusing almost exclusively on HIV testing and counseling. More recently, comprehensive HIV prevention has involved both primary and secondary prevention activities to decrease the number of new HIV infections and associated complications, respectively (Marks et al., 2006; O'Leary and Wolitski, 2009). Psychiatric factors both complicate and perpetuate the HIV pandemic as a result of unsafe sexual practices and substance use disorders. In this chapter, we describe some of the psychiatric and psychodynamic factors that lead to HIV transmission and present novel strategies to assist clinicians and health-care policymakers in prevention efforts.

PRIMARY HIV PREVENTION STRATEGIES

Primary prevention is defined as any activity that reduces the burden of morbidity or mortality from disease; it is to be distinguished from secondary prevention, in which activities are designed to prevent the complications of already existing disease. In the case of HIV, primary prevention efforts focus on strategies designed to prevent the transmission of HIV—keeping seronegative people seronegative. In the HIV pandemic, however, many prevention strategies share characteristics of both primary and secondary efforts, so the distinction is somewhat artificial. Multiple prevention strategies have been devised, and these center around HIV counseling, substance abuse programs, and HIV prevention and intervention programs for children.

Counseling healthy pregnant women, uninfected children, adolescents, adults, and older persons about HIV risk reduction and providing information about sexual health are important components to primary prevention strategies, but few physicians and other clinicians actually do this unless it is a part of a program specifically designed to prevent HIV transmission. Therefore, comfort and experience in discussing sensitive issues in a primary care setting are of vital importance (Makadon and Silin, 1995). Similarly, screening for sexually transmitted diseases (STDs) is an important HIV prevention intervention given that the presence of an STD both increases the chance of contracting HIV upon exposure to the virus and serves as a marker for unsafe sexual practices (Wasserheit, 1992). Prescribing condoms and encouraging free access to condoms has also been regarded as a primary prevention activity, as condom use cannot be underestimated in preventing spread of HIV disease.

Primary prevention of HIV has expanded in recent years to include specialized intervention among vulnerable populations, including women and children. Neonatal primary prevention has long been a primary focus of prevention efforts and is one of the more successful prevention programs worldwide. Nonetheless, neonatal transmission continues to occur at alarming rates in resource-limited countries without access to antiretroviral therapy (ART).

In industrialized countries, mother-to-child HIV transmission has been virtually eliminated, yet 500,000 children worldwide were infected via this vector in 2007 alone. Reasons for this failure to prevent HIV transmission include inadequate HIV counseling and testing, continued postnatal transmission through breastfeeding, and the lack of family planning resources and availability of ART therapy. Political will has also been identified as a key factor for the implementation of these prevention strategies, with Thailand and South Africa serving as good models. The reader is referred to an excellent review on this topic by McIntyre and Lallemant (2008). For prevention to be effective, however, it is clear that increased access to ART therapy for longer periods of time surrounding the postnatal period will be required to have a significant impact on the HIV transmission rate in countries dependent on postnatal breastfeeding (Six Week Extended-Dose Nevirapine (SWEN) Study Team, 2008).

Childhood trauma is also an important primary prevention area, in that childhood trauma is a powerful predictor of future unsafe sexual practices, increased numbers of sexual partners, and increased frequency of risky sexual behavior (Kalichman et al., 2004; Arreola et al., 2008). Children exposed to chaotic homes and to early childhood trauma are less likely to internalize a strong sense of self-worth and integrate the value of their bodies and their personhood. Children exposed to parental role models who abuse drugs and alcohol or have nonmonogamous relationships are subsequently at risk of emotional, physical, and sexual abuse as well as neglect and abandonment. These children are then more likely to repeat what they have witnessed and experienced. Strategies directed toward addressing risk behavior prevention include carefully designed educational curriculum from elementary school through college.

Effective strategies used in childcare settings include parent effectiveness education and child abuse prevention strategies as well as early childhood and adolescent age-appropriate sex education. Such programs are designed to bolster parental and child coping as well as raise awareness of safe and appropriate partner choice and safer sexual practices. However, as ART becomes more available, preventative services should evolve to provide a package of broader resources for affected individuals. Prevention strategies for tuberculosis, diarrhea, and malaria as well as for depression and cervical cancer should be introduced into clinic resources. Similarly, attention to cardiovascular disease prevention strategies, including those focusing on dietary health, exercise, and smoking cessation, should come to play a larger role in the future, instead of just focusing on HIV prevention in a narrow definition. It has been argued convincingly that the repackaging of preventative services in such a manner would lend itself to the standardization of care as well as ensuring broad access to preventative programs (Tolle, 2009).

Cervical cancer is the only human cancer that is almost entirely preventable through regular screening for the disease. Prevention efforts in this area contain both primary and secondary roles because women with HIV are also at higher risk for development of cervical cancer. Risk of cervical cancer among women with HIV remains high and does not appear to be affected by CD4 levels or access to antiviral therapy. Recently approved human papilloma virus (HPV) vaccines appear to decrease the risk of primary cervical cancer, although their effect on cohorts of immunocompromised women with multiple and persistent strains of HPV has been questioned. More attention to this topic is needed to improve detection and treatment in at-risk groups (Heard, 2009). Obstetricians and gynecologists have a good opportunity to offer this primary- and secondary-prevention care as they already provide preventative care to this at-risk and growing population. Guidelines for the provision of HIV screening and care to women have recently been published (Clark et al., 2008).

TABLE 5.1 Role of Psychiatric Disorders in HIV Transmission

- Cognitive impairment: disinhibition and poor judgment
- Mania: disinhibition and hypersexuality
- Psychosis: regression, inappropriate partner choice
- PTSD: sense of foreshortened future, problems with caring for self and body
- Depression: problems with self-worth
- Substance use disorders: sharing of needles and injection drug use, hypersexuality, disinhibition, intoxication, exchange of sex for drugs

Some psychiatric disorders, including substance use disorders, are associated with unsafe sex. Substance use disorder is both a direct and indirect vector of HIV transmission. While injection drug use can lead directly to HIV transmission through sharing of needles, syringes, and other drug paraphernalia, intoxication with alcohol and other drugs can also make individuals vulnerable to perpetuating infection. Disinhibition, inappropriate partner choice, exchange of sex for drugs, and unsafe sexual practices are prevalent during both intoxication and withdrawal states. Other psychiatric disorders, such as cognitive impairment, hypersexuality, and disinhibition, along with the high prevalence of multimorbid substance abuse disorders in persons with severe mental illness, can play a role in the transmission of HIV. Early recognition and treatment of psychiatric disorders can prevent HIV transmission through reduction in risky behaviors. A summary of the role of psychiatric disorders in HIV transmission is presented in Table 5.1.

Educational programs and ready availability of HIV testing and of condoms in psychiatric inpatient and ambulatory settings can help prevent transmission of HIV and other sexually transmitted diseases. Detailed descriptions of psychiatric disorders and their treatments as well as preventions strategies can be found in Chapters 1, 6, 7, and 8 of this handbook.

Other education focusing on strategies to reduce alcohol and drug abuse and harm, such as needle-exchange programs, are also of vital importance, even though they are politically and socially controversial in some settings. Methadone maintenance programs and buprenorphine programs are effective strategies to prevent HIV transmission; both require expansion and increased access to resources for dealing with what remains an epidemic of HIV.

SECONDARY HIV PREVENTION STRATEGIES

Secondary HIV prevention refers to activities designed to minimize consequences of HIV in a person who is already seropositive for the disease. HIV and other primary care settings are ideal for secondary prevention (King-Spooner, 1999; Janssen et al., 2001; CDC, 2003; King et al., 2009). Goals of secondary HIV prevention include ensuring continued health, reducing the risk for re-infection, and reducing the risk of spread to other noninfected groups. To ensure continued health in this population, effective programs have been designed to increase ART adherence and access to ART therapy. In addition, it is important to prevent multimorbid medical illnesses secondary to HIV, including cardiac disease, endocrine disturbances, pulmonary issues, opportunistic infection, and pain. A further discussion of medical complications can be found in Chapter 10. Pain is especially common in patients with HIV/AIDS and ranges in prevalence from 28% to 97% across various studies (Schofferman, 1988; Lebovits et al., 1989, 1994; Singh et al., 1992; Zarowny et al., 1992, and Reiter and Kudler, 1996). Untreated pain leads to an increase in psychological distress and a reduction in quality of life. Sources of pain are varied and range from neuropathic pain to chronic pain of malignancy, and all types of pain are associated with increased suicidal risk. Pain is commonly undertreated, in part because of the common prevalence of substance abuse disorder in patients with HIV/AIDS. Nonetheless, attention to minimizing the consequences of pain from HIV in substance users is important to maintain quality of life.

Education about high-risk sexual activities and harm reduction strategies and treatment for patients abusing drug and alcohol are also secondary prevention factors. Patients with HIV are at high risk of acquiring other blood-born pathogens such as hepatitis C. Involvement in needle exchange programs mitigates this risk as well as the risk of spreading HIV to other seronegative individuals. Similarly, drug and alcohol abuse treatment has been demonstrated to significantly reduce both morbidity from the direct effects of substance abuse (cirrhosis, infections) and the rate of progression of concurrent disease (e.g., use of alcohol in patients with comorbid HIV and HCV). Psychoeducational support groups designed to encourage and maintain healthy lifestyle choices are also important secondary prevention tools.

OBSTACLES TO HIV PREVENTION AND THE ROLE OF PHYSICIANS

While there are still many obstacles to carrying out HIV prevention, physicians can play an important role in recognizing and removing these barriers (Makadon and Silin, 1995). Four major barriers to providing clinical prevention information have been identified. First, many physicians do not focus on prevention. Second, physicians are taught mainly to respond to patient-generated complaints, rather than automatically taking a holistic approach and initiating preventative care when possible (Kottke et al., 1993). This highly focused perspective has failed to address the complexities of clinical prevention and have placed continued effort at treating illness rather than preventing it.

Another obstacle to providing clinical prevention is that physicians are uncomfortable with issues raised by HIV and AIDS—transmission of the virus involves socially unacceptable behaviors such as illicit drug use and unsafe sexual practices. It is imperative that health-care providers create an atmosphere that is nonjudgmental, trusting, and confidential for patients to discuss risky behavior. There are also practical constraints of time and resources; sensitive discussions take considerable time and are not generally amenable to standard medical billing practices of 10- to 15-minute time slots. AIDS psychiatrists have a unique role here, for it is often possible for them to spend more time with patients and offer counseling and psychoeducation regarding care and risk alternatives. It has also been shown that discussions regarding HIV risk reduction need not take extensive amounts of time and are amenable to primary care settings (Epstein et al., 1998).

Finally, there continues to be significant ambiguity among physicians about the risks of multiple sex partners, oral sex, intercourse with condoms, and risk of transmission between women. Patients often receive unclear messages regarding these topics (Makadon and Silin, 1995), which can communicate disinterest, uncertainty, or low risk where some risk actually exists. Practice guidelines based on available data are needed to better standardize clinical prevention messages in clinical and community settings (Makadon and Silin, 1995).

Conclusions

Psychiatrists and other mental health clinicians can play an important role in HIV prevention. They can contribute to both the recognition and treatment of psychiatric disorders that can render patients vulnerable to the transmission of HIV and can help develop strategies for HIV prevention. Prevention remains the most effective strategy to decrease HIV transmission and arrest the AIDS pandemic. While effective treatment exists for the AIDS in the form of comprehensive medical care and ART, no cure exists and none is on the horizon. The development and implementation of primary prevention strategies can assist in preventing further cases, especially among the most vulnerable—in neonates—and more efforts are needed in this area. For persons already infected with HIV, ART has transformed both care and life expectancy into that of any other chronic illness. Current and additional secondary prevention strategies for persons with HIV will work to minimize the role of metabolic disorders, cardiovascular disease, malignancy, and other complications of HIV and multimorbid medical conditions that pose a significant or greater threat to longevity than HIV itself.

REFERENCES

Arreola S, Neilands T, Pollack L, Paul J, Catania J (2008). Childhood sexual experiences and adult health sequelae among gay and bisexual men: defining childhood sexual abuse. *J Sex Res* 45(3):246–252.

[CDC] Centers for Disease Control and Prevention (2003). Incorporating HIV prevention into the medical care of persons living with HIV. Recommendations of CDC, the Health Resources and Services Administration, the National Institute of Health, and the HIV Medicine Association of the infectious Diseases Society of America. *Recommendations and Reports* 52(RR12):1–24.

[CDC] Centers for Disease Control and Prevention (2008). HIV prevalence estimates—United States, 2006. *MMWR Morb Mortal Wkly Rep* 57 (39):1073–1076.

[CDC] Centers for Disease Control and Prevention (2009). HIV prevention in the United States at a critical crossroads. Retrieved September 11, 2009, from http://www.cdc.gov/hiv/resources/reports/hiv_prev_us.htm

Clark J, Lampe MA, Jamieson DJ (2008). Testing women for human immunodeficiency virus infection: who, when, and how? *Clin Obstet Gynecol* 51:507–517.

Epstein RM, Morse DS, Frankel RM, et al. (1998). Awkward moments in patient–physician communication about HIV risk. *Ann Intern Med* 128:435–442.

Hall HI, Song R, Rhodes P, et al. (2008). Estimation of HIV incidence in the United States. *JAMA* 300(5):520–529.

Heard I (2009). Prevention of cervical cancer in women with HIV. *Curr Opin HIV AIDS* 4:68–73.

Janssen RS, Holtgrave DR, Valdisseri R, et al. (2001). The serostatus approach to fighting the HIV epidemic: prevention strategies for infected individuals. *Am J Public Health* 91(7):1019–1024.

Kalichman SC, Gore-Felton C, Benotsch E, Cage M, Rompa D (2004). Trauma symptoms, sexual behaviors, and substance abuse: correlates of childhood sexual abuse and HIV risks among men who have sex with men. *J Child Sex Abuse* 13(1):1–15.

King R, Lifshay J, Nakayiwa S, et al. (2009). The virus stops with me: HIV-infected Ugandans' motivations in preventing HIV transmission. *Soc Sci Med* 68(4):749–757.

King-Spooner S (1999). HIV prevention and the positive population. *Int J STD AIDS* 10(3):141–150.

Kottke TE, Brekke ML, Solberg LI (1993). Making "time" for preventive services. *Mayo Clin Proc* 68(8):785–791.

Lebovits AH, Lefkowitz M, McCarthy D, Simon R, Wilpon H, Jung R, Fried E (1989). The prevalence and management of pain in patients with AIDS: a review of 134 cases. *Clin J Pain* 5:245–248.

Lebovits AH, Smith G, Maignan M, Lefkowitz M (1994). Pain in hospitalized patients with AIDS: analgesic and psychotropic medications. *Clin J Pain* 10:156–161.

Makadon HJ, Silin JG (1995). Prevention of HIV infection in primary care: current practices, future possibilities. *Ann Intern Med* 123(9):715–719.

Marks G, Crepaz N, Janssen RS. (2006). Estimating sexual transmission of HIV from persons aware and unaware that they are infected with the virus in the USA. *AIDS* 20(10):1447–1450.

McIntyre J, Lallemant M (2008). The prevention of mother-to-child transmission of HIV: are we translating scientific success into programmatic failure? *Curr Opin HIV AIDS* 3:139–145.

O'Leary A, Wolitski RJ (2009). Moral agency and the sexual transmission of HIV. *Psychol Bull* 135(3):478–494.

Reiter GS, Kudler NR (1996). Palliative care and HIV: systemic manifestations and late-stage issues. *AIDS Clin Care* 8:27–36.

Schofferman J (1988). Pain: diagnosis and management in the palliative care of AIDS. *J Palliat Care* 4:46–49.

Singh S, Fermie P, Peters W (1992). Symptom control for individuals with advanced HIV in a subacute residential unit: which symptoms need palliation? *Int Conf AIDS* PoB D428 (abst.).

Six Week Extended-Dose Nevirapine (SWEN) Study Team, Bedri A, Gudetta B, Isehak A, Kumbi S, Lulseged S, Mengistu Y, Bhore AV, Bhosale R, Varadhrajan V, Gupte N, Sastry J, Suryavanshi N, Tripathy S, Mmiro F, Mubiru M, Onyango C, Taylor A, Musoke P, Nakabiito C, Abashawl A, Adamu R, Antelman G, Bollinger RC, Bright P, Chaudhary MA, Coberly J, Guay L, Fowler MG, Gupta A, Hassen E, Jackson JB, Moulton LH, Nayak U, Omer SB, Propper L, Ram M, Rexroad V, Ruff AJ, Shankar A, Zwerski S (2008). Extended-dose nevirapine to 6 weeks of age for infants to prevent HIV transmission via breastfeeding in Ethiopia, India, and Uganda: an analysis of three randomised controlled trials. *Lancet* 372:300–313.

Tolle MA (2009). A package of primary health care services for comprehensive family-centred HIV/AIDS care and treatment programs in low-income settings. *Trop Med Int Health* 14(6):663–672.

Wasserheit JN (1992). Epidemiological synergy. Interrelationships between human immunodeficiency virus infection and other sexually transmitted diseases. *Sex Transm Dis* 19(2):61–77.

Zarowny D, McCormack J, Li R, Singer J (1992). Incidence of pain in ambulatory HIV patients. *Int Conf AIDS* 8:B178 (abstract no. PoB 3551).

6

DIAGNOSIS OF PSYCHIATRIC DISORDERS

Sharon M. Batista, Harold W. Goforth, and Mary Ann Cohen

As we enter the third decade of the AIDS pandemic, persons with AIDS are living longer and healthier lives as a result of appropriate medical care and advances in antiretroviral therapy. In the United States and throughout the world, however, some men, women, and children with AIDS are unable to benefit from this medical progress because of inadequate access to care. A multiplicity of barriers involving economic, social, political, and psychiatric factors contribute to this lack of access. For this and other reasons, psychiatric factors take on new relevance and meaning in this stage of the pandemic (Cohen, 2008).

Psychiatric disorders and distress play a significant role in the transmission of, exposure to, and infection with HIV. They are thus relevant to HIV prevention, clinical care, and adherence to treatment throughout every aspect of illness from the initial risk behavior to death. Psychiatric disorders can result in considerable suffering, from diagnosis to end-stage illness. Persons with HIV and AIDS may have no psychiatric diagnosis at all or any diagnosis described in psychiatric nomenclature (Cohen and Alfonso, 2004; Cohen, 2008). In this chapter, we provide guidelines for the diagnosis of those psychiatric disorders that are most likely to complicate and perpetuate the HIV pandemic and pose diagnostic dilemmas for clinicians. Although we introduce aspects of treatment of each disorder, please see Chapters 7, 8, 9, 10, 11, and 12 for detailed descriptions of psychotherapeutic and psychopharmacological treatment approaches to AIDS psychiatry.

Differential Diagnosis

Consideration of a broad differential diagnosis is paramount in evaluating behavioral disorders in persons with HIV, especially when investigating medical and neuropsychiatric etiological factors related to HIV illness and its treatment. Since few persons with HIV have access to psychiatrists or other mental health clinicians, and even fewer have access to an AIDS psychiatrist, a summary of suggested key questions is provided here to aid HIV clinicians in detecting the underlying psychiatric diagnoses most frequently encountered in persons with HIV and AIDS. While these questions are by no means a substitute for comprehensive psychiatric evaluation (described in detail in Chapter 2 of this handbook), they can inform clinicians of the need for further assessment, emergency intervention, or referral to a psychiatrist. These questions address the most prevalent diagnoses that complicate and perpetuate the HIV pandemic and are summarized in Table 6.1.

TABLE 6.1 Diagnosing Psychiatric Disorders that Complicate and Perpetuate the HIV Pandemic—Key Questions for HIV Clinicians

Cognitive Disorders

- Dementia: Have you had any problems with your memory?
- Delirium: Do you feel confused?

Substance-Related Disorders

- What is the most alcohol (or other drugs) that can you hold in a day?

Posttraumatic Stress Disorder

- Do you have frightening dreams or intrusive thoughts?

Bereavement

- Are you preoccupied with your loss?

Mood Disorders

- Due to medical condition, with depressed features: Are you depressed or suicidal?
- Due to medical condition, with manic features: Do you feel irritable?
- Major depressive disorder: Are you depressed or suicidal?
- Bipolar disorder: Do you have a history of having periods of being up or being down?

Psychotic Disorders and Schizophrenia

- Does your mind play tricks on you sometimes?

Table 6.2 presents an overview of differential diagnostic considerations in neuropsychiatric manifestations of HIV infection; it does not include the psychiatric manifestations of other associated medical illnesses or of medications. Differential diagnostic categories include behavioral presentations due to medical illness, cognitive disorders, mood disorders, anxiety

TABLE 6.2 Differential Diagnosis of Neuropsychiatric Manifestations of HIV Infection: Signs and Symptoms that Can Overshadow, Overlap, or Masquerade as Each Other

Substance-Induced Disorders	Psychiatric Disorders with Similar Symptoms, Signs, and Behaviors	HIV-Related Neuropsychiatric Disorders with Similar Symptoms, Signs, and Behaviors
Intoxication from alcohol or benzodiazepines: sedation, slurred speech, psychomotor retardation, memory impairment, disinhibition, agitation	Mania: irritability, agitation Dementia: memory impairment, disinhibition	HIV-associated dementia (HAD): memory impairment, disinhibition, slow speech Intrinsic involvement of the brain with HIV or opportunistic infections such as toxoplasmosis, or lymphoma and progressive multifocal leukoencephalopathy (PML) or cancers such as CNS lymphoma Mental status changes secondary to antiretroviral therapies
Withdrawal from alcohol: irritability, loss of appetite, tremor, hallucinations, paranoia	Major depressive disorder: depression, insomnia, loss of appetite, psychomotor retardation, withdrawal	Treatment for opportunistic infections and cancers: depression, mania Drug toxicity, e.g., treatment for comorbid hepatitis C virus infection with interferon and ribavirin: depression, fatigue, loss of appetite
Withdrawal from benzodiazepines: anxiety, insomnia, hypervigilance, tremors	Major depressive disorder: depression, insomnia, loss of appetite, psychomotor retardation, withdrawal Adjustment disorder: depression, anxiety	HIV-induced mood disorder: depression, insomnia

(continued)

TABLE 6.2 (Continued)

Substance-Induced Disorders	Psychiatric Disorders with Similar Symptoms, Signs, and Behaviors	HIV-Related Neuropsychiatric Disorders with Similar Symptoms, Signs, and Behaviors
Substance-induced mood disorders: depression or mania	Bipolar disorder: depression, mania	HIV-induced mood disorder: depression, mania, insomnia "AIDS mania": irritability HCV infection: depression, fatigue, loss of appetite
Substance-induced psychosis with delusions or hallucinations	Schizoaffective disorder Schizophrenia	HIV-induced psychosis Mental status changes secondary to antiretroviral therapies
Amnestic disorders	Dementia Delirium	HAD
Anxiety	Generalized anxiety disorder PTSD: hypervigilance, hyperarousal, insomnia	
Sleep disorders	Sleep disorders Dementia: reversal of sleep/wake cycle	HIV-induced sleep disorders
Sexual dysfunction	Major depressive disorder	HIV-induced mood disorder: depression
Delirium: hallucinations, somnolence, withdrawal, confusion, insomnia, agitation	Dementia: paranoia, delusions, agitation, memory impairment, reversal of sleep/wake cycle Schizophrenia	HIV-induced psychosis HAD Mental status changes secondary to antiretroviral therapies
Dementia: paranoia, delusions, agitation	Schizophrenia	HAD Mental status changes secondary to antiretroviral therapies

disorders, and substance abuse disorders. Table 6.3 provides an example of the complexity involved in the differential diagnosis of a person with AIDS who presents with visual hallucinations. The reader is referred to Chapter 10 for a more thorough discussion of comorbid medical illness in HIV and AIDS.

TABLE 6.3 Differential Diagnosis of Causes of Visual Hallucinations in Persons with AIDS with CD4 Count <200

Medical Causes

Infectious

- Cytomegalovirus (CMV) retinopathy
- Sepsis
- Fungemia

Neurological Causes

- Space-occupying lesions of brain: CNS lymphomas, toxoplasmosis, progressive multifocal leukoencephalopathy (PML)
- Seizures: ictal, interictal, and postictal states

Psychiatric Causes

Substance use disorders

- Alcohol withdrawal
- Benzodiazepine withdrawal
- Hallucinogens
- Amphetamine and other stimulants

Delirium—see Table 6.5 for specific causes of delirium

- Metabolic encephalopathy
- Medications that cause delirium such as anticholinergics

Psychotic disorders

- Schizophrenia
- Schizoaffective disorder

Mood disorders

- Major depressive disorder with psychotic features
- Mania

Anxiety disorders

- Posttraumatic stress disorder with psychotic features

COGNITIVE DISORDERS IN HIV AND AIDS: DELIRIUM AND DEMENTIA

HIV infection is associated with a range of cognitive and behavioral symptoms that can occur during the early stages of infection but become more frequent and severe as the immune system declines and symptomatic illness and AIDS ensue. The cognitive disorders are delirium and dementia.

Delirium

Delirium is a cognitive disorder that is highly prevalent but is frequently unrecognized or misdiagnosed in persons with AIDS. Delirium as a disorder

TABLE 6.4 Diagnosis of Delirium in Persons with HIV

Confusion
Hypoactive delirium—quiet, withdrawn
Hyperactive delirium—agitated
Cognitive impairment in ability to do the following:

- Process
- Retain
- Retrieve
- Apply information about environment, body, and self

Impairment of the following:

- Thought process
- Memory
- Perception, as manifested by hallucinations and illusions
- Awareness
- Attention
- Orientation

Rapid fluctuations in the following over the course of minutes, hours, or days:

- Level of consciousness
- Behavior
- Mood
- State of alertness to falling asleep mid-sentence
- "Nodding out"

of cognition includes global cognitive impairment with concurrent deficits in memory, thinking, orientation, or perception; disturbances of the sleep–wake cycle; and a characteristic course marked by rapid onset, relatively brief duration, and fluctuations in the severity of the disturbance. The signs and symptoms of delirium are summarized in Table 6.4.

Causes of delirium in persons with AIDS

Delirium is 100% reversible when an underlying cause can be identified. Factors predisposing to delirium in AIDS include addiction to alcohol or drugs, brain damage, and chronic illness. Facilitating factors are psychological stress, sleep deprivation, and sensory deprivation during intensive care unit admission. See Table 6.5 for causes of delirium in persons with HIV and Table 6.6 for medications that may cause delirium.

Although it is not always easy to identify the cause of delirium in persons with HIV, it is important to consider a careful evaluation including history, physical examination, laboratory studies, and imaging studies where indicated. A decrease in frequency of electroencephalogram (EEG) background activity is indicative of delirium, possibly as a result of a reduction of brain metabolism. EEG changes virtually always accompany delirium and make

TABLE 6.5 Causes of Delirium in Persons with HIV and AIDS

Toxic or Drug-Induced Delirium

- Intoxication: sedative-hypnotics, alcoholic hallucinosis, opiates
  Drugs: antibiotics, anticholinergics, anticonvulsants, antineoplastic drugs, antiretrovirals, ketamine, lithium, narcotic analgesics
- Withdrawal: alcohol, sedative-hypnotics

Metabolic Encephalopathy

- Hypoxia
- Hepatic, renal, pulmonary, or pancreatic insufficiency
- Hypoglycemia

Disorders of Fluid, Electrolyte, and Acid–Base Imbalance

- Dehydration
- Lactic acidosis (secondary to antiretroviral treatment)
- Hypernatremia, hypokalemia, hypocalcemia, hypercalcemia, alkalosis, acidosis

Endocrine Disorders

- Hypothyroidism
- Pancreatitis and diabetes mellitus

Infections

- Systemic: bacteremia, septicemia, infective endocarditis, bacterial pneumonia,
- *Pneumocystis jerovici* pneumonia, cryptococcal pneumonia
- Herpes zoster
- Disseminated *Mycobacterium avium-intracellulare* (MAC) complex
- Disseminated candidiasis
- Intracranial: cryptococcal meningitis, HIV encephalitis, tuberculous meningitis, toxoplasmosis

Malnutrition and Vitamin Deficiency

- Protein energy undernutrition
- Vitamin B_{12} deficiency
- Thiamine deficiency and Wernicke's encephalopathy
- Wasting and failure to thrive

Neoplastic

- Space-occupying lesions: CNS lymphoma, CNS metastases, cryptococoma, toxoplasmosis
- Paraneoplastic syndromes associated with lung and other neoplasms

(*continued*)

TABLE 6.5 (Continued)

Neurological

- Seizures: ictal, interictal, postictal states
- Head trauma
- Space-occupying lesions of the brain: CNS lymphomas, toxoplasmosis, cytomegalovirus infection, abscesses, cryptococcoma

Hypoxia

- *Pneumocystis jerovici* pneumonia
- Pulmonary hypertension
- Cardiomyopathy
- Coronary artery disease
- End-stage pulmonary disease
- Anemia

TABLE 6.6 Selected Medications Associated with Delirium in Persons with HIV

Antiretrovirals

- Efavirenz
- Nevirapine
- Zidovudine

Antivirals

- Interferon
- Gancyclovir

Antibiotics

- Aminoglycosides
- Amodiaquine
- Cephalosporins
- Gentamycin
- Rifampin
- Sulfonamides
- Vancomycin

Anticholinergics

- Diphenhydramine
- Benztropine

Narcotic Analgesics

the EEG a useful diagnostic tool in persons with AIDS who manifest a change in mental status. EEG changes can aid in identifying the specific etiology of delirium. Triphasic waves are characteristic of hepatic encephalopathy and generalized fast-wave activity may be indicative of delirium tremens. EEG testing may also be helpful in evaluating and monitoring the course of HIV dementia (Parisi et al., 1989) or diagnosing seizure-related behavior changes. A controlled study (Koralnik et al., 1990) of men with asymptomatic HIV infection showed that EEG and other electrophysiologic tests were the most sensitive indicators of subclinical neurological impairment.

Treatment of delirium in AIDS

Treatment of delirium consists of first identifying and treating the underlying cause and then providing supportive care, such as maintaining hydration, electrolyte balance, and nutrition. In addition, it is important to provide an optimal environment for the patient: a quiet, well-lit room with a dim light at night, radio or television, a large calendar with the date marked clearly each day, an easy-to-read clock, photographs and familiar objects, soothing favorite music, and, if possible, visits from familiar people. Medical and nursing support should be directed toward orientation and companionship as well as to adequate sleep and sedation.

The atypical antipsychotic medications olanzapine, 2.5 mg, or quetiapine 25 mg may be recommended as a standing order at bedtime until identification and treatment of the underlying cause have been accomplished. The dosage can be increased gradually in divided doses if necessary to control agitation. For extreme agitation, olanzapine or quetiapine can be given in divided doses every 1 to 6 hours. While other antipsychotic medications are used to treat delirium, most cause severe extrapyramidal side effects in persons with HIV and AIDS and can complicate the course. If agitation is severe, lorazepam can be added to the antipsychotic for additional sedation as needed (Cohen and Alfonso, 2004). This medication is advantageous because it may be administered intravenously or intramuscularly in severely agitated patients with low risk of adverse effects. For patients with HIV who may be more sensitive to extrapyramidal symptoms, avoidance of typical neuroleptics such as haloperidol is preferable.

HIV-associated dementia

HIV infection is associated with a range of cognitive and behavioral symptoms that can occur during the early stages of infection but become more frequent and severe as the immune system declines and symptomatic illness and AIDS ensue. HIV infects and destroys subcortical white matter, disrupting neural networks, signal transmission, and frontal lobe function (Gendelman et al., 1998; Reynolds et al., 2008). HIV-associated dementia (HAD) is one of the subcortical dementias characterized by cognitive and psychomotor slowing and impaired attention, concentration, judgment, impulse control, and executive function. See Table 6.7 for a summary of

TABLE 6.7 Symptoms and Signs of HIV-Associated Dementia (HAD)

Symptoms	Signs
Early	
Word-finding difficulty	Cognitive impairment
Forgetfulness	Apathy
Poor concentration	Regression
Confusion	Psychosis
Slowed thinking	Psychomotor retardation
Difficulty performing complex learned tasks	Difficulty with abstract thinking
Loss of balance	Ataxia
Change in or decreased quality of handwriting	Tremor
Leg weakness	Paresis
Impairment of coordination	Slow speech
Dropping things	
Late	
Disorientation	Mutism
Severe confusion	Incontinence
Seizures	Perseveration
	Severe regression
	Carphologia (picking)

symptoms and signs of HAD. These deficits profoundly impact function (Clifford, 2002; Boisse et al., 2008) and adherence to antiretroviral therapy (ART) (Arlt et al., 2008) and increase the need for psychosocial support. Neuropsychological deficits in HIV-associated neurocognitive disorders also reflect underlying subcortical–frontal pathology (Heaton et al., 1995). Other neuropsychiatric symptoms associated with HAD include apathy, depression, mania, and psychosis.

Epidemiology

Since the development of new classes of antiretroviral medications in 1996 (such as protease inhibitors and non-reverse transcriptase inhibitors in addition to the pre-existing reverse transcriptase inhibitors) and the advent of the use of combinations of these antiretroviral medications (initially termed highly active antiretroviral therapy, or HAART, then combination antiretroviral therapy, or CART, and currently antiretroviral therapy, or ART), the overall incidence of HIV-associated dementia has declined in areas with access to treatment. However, while HIV patients taking ART may have enhanced immune function and survive longer without HIV-associated cognitive decline, the prevalence of all-cause dementia in HIV-infected patients likely has remained stable or increased. HAD can occur at any age and is a treatable cause of dementia in young persons with HIV. The combination of HAD, older age, and functional impairment are predictors of AIDS progression and death (Dougherty et al., 2002; Shen et al., 2005; Sevigny et al., 2007; Tozzi et al., 2007; Uthman and Abdulmalik, 2008).

When patients present with cognitive complaints, it is important to assess for depression, anxiety, substance use disorders, and other psychiatric disorders as well as for reversible medical causes of cognitive impairment. See Table 6.8 for a summary of the clinical and laboratory assessments of neurocognitive disorders. A minimal basic workup should include complete blood count (CBC) with differential, CD4 lymphocyte count, HIV-1 viral load, serum chemistries, a toxicology screen, thyroid function tests, and serological tests for syphilis. Magnetic resonance imaging (MRI) of the brain with gadolinium is preferred over computed tomography (CT) as it provides better visualization of subcortical and posterior fossa structures and focal lesions; however, MRI may be less feasible in agitated patients.

Treatment of HIV-associated dementia

It is important to diagnose HIV as early as possible after infection so that ART can be initiated, since there is evidence that HIV begins to damage the brain within months of infection (Koutsilieri et al., 2001; Meehan and Brush 2001), causing subtle neurocognitive deficits that increase the risk of later HAD (Silberstein et al., 1993). ART may

---

TABLE 6.8 Clinical and Laboratory Evaluation of Patients with HIV and Neurocognitive Symptoms

- Medical evaluation with screening laboratories: complete blood count, chemistry screen (including liver and renal function tests), urinalysis, chest X-ray, electrocardiogram, blood and urine cultures (when applicable)
- CD4 lymphocyte count, HIV-1 plasma viral load
- Psychiatric diagnostic interview including personal and family history
- Cognitive screen (HIV Dementia Scale)
- Additional laboratories when applicable: illicit-drug toxicology screen, serum psychotropic drug levels, thyroid function tests, antithyroid antibodies, vitamin B_{12} and B_6 levels, total or bioavailable testosterone, dehydroepiandrosterone sulfate, adrenocorticotropic stimulation test, 24-hour urine cortisol
- Evaluation for hepatitis C (including viral load)
- Review of antiretroviral regimen for neuropsychiatric side effects
- Review of psychotropic mediations for efficacy, neuropsychiatric side effects, drug interactions
- Neuroimaging (MRI, MR spectroscopy, diffusion tensor imaging)
- Lumbar puncture (including cerebrospinal fluid HIV-1 viral load if available)
- Review of antiretroviral medication for CNS penetrance

---

reduce the severity of HAD, slow its progression, and even induce full recovery in some people (Chang et al., 1998; Cohen and Jacobson, 2000; McArthur et al., 2004; Cysique et al., 2006; Price and Spudich, 2008). However, most patients with HAD are left with persisting, mild neuropsychiatric deficits despite ART (Ferrando et al., 1998b, Tozzi et al., 2007), and in some instances, ART can accelerate HAD associated with immune reconstitution inflammatory syndrome (IRIS) (Alisky, 2007; Chang et al., 2008; Nath, et al., 2008).

Effective ART therapy remains the primary treatment modality for HIV-related cognitive decline. In cases where cognitive decline is present, evaluation by viral genotype may be beneficial to ensure continued viral sensitivity to the selected ART regimen. The treatment of HAD with agitation or psychotic features is with atypical antipsychotic medications such as olanzapine or quetiepine in low doses. Psychostimulants, particularly methylphenidate, dextroamphetamine, and modafinil, have been used for apathy and withdrawal in late-stage HAD (Holmes et al., 1989; Rabkin et al., 2004b). Most importantly, none of these options has shown the magnitude of benefit of ART in reducing associated morbidity.

Mood Disorders

Mood disorders have complex synergistic and catalytic interactions with HIV infection and are significant factors in nonadherence to risk reduction and to medical care. Mood disorders associated with HIV include illness- and treatment-related depression and mania, responses to diagnoses of HIV, and comorbid primary mood disorders such as major depressive disorder and bipolar disorder.

Mood disorders as responses to HIV diagnosis, illness, and treatment

Bereavement

Persons with HIV and AIDS may experience not only the losses of loved ones, children, partners, parents, and friends, but also losses related to illness. Early intervention at the time of bereavement is an effective and worthwhile strategy to optimize wellness in HIV-infected groups and may impact long-term immunity. Brief group interventions such as bereavement support groups and interpersonal therapy have been shown to significantly reduce overall distress and accelerate grief resolution (Goodkin et al., 1999, 2001; Sikkema et al., 2004, 2005; Goforth et al., 2009).

Adjustment disorder with depressive features

Adjustment disorders are defined as brief, maladaptive reactions to significant psychosocial stressors within 3 months of the stressor's onset (DSM-IV-TR; American Psychiatric Association, 2000). The prevalence of these disorders is estimated at between 2% and 8% of the general population, with women diagnosed twice as often as men, and is likely the most common Axis I disorder in HIV patients (O'Dowd et al., 1991).

The clinical picture of adjustment disorders can be varied, with depression, anxiety, conduct disturbance, and mixed subtypes. Adjustment disorders can also be associated with severe reactions, including suicidality, and may be a frequent concomitant of HIV testing with either negative or positive test results. Please refer to the section on suicide later in this chapter for information about suicide assessments in patients with mood disorders.

Ideally, adjustment disorders should be treated conservatively with supportive and other appropriate forms of psychotherapy. A psychoeducational approach should be used to dispel misconceptions and increase or sustain healthy behavior as well as bolster existing psychological support. Identification of elements over which the patient has control can help the patient have a sense of empowerment and maintain an internal locus of control. Given that adjustment disorders typically resolve within several months, medications should likely be reserved as augmentation strategies rather than as a primary treatment modality.

Major depressive disorder and mood disorders with depressive features due to HIV and AIDS

Depressive illness is a major cause of distress in patients with HIV and AIDS and has a severe impact on the quality of life and on medication adherence. Depression is a debilitating condition; its symptoms include sadness, pessimism, anhedonia, guilt, and suicidality in addition to neurovegetative changes such as impaired sleep and appetite. These latter signs can often be confused with the primary illness, as HIV and AIDS often produce fatigue, anorexia, and wasting syndromes, making the diagnosis of depression challenging in this patient group. Additionally, somatic symptoms of depression may be confused with opportunistic infections, further complicating the differential diagnosis and increasing utilization of physicians' time and services. Table 6.9 summarizes significant diagnostic features of major depressive disorder and mood disorder due to medical illness with depressive features.

Major depressive disorder is frequently underdiagnosed and undertreated (Evans et al., 1996–97) in persons with HIV and AIDS. Depression

Table 6.9 Diagnostic Features of Major Depressive Disorders and Mood Disorders with Depressive Features in Persons with HIV and AIDS

Symptoms and Signs Distinguishing Depression from Other Psychiatric, Medical, or Other Factors

- Depression
- Sadness
- Crying frequently
- Pessimism
- Anhedonia
- Anergia
- Low self-esteem and self-worth
- Feelings of profound guilt

Symptoms and Signs that May Be Confused with Other Disorders

- Psychomotor retardation or agitation
- Loss of or increase in appetite
- Loss of or increase in weight
- Loss of libido
- Impairment of concentration
- Delusions and hallucinations of a derogatory nature
- Suicidal ideation

in HIV can be either primary or secondary in nature. When depression develops during the course of HIV infection, it is described typically as a mood disorder due to a medical condition if it is etiologically related to HIV infection, opportunistic disease, antiviral treatments, or comorbid medical conditions. Growing evidence points toward a substantial link with chronic depression and immune suppression (Goforth et al., in press). When a person with HIV or AIDS has a longstanding history of depression or family history of depression or bipolar disorder, however, major depressive disorder is a more likely diagnosis.

Mood disorders with depressive features or secondary depression

Common aspects of HIV illness that directly impact the emergence of depressive symptoms include endocrine abnormalities, opportunistic disease, nutritional states, comorbid illness, and medication effect. Significant factors and causes of secondary depression are summarized in Table 6.10. Further discussion of comorbid medical conditions presenting as major affective disorders is found in Chapter 10.

Antiretroviral therapy (ART) has revolutionized the treatment of HIV and has led to increased quality of life and longer lives for those affected. However, ART-related medications are highly toxic and can produce neurobehavioral disturbances and changes. The antiviral agent most frequently

TABLE 6.10 Significant Factors and Causes of Secondary Depression in HIV and AIDS

Psychiatric Disorders

Substance use disorders

- Cocaine-induced mood disorder
- Sedative-hypnotic–induced mood disorder
- Alcohol-induced mood disorder

HIV-associated dementia

Medical Illness

Infections

- Hepatitis C
- HIV-induced mood disorder
- HIV-associated nephropathy and end-stage renal disease
- Cirrhosis of the liver

Endocrine disorders

- Hypothyroidism
- Diabetes mellitus
- Hypotestosteronism
- Adrenal insufficiency

Medications

Source: Goforth HW, Cohen MA, Murrough J (2008). Mood disorders. In MA Cohen and JM Gorman (eds.), *Comprehensive Textbook of AIDS Psychiatry* (pp. 97–108). New York: Oxford University Press.

found to produce such changes is efavirenz, which has been linked through case reports to episodes of suicidal ideation, cognitive changes, headache, dizziness, insomnia, and nightmares. Its neuropsychiatric profile has been shown to be related to blood levels (Gutierrez et al., 2005), but the neuro-behavioral symptoms appear to abate gradually as patients continue to receive the agent over time with almost complete resolution expected after 3 months (Clifford et al., 2005) unless there is a longstanding history of underlying mood disorder.

Hepatitis C virus (HCV) coinfection among HIV-infected populations is problematic and poses a unique set of challenges for the practitioner. Treatment of HCV with interferon-based therapies dramatically increases the risk of depressive symptoms to near 80% (Laguno et al., 2004; Reichenberg et al., 2005; Scalori et al., 2005). These effects on mood, increased fatigue, and worsened quality of life are even greater in patients with concurrent, advanced HIV disease (Ryan et al., 2004). We would recommend using antidepressants such as citalopram, escitalopram, or bupropion for persons with depression and HIV/HCV coinfection as well as maintaining a low threshold for treatment of emerging depressive or psychotic symptoms (Hoffman et al., 2003) in persons undergoing interferon treatment regardless of prior history of depressive illness.

Secondary Mania

Although secondary manic syndromes due to late-stage AIDS have become less prevalent with the use of ART, they can have disastrous consequences for the patient when they do occur. In a chart review, Lyketsos and colleagues (1993) reported that manic syndromes affected approximately 8% of the examined population across a 17-month period. These patients were less likely to have a family history of bipolar disorder but more likely to have concurrent dementia than patients with manic episodes early in the non-AIDS stage of their disease. Ellen and colleagues (1999) identified mania in 1.2% of HIV-seropositive patients and in 4.3% of those with AIDS-defining illness, which is suggestive of disease progression. Other etiologies of secondary mania include opportunistic infections such as cryptococcal meningitis (Thienhaus and Khosla, 1984; Johannesen and Wilson, 1988), treatment with zidovudine (Maxwell et al., 1988) or didanosine (Brouillette et al., 1994), efavirenz in overdose (Blanch et al., 2002), and clarithromycin (Nightingale et al., 1995) or ethambutol treatment (Pickles and Spelman, 1996). Treatment is directed toward both symptom control and the underlying disease, since mania most commonly presents in advanced illness.

Suicidality

Like persons with other chronic medical conditions, persons with HIV and AIDS are at an increased risk of suicide (Cote et al., 1992). Depression and suicidality are two of the most common reasons for consultation requests in HIV-positive patients. Current guidelines indicate that patients should be assessed for suicidality at least annually (New York State Department of Health AIDS Institute Guidelines, 2009) and more frequently for patients with somatic complaints, changes in health status, or changes in significant relationships.

Most of the data about suicide are from the pre-ART era when HIV was considered a death sentence. While there is no way to know all of the reasons for suicide, one factor that cannot be ignored is the reaction to receiving a life-threatening diagnosis. Common suicide methods are similar to those used in the general population: medication overdoses, firearms, and suffocation. Kalichman and colleagues (2000) found that thoughts of suicide are prevalent in the population of persons infected with HIV, with rates of up to

27% of persons indicating suicidal ideation within the week of their survey. Older individuals, women, and racial minorities are at particular risk of suicide (Marzuk, 1997; Kalichman, 2000). Psychosocial factors include interpersonal rejection, lack of social supports, and AIDS-related stigma (Heckman, 2002).

Patients with depressive complaints should be assessed for suicidality frequently, as well as for acute changes in their impulsivity or acute stressors. While it is common practice to make a safety contract with a patient, there is no evidence that this is associated with improved outcomes, although we have found it useful in helping patients to plan for their safety and maintain rapport with them despite impairing levels of distress. Practitioners are often anxious about the implications for the therapeutic alliance should they recommend acute hospitalization of a patient with thoughts of death, but emphasis must always be placed on the safety of the patient, especially if the patient is able to enumerate a specific and accessible suicide plan. More often than not, patients are able to come to appreciate that preventive measures were taken, and the suggestion of voluntary or involuntary hospitalization can be used as a positive intervention demonstrating that the patient's feelings and behaviors are being taken seriously. If a patient is indeed hospitalized, this can be an important opportunity to enhance supports, which can be a crucial mitigating factor, as well as to improve assess to medical care, psychiatric services, and psychotherapy.

For further information about suicide assessment please refer to Chapter 2.

Bipolar disorder

Mania can occur at any point along the course of HIV illness, but the occurrence generally clusters into two categories: (a) a preexisting bipolar disorder that predated HIV seroconversion or is not directly related to the disease, which can occur at any point during the course of the disease; and (b) the late-stage manic syndrome that occurs most commonly but not exclusively in the context of HAD (Lyketsos et al., 1997; Treisman et al., 1998). Primary bipolar disorder is more likely to appear consistent with the usual course of the illness, including euphoric mood, expansiveness, and signs or symptoms of poor judgment. In addition, the presence of a family history of bipolar disorder is more common in this category, and it is less likely to be associated with a preexisting condition. AIDS mania has been noted to be associated with marked cognitive deficits, a pronounced irritable mood, and greater severity coupled with a rather dismal prognosis (Lyketsos et al., 1993, 1997).

The choice of an effective mood stabilizer in treating patients with bipolar disorder and concurrent HIV disease is complex and is based on both available supporting evidence of primary efficacy and the potential for pharmacological interactions and potential adverse events. Olanzapine and quetiepine are recommended. Lithium has been a mainstay of mania treatment and is the oldest and best characterized mood stabilizer. Its use in HIV and AIDS patients, however, is commonly precluded because of its expansive list of adverse events. The major problem with lithium in treating AIDS patients is the unpredictable fluctuations in serum blood levels due to a variety of mechanisms, making toxicity an ever-present consideration. Shifts in electrolyte balance via sweating, vomiting, diarrhea, or metabolic alkalosis can lead to dangerously elevated lithium levels, as can failure to adequately excrete the drug due to renal impairment from HIV-related nephropathy and heroin nephropathy. Thus, the use of lithium in persons with HIV or AIDS should be exercised with caution after an appropriate medical evaluation (Cohen and Jacobson, 2000). More details about treatment are found in Chapter 7.

ANXIETY DISORDERS

Anxiety is a painful and ubiquitous concomitant of most severe medical illnesses, and AIDS is no exception. In reviewing the specific anxiety disorders commonly seen in persons with HIV and AIDS, it is important to recognize that these are often superimposed on the anxiety that is experienced in the general population and commonly in the population with chronic symptomatic medical illness (Wells et al., 1988, 1989). HIV-positive persons suffer from anxiety symptoms (Sewell et al., 2000) and anxiety disorders at increased rates (Morrison et al., 2002). The lifetime prevalence of anxiety disorders in the general population is about 25% (Kessler et al., 1994, 2005) and is an especially common complaint in the ambulatory medical setting (Schurman et al., 1985; Spitzer et al., 1999). The prevalence of anxiety in the waiting-room population of an urban HIV clinic was 70% (Cohen et al., 2001).

Given that anxiety disorders in HIV patients can masquerade as physical illness (Pollack et al., 2004), when evaluating a patient for diagnosis and treatment of an anxiety disorder it is important to exclude potential medical etiologies. Upon initial evaluation, a thorough medical history, physical exam, and appropriate basic screening tests (EKG, CBC, thyroid function test, blood chemistry, urinalysis, RPR/VDRL, urine toxicology) should be performed to aid in diagnosis and to rule out contributing medical illness (Basu et al., 2005). Rarely, endocrine dysfunction, cardiovascular illness, or drug intoxication or withdrawal may be mistaken for an anxiety disorder (Pollack et al., 2004). The reader is referred to Chapter 10 for further information regarding medical etiologies.

Posttraumatic stress disorder (PTSD)

The prevalence of PTSD in persons with HIV and AIDS ranges from 30% (Kelly et al., 1998) to 42% (Cohen et al., 2002). Intimate-partner violence, history of childhood trauma, and childhood sexual trauma are all risk factors for HIV infection as well as for PTSD. The severity of HIV-related PTSD symptoms is associated with a greater number of HIV-related physical symptoms, extensive history of pre-HIV trauma, decreased social support, increased perception of stigma, and negative life events (Katz and Nevid, 2005).

Posttraumatic stress disorder is often multimorbid with other psychiatric and medical disorders, pain (Smith et al., 2002; Tsao et al., 2004), and depressive symptoms (Sledjeski et al., 2005). PTSD is associated with non-adherence to risk reduction and medical care (Cohen et al., 2001; Ricart et al., 2002). It is often difficult to diagnose PTSD in persons with HIV since its symptoms may be overshadowed by associated psychiatric disorders including substance use disorder, mood disorders, and HIV-associated dementia, and delirium. Diagnosis is further complicated by repression or retrograde amnesia for traumatic events, difficulties with forming trusting relationships and disclosing trauma if it is recalled, and nonadherence to care. Diagnosis and signs and symptoms of PTSD are presented in Table 6.11.

Treatment of anxiety disorders

Psychotherapy is an excellent first-line therapy for patients with mild anxiety symptoms or can be used in combination with medication for those in need of more immediate relief or those suffering from more severe symptoms. Group therapy ameliorates symptoms of depression, anxiety, and distress, and enhances coping in persons with chronic illnesses, including HIV (Mulder et al., 1994; Sherman et al., 2004). The reader is referred to Chapter 8 for further details on psychotherapeutic techniques used in HIV illness.

Psychodynamic therapy of PTSD alleviates symptoms, decreases suffering, and enables persons with HIV and AIDS to cope better and to adhere to risk reduction and medical care. Psychiatric treatment of PTSD not only reduces morbidity and mortality but also HIV transmission by improving adherence. Selective serotonin reuptake inhibitors (SSRIs) are useful as first-line therapies for treating chronic anxiety disorders (Ferrando and Wapenyi, 2002, Pollack et al., 2004). Benzodiazepines are useful as an adjunct to SSRIs for those who cannot wait for several weeks while an SSRI is titrated to an effective dose, or for those patients who require acute relief of distressing symptoms such as panic. Chapter 7 discusses pharmacological treatment and potential drug–drug interactions more extensively.

TABLE 6.11 Diagnosis of Posttraumatic Stress Disorder in Persons with HIV and AIDS

History of Exposure to Trauma

- Early childhood emotional, physical, or sexual trauma and/or profound neglect
- Adulthood trauma such as assault, rape, or intimate-partner violence
- Events involved or witnessed involving actual or threatened death
- Response that involved intense fear, horror, or helplessness

Persistent Re-experience of Trauma

- Intrusive thoughts
- Recurrent nightmares
- Reliving the experience
- Severe distress with exposure to reminders
- Hyperarousal upon exposure

Avoidance and Numbing

- Avoidance of thoughts, feelings, or reminders of trauma
- Avoidance of persons, places, and things reminiscent of trauma
- Retrograde amnesia
- Decreased interest in activities
- Detachment
- Restricted range of affect or numbing
- Sense of a foreshortened future

Associated Manifestations

- Insomnia
- Irritability
- Difficulty with concentration
- Hypervigilance
- Easy startle

SUBSTANCE USE, ABUSE, AND DEPENDENCE

Substance use disorders are of particular concern to clinicians caring for persons with HIV because of the prevalence of substance use in persons with HIV and among persons with other psychiatric disorders. Historically, both injection drug use (IDU) and commercial sex have been major vectors of HIV transmission worldwide. Other noninjectable substances of abuse pose increased risk for HIV infection through enabling high-risk sexual behavior (Ferrando et al., 1998a) that is associated with transmission of HIV (Chesney et al., 1998; Woody et al., 1999; Venable et al., 2004). These substances include alcohol, sedative-hypnotics, cocaine, amphetamines, and all substances of abuse. It is important to assess all patients for substance use as this

TABLE 6.12 Modification of the CAGE Questionnaire to Include Alcohol and Other Drugs

- Have you ever felt the need to *cut* down on your use of alcohol or drugs?
- Has anyone *annoyed* you about the way you use of alcohol or drugs?
- Have you ever felt *guilty* about your use of alcohol or drugs?
- Have you ever used alcohol or drugs to steady your nerves or as an *eye-opener*?

can have an impact on adherence to risk reduction and safer sex practices as well as to adherence to medical care and ART.

A substance abuse history should begin with asking specific questions about a variety of substances including alcohol, cocaine, opiates, marijuana, and club drugs. Also, a thorough history of prescription drug abuse is necessary. A modification of the CAGE questionnaire, a screening device for alcohol use (Ewing, 1984), to screen for both alcohol and drug dependence is presented in Table 6.12.

A more complete evaluation for substance use disorders can be found in Chapter 2 and includes the age and situation when the substance was first used; patterns, amount, and frequency of use; and routes of administration and reactions to the use. The time of last use is important to know to determine the risk for withdrawal. A history of past substance use treatment and response to this treatment with the longest periods of abstinence are also important elements of a substance abuse history. Urine toxicology, basic blood testing, and collateral information all assist in the assessment and counteract the effects of denial and minimization when discussing drug history.

Heroin and other opiates

Heroin reaches peak serum concentration within 1 minute when taken intravenously but actually begins crossing the blood–brain barrier within 15–20 seconds. Signs and symptoms of intoxication and withdrawal are summarized in Table 6.13.

Heroin withdrawal usually begins within 4 to 8 hours after last use, whereas with methadone, with its longer elimination half-life, withdrawal may not begin until 24 to 48 hours after last use. Intoxication and withdrawal with other opiates are similar in presentation but differ in onset as half-lives vary with each substance.

Cocaine and other stimulants

Intoxication with cocaine and other stimulants including methamphetamine produces euphoria, cardiovascular symptoms (palpitations, hypertension),

TABLE 6.13 Signs and Symptoms of Opiate Intoxication and Withdrawal

Opiate Intoxication

- Euphoria and tranquility
- Sedation
- Slurred speech
- Impaired memory and attention
- Miosis

Opioid Withdrawal—Objective Signs

- Rhinorrhea and lacrimation
- Nausea, vomiting, diarrhea
- Piloerection
- Mydriasis
- Yawning

Opioid Withdrawal—Subjective Signs

- Body aches
- Cravings
- Irritability
- Dysphoria
- Anxiety
- Hot and cold flashes
- Anorexia

---

autonomic symptoms (diaphoresis), and behavioral manifestations (anxiety, agitation, psychosis, paranoia). Post-intoxication, the patient experiences irritability, tiredness, depression, and somnolence. While there is no specific withdrawal syndrome, chronic use leads to depression and frank neuropsychological impairment, as well as enhancing neurotoxicity in HIV patients (Urbina and Jones, 2004). These drugs are associated with hypersexuality and unsafe sex as well as disinhibition and exchange of sex for drugs. No specific treatments have been shown to be effective in decreasing stimulant use among persons with HIV. Bupropion or modafinil may help decrease amphetamine use. The best treatment approach may be to establish rapport, develop a support network, and help the patient to attend a drug treatment and/or 12 Step program.

Alcohol and benzodiazepines

Among HIV-positive persons, alcohol abuse leads to increased medical comorbidities and reduced adherence to treatment (Brathwaite et al., 2005). Additionally, alcohol use is associated with risky sexual behaviors

TABLE 6.14 Symptoms of Alcohol and Benzodiazepine Intoxication and Withdrawal

Alcohol	Benzodiazepines
Intoxication	
Decreased coordination, ataxia	Sedation, ataxia
Confusion, nystagmus, dysarthria	Psychomotor retardation
Disinhibition	Disinhibition
Memory impairment	Memory impairment
Nausea, vomiting, diarrhea, diplopia	Respiratory depression
Hypothermia, sweats, stupor, coma	
Withdrawal	
Tremors, sweats, anxiety, restlessness, vomiting, diarrhea, agitation, tachycardia	Tremors, anxiety, restlessness, insomnia, headache, insomnia, nightmares, nausea
	Headache
Severe withdrawal	
Delirium tremens	
Confusion, elevated vital signs, agitation, tremor, diaphoresis, hallucinations, seizures	Seizures and death
Death can occur if untreated and rarely if treated	

and intravenous drug use, both of which lead to higher rates of HIV transmission (Petry, 1999; Szerlip et al., 2005). Symptoms of intoxication and withdrawal are presented in Table 6.14.

Club drugs

Stimulants and hallucinogens such as LSD and 3,4-methylenedioxymethamphetamine (MDMA), also known as Ecstasy, are common examples of club drugs whose use has tended to cluster with young to middle-aged gay men and in close association with sexual activity. Other examples include ketamine and gamma-hydroxybutyric acid (GHB) (Bialer, 2002). The club drugs of most concern in relation to HIV/AIDS are MDMA and GHB. Although MDMA is considered a benign drug by many, there are now numerous reports of severe toxic, sometimes fatal, reactions (McCann et al., 1996). Chronic use may lead to mood instability and cognitive impairment, which are particular problems for people with HIV (Bolla et al., 1998; McCann and Ricuarte, 2000; Kalant, 2001).

In the club scene, GHB is taken for its sedating and euphoric effects. It has also been used as a date-rape drug, leading to concerns of HIV exposure through unprotected sexual intercourse. It has potent amnestic effects and a relatively narrow therapeutic range with toxicity presenting as seizures, coma, and death. In addition, a severe withdrawal syndrome among chronic users has been reported (Bialer, 2002). GHB may induce psychosis with delusions that may persist for months after last use.

Treatment and management of substance use disorders

Current guidelines recommend that all HIV-positive patients be screened regularly for substance use and symptoms of mental illness. Guidelines also indicate that mental health professionals should not delay treatment for a mental illness while waiting for a patient to become abstinent from substances (New York State Department of Health AIDS Institute Guidelines, 2009).

The initial phase of addiction treatment is usually concerned with providing safe and humane detoxification from the substance of abuse. Benzodiazepines are recommended as the treatment of choice in management of alcohol or sedative-hypnotic withdrawal (Mayo-Smith, 1997), although some clinicians have also advocated the use of anticonvulsants (Pages and Ries, 1998; Malcolm et al., 2001). Detoxification can generally be done at the same dosages as those for seronegative patients until the later stages of HIV illness, when lower doses may be necessary. Methadone detoxification or replacement therapy remains the preferred method of managing opioid dependence in an HIV population, but other options include buprenorphine replacement therapy and clonidine detoxification (NIH Consensus Development Conference, 1998). After medical stabilization and detoxification, the goals of treatment should include maintenance of abstinence, when possible, and rapid treatment of relapse. Substance abuse treatment is usually provided on an outpatient basis, although treatment communities afford a higher level of care for those with a more severe and refractory substance use disorder.

Harm reduction is a strategy that is applicable to the addicted, HIV-positive patient (Ferrando and Batki, 2000) and focuses on reducing behavior that has potentially harmful consequences, such as the sharing of needles or illicit activities to pay for substance use, rather than the traditional abstinence model. Such risk-reduction programs have not only been effective in decreasing risk-taking behaviors, but some studies and meta-analyses indicate that they may have also contributed to a significant decrease in HIV seroconversion among the IDU population (Cochrane Collaborative Review Group, 2004; Des Jarlais et al., 2005).

For patients who have history of alcohol dependence but are abstinent, treatment focuses on renewing commitment to abstinence and enhancing the ability to tolerate stressors and cravings without relapse. Naltrexone may be recommended to reduce alcohol use and has been considered for reducing cocaine use, but there are no published studies in HIV-positive patients. Careful monitoring of liver function tests is recommended. Please refer to Chapter 14 for resources regarding substance use and medication interactions as well as treatment guidelines.

Smoking and nicotine dependence

Smoking prevalence among HIV-seropositive persons is higher than that of the general population, and more than 50% of HIV-seropositive patients actively use tobacco products. This rate increases to greater than 75% in substance-abusing populations (Burns et al., 1996; Niaura et al., 2000). Tobacco use places HIV-infected patients at increased risk of pulmonary infections, oropharyngeal carcinomas, and AIDS-defining malignancies (Shiboski et al., 1999; Castle et al., 2002; Miguez-Burbano et al., 2003). Smoking cessation is an important primary care component when dealing with an HIV-seropositive population, and tobacco cessation at any age is associated with improved health (New York State Department of Health AIDS Institute Guidelines, 2009).

Patients who are interested in tobacco cessation should be given encouragement and provided opportunities for counseling and pharmacotherapy designed to assist them in this endeavor. Nicotine substitution (through inhalers, patches, or gum), bupropion, and varenicline are all approved by the U.S. Food and Drug Administration (FDA) for smoking cessation, and all appear to be essentially equivalent in effectiveness (Hughes et al., 1999; Gonzales et al., 2006; Jorenby et al., 2006; New York State Department of Health AIDS Institute Guidelines, 1999).

When using these agents in patients on ART, it is important to be aware of potential drug–drug interactions—especially with use of bupropion and ritonavir. The majority of varenicline is excreted renally unchanged (Chantix Prescribing Information, 2009), but it has been linked with serious neuropsychiatric symptoms, making its use in patients with a psychiatric history difficult given other options (U.S. FDA Public Health Advisory on Chantix, 2008).

PSYCHOTIC DISORDERS

Schizophrenia has a worldwide prevalence of about 1% and is a lifelong disorder characterized by both positive and negative features. The more chronic and disabling negative features are often those that are least well understood but that profoundly influence social interactions and coping mechanisms. In diagnosing a psychotic disorder, it is important to rule out substance use as a potential etiology of the disorder. HIV-related cognitive impairment may also present with mild psychotic symptoms; often the life history of the patient can provide clues to differentiate this from a psychotic disorder, such as the relationship between HIV infection to the onset of the symptoms. Corroborative information from family members can be essential in making the diagnosis, as a family member may be able to describe the patient's baseline and change in function over time, as well as provide essential additional family history.

Currently there is no significant difference between the pharmacological treatment of schizophrenia in an HIV-infected individual and the treatment of an uninfected person other than to consider potential adverse reactions and interactions between ART medications and antipsychotics. This is discussed in Chapter 7. Studies have shown that adequate treatment of positive symptoms leads to significant reductions in HIV risk behaviors (McKinnon et al., 1996). The treatment of negative symptoms may help to motivate and engage the patient in treatment. Reality testing should be supported at all times, and the confrontation of delusional thoughts should be gentle and appropriately timed.

There are no published studies of schizoaffective disorder in persons with HIV. We recommend that treatment of a patient with schizoaffective disorder follow guidelines for treatment of nonmedically ill patients, with the caveat that attention must be paid to the toxicity of various mood stabilizers in the HIV patient.

CONCLUSION

Diagnostic uncertainty is common when examining a person with HIV and comorbid mental illness. Multimorbid medical conditions can masquerade as primary psychiatric disorders, and HIV-related illness can present as psychiatric illness. The treatment of a person with HIV or AIDS requires a comprehensive assessment for potential psychiatric complaints—depression and suicidality, anxiety disorders, and substance use—because these all increase mortality and are associated with poor outcomes. Likewise, psychiatric illness can be a barrier to successful treatment of any medical condition a patient may have. For these reasons, we recommend frequent assessment for psychiatric complaints and that primary practitioners maintain a low threshold for referral to a mental health provider should concerning symptoms arise.

REFERENCES

Alisky JM (2007). The coming problem of HIV-associated Alzheimer's disease. *Med Hypotheses* 69(5):1140–1143.

American Psychiatric Association (2000). *Diagnostic and Statistical Manual of Mental Disorders*, fourth edition, text revision (DSM IV-TR). Washington, DC: American Psychiatric Association.

Arlt S, Lindner R, Rösler A, von Renteln-Kruse W (2008). Adherence to medication in patients with dementia: predictors and strategies for improvement. *Drugs Aging* 25:1033–1047.

Basu S, Chwastiak LA, Bruce RD (2005). Clinical management of depression and anxiety in HIV-infected adults. *AIDS* 19(18):2057–2067.

Bialer PA (2002). Designer drugs in the general hospital. *Psychiatr Clin North Am* 25:231–243.

Blanch J, Rousaud A, Hautzinger M, Martinez E, Peri JM, Andres S, Cirera E, Gatell JM, Gasto C (2002). Assessment of the efficacy of a cognitive-behavioural group psychotherapy programme for HIV-infected patients referred to a consultation-liaison psychiatry department. *Psychother Psychosom* 71(2):77–84.

Boisse L, Gill MJ, Power C (2008). HIV infection of the central nervous system: clinical features and neuropathogenesis. *Neurol Clin* 26(3):799–819.

Bolla KI, McCann UD, Ricuarte GA (1998). Memory impairment in abstinent MDMA ("ecstasy") users. *Neurology* 51:1532–1537.

Braithwaite RS, McGinnis KA, Conigliaro J, et al. (2005). A temporal and dose–response association between alcohol consumption and medication adherence among veterans in care. *Alcohol Clin Exp Res* 29:1190–1197.

Brouillette MJ, Chouinard G, Lalonde R (1994). Didanosine-induced mania in HIV infection. *Am J Psychiatry* 151(12):1839–1840.

Burns DN, Hillman D, Neaton JD, Sherer R, Mitchell T, Capps L, Vallier WG, Thurnherr MD, Gordin FM (1996). Cigarette smoking, bacterial pneumonia, and other clinical outcomes in HIV-1 infection. Terry Beirn Community Programs for Clinical Research on AIDS. *J Acquir Immune Defic Syndr Hum Retrovirol* 13:374–383.

Castle PE, Wacholder S, Lorincz AT, Scott DR, Sherman ME, Glass AG, Rush BB, Schussler JE, Schiffman M (2002). A prospective study of high-grade cervical neoplasia risk among human papillomavirus–infected women. *J Natl Cancer Inst* 94:406–1414.

Chang L, Ernst T, Leonido-Yee M, et al. (1999). Highly active antiretroviral therapy reverses brain metabolite abnormalities in mild HIV dementia. *Neurology* 53:782–789.

Chang L, Yakupov R, Nakama H, Stokes B, Ernst T (2008). Antiretroviral treatment is associated with increased attentional load-dependent brain activation in HIV patients. *J Neuroimmune Pharmacol* 3(2):95–104.

Chantix Prescribing Information. Retrieved April 19, 2009, from http://www.pfizer.com/files/products/uspi_chantix.pdf

Chesney MA, Barrett DC, Stall R (1998). Histories of substance use and risk behavior: precursors to HIV seroconversion in homosexual men. *Am J Public Health* 88:113–116.

Clifford DB (2002). AIDS dementia [review]. *Med Clin North Am* 86(3):537–550.

Clifford DB, Evans S, Yang Y, Acosta EP, Goodkin K, Tashima K, Simpson D, Dorfman D, Ribaudo H, Gulick RM (2005). Impact of efavirenz on neuropsychological performance and symptoms in HIV-infected individuals. *Ann Intern Med* 143(10):714–721.

Cochrane Collaborative Review Group on HIV Infection and AIDS (2004). Evidence assessment strategies for HIV/AIDS prevention treatment and care. University of California, San Francisco, Institute for Global Health. Retrieved January 10, 2006, from www.igh.org/Cochrane/pdfs/Evidence Assessment.pdf.

Cohen MA (2008). History of AIDS psychiatry—a biopsychosocial approach—paradigm and paradox. In MA Cohen and JM Gorman (eds.) (pp. 3–14). *Comprehensive Textbook of AIDS Psychiatry*. New York: Oxford University Press.

Cohen MA, Alfonso CA (2004). AIDS psychiatry: psychiatric and palliative care, and pain management. In GP Wormser (ed.), *AIDS and Other Manifestations of HIV Infection*, fourth edition (pp. 537–576). New York: Elsevier.

Cohen MA, Alfonso CA, Hoffman RG, Milau V, Carrera G (2001). The impact of PTSD on treatment adherence in persons with HIV infection. *Gen Hosp Psychiatry* 23:294–296.

Cohen MA, Hoffman RG, Cromwell C, Schmeidler J, Ebrahim F, Carrera G, Endorf F, Alfonso CA, Jacobson JM (2002). The prevalence of distress in persons with human immunodeficiency virus infection. *Psychosomatics* 43(1):10–15.

Cohen MA, Jacobson JM (2000). Maximizing life's potentials in AIDS: a psychopharmacologic update. *Gen Hosp Psychiatry* 22:375–388.

Coté TR, Biggar RJ, Dannenberg AL (1992). Risk of suicide among persons with AIDS. A national assessment. *JAMA* 268(15):2066–2068.

Cysique LAJ, Maruff P, Brew BJ (2006). Variable benefit in neuropsychological function in HIV-infected HAART-treated patients. *Neurology* 66: 1447–1450.

Des Jarlais DC, Perlis T, Arasteh K, et al. (2005). HIV incidence among injection drug users in New York City, 1990 to 2002: use of serologic test algorithm to assess expansion of HIV prevention services. *Am J Public Health* 95: 1439–1444.

Dougherty RH, Skolasky RL Jr, McArthur JC (2002). Progression of HIV-associated dementia treated with HAART. *AIDS Reader* 12(2):69–74.

Ellen SR, Judd FK, Mijch AM, Cockram A (1999). Secondary mania in patients with HIV infection. *Aust N Z J Psychiatry* 33(3):353–360.

Evans DL, Staab J, Ward H, Leserman J, Perkins DO, Golden RN, Petitto JM (1996–97). Depression in the medically ill: management considerations. *Depress Anxiety* 4(4):199–208.

Ewing J (1984). The CAGE questionnaire. *JAMA* 252:1903–1907.

Ferrando SJ, Batki SL (2000). Substance abuse and HIV infection. *New Dir Ment Health Serv* 87:57–67.

Ferrando S, Goggin K, Sewell M, et al. (1998a). Substance use disorders in gay/bisexual men with HIV and AIDS. *Am J Addict* 7:51–60.

Ferrando S, van Gorp W, McElhiney M, Goggin K, Sewell M, Rabkin J (1998b). Highly active antiretroviral treatment in HIV infection: benefits for neuropsychological function. *AIDS* 1(2):F65–F70.

Ferrando SJ, Wapenyi K (2002). Psychopharmacological treatment of patients with HIV and AIDS. *Psychiatr Q* 73(1):33–49.

Gendelman HE, Zheng J, Coulter CL, Ghorpade A, Che M, Thylin M, Rubocki R, Persidsky Y, Hahn F, Reinhard J Jr, Swindells S (1998). Suppression of inflammatory neurotoxins by highly active antiretroviral therapy. Human immunodeficiency virus–associated dementia. *J Infect Dis* 178:1000–1007.

Goforth HW, Lowery J, Cutson TM, Kenedi C, Cohen MA (2009). Impact of bereavement on progression of AIDS and HIV infection: a review. *Psychosomatics*.50:433–439

Goforth HW, Cohen MA, Murrough J (2008). Mood disorders. In MA Cohen and JM Gorman (eds.), *Comprehensive Textbook of AIDS Psychiatry* (pp. 97–108). New York: Oxford University Press.

Gonzales D, Rennard SI, Nides M, Oncken C, Azoulay S, Billing CB, Watsky EJ, Gong J, Williams KE, Reeves KR (2006). Varenicline Phase 3 Study Group. Varenicline, an $\alpha_4\beta_2$ nicotinic acetylcholine receptor partial agonist, vs. sustained-release bupropion and placebo for smoking cessation: a randomized controlled trial. *JAMA* 296:47–55.

Goodkin K, Baldewicz TT, Asthana D, Khamis I, Blaney NT, Kumar M, Burkhalter JE, Leeds B, Shapshak P (2001). A bereavement support group intervention affects plasma burden of human immunodeficiency virus type 1. Report of a randomized controlled trial. *J Hum Virol* 4 (1):44–54.

Goodkin K, Blaney NT, Feaster DJ, Baldewicz T, Burkhalter JE, Leeds B (1999). A randomized controlled clinical trial of a bereavement support group intervention in human immunodeficiency virus type 1-seropositive and -seronegative homosexual men. *Arch Gen Psychiatry* 56(1):52–59.

Gutierrez F, Navarro A, Padilla S, Anton R, Masia M, Borras J, Martin-Hidalgo A (2005). Prediction of neuropsychiatric adverse events associated with long-term efavirenz therapy, using plasma drug level monitoring. *Clin Infect Dis* 41(11):1648–1653.

Heaton RK, Grant I, Butters N, et al. (1995). The HNRC 500—neuropsychology of HIV infection at different disease stages. HIV Neurobehavioral Research Center. *J Int Neuropsychol Soc* 1:231–251.

Heckman TG, Miller J, Kochman A, Kalichman SC, Carlson B, Silverthorn M (2002). Thoughts of suicide among HIV-infected rural persons enrolled in a telephone-delivered mental health intervention. *Ann Behav Med* 24(2): 141–148.

Hoffman RG, Cohen MA, Alfonso CA, Weiss JJ, Jones S, Keller M, Condemarin JR, Chiu NM, Jacobson JM (2003). Treatment of interferon-induced psychosis in patients with comorbid hepatitis C and HIV. *Psychosomatics* 44 (5):417–420.

Holmes VF, Fernandez F, and Levy JK (1989). Psychostimulant response in AIDS-related complex patients. *J Clin Psychiatry* 50:5–8.

Hughes JR, Goldstein MG, Hurt RD, Shiffman S (1999). Recent advances in the pharmacotherapy of smoking. *JAMA* 281:72–76.

Johannesen DJ, Wilson LG (1988). Mania with cryptococcal meningitis in two AIDS patients. *J Clin Psychiatry* 49:200–201.

Jorenby DE, Hays JT, Rigotti NA, Azoulay S, Watsky EJ, Williams KE, Billing CB, Gong J, Reeves KR; Varenicline Phase 3 Study Group (2006). Efficacy of varenicline, an $\alpha_4\beta_2$ nicotinic acetylcholine receptor partial agonist, vs placebo or sustained-release bupropion for smoking cessation: a randomized controlled trial. (Published Erratum in: *JAMA* 2006;296:1355). *JAMA* 296:56–63.

Kalant H (2001). The pharmacology and toxicology of "ecstasy" (MDMA) and related drugs. *CMAJ* 165:917–928.

Kalichman SC, Heckman T, Kochman A, Sikkema K, Bergholte J (2000). Depression and thoughts of suicide among middle-aged and older persons living with HIV-AIDS. *Psychiatr Serv* 51(7):903–907.

Katz S, Nevid JS (2005). Risk factors associated with posttraumatic stress disorder symptomatology in HIV-infected women. *AIDS Patient Care STDS* 19(2):110–120.

Kelly B, Raphael B, Judd F, Perdices M, Kernutt G, Burnett P, Dunne M, Burrows G (1998). Posttraumatic stress disorder in response to HIV infection. *Gen Hosp Psychiatry* 20(6):345–352.

Kessler RC, Demler O, Frank RG, Olfson M, Pincus HA, Walters EE, Wang P, Wells KB, Zaslavsky AM (2005). Prevalence and treatment of mental disorders, 1990 to 2003. *N Engl J Med* 352(24):2515–2523.

Kessler RC, McGonagle KA, Zhao S, Nelson CB, Hughes M, Eshleman S, Wittchen HU, Kendler KS (1994). Lifetime and 12-month prevalence of DSM-III-R psychiatric disorders in the United States. Results from the National Comorbidity Survey. *Arch Gen Psychiatry* 51(1):8–19.

Koralnik IJ, Beaumanoir A, Hausler R, Kohler A, Safran AB, Delacoux R, et al. (1990). A controlled study of early neurologic abnormalities in men with asymptomatic human immunodeficiency virus infection. *N Engl J Med* 32 3:864–870.

Koutsilieri E, ter Meulen V, Riederer P (2001). Neurotransmission in HIV associated dementia: a short review. *J Neural Transm* 108:767–75.

Laguno M, Blanch J, Murillas J, Blanco JL, Leon A, Lonca M, Larrousse M, Biglia A, Martinez E, Garcia F, Miro JM, de Pablo J, Gatell JM, Mallolas J (2004). Depressive symptoms after initiation of interferon therapy in human immunodeficiency virus–infected patients with chronic hepatitis C. *Antivir Ther* 9(6):905–909.

Lyketsos CG, Hoover DR, Guccione M, Senterfitt W, Dew MA, Wesch J, VanRaden MJ, Treisman GJ, Morgenstern H (1993). Depressive symptoms as predictors of medical outcomes in HIV infection. Multicenter AIDS Cohort Study. *JAMA* 270(21):2563–2567.

Lyketsos CG, Schwartz J, Fishman M, Treisman G (1997). AIDS mania. *J Neuropsychiatry Clin Neurosci* 9(2):277–279.

Malcolm R, Myrick H, Brady KT, Ballenger JC (2001). Update on anticonvulsants for the treatment of alcohol withdrawal. *Am J Addict* 10(Suppl.):16–23.

Marzuk PM, Tardiff K, Leon AC, Hirsch CS, Hartwell N, Portera L, Iqbal MI (1997). HIV seroprevalence among suicide victims in New York City, 1991–1993. *Am J Psychiatry* 154(12):1720–1725.

Maxwell S, Scheftner WA, Kessler HA, Busch K (1988). Manic syndrome associated with zidovudine treatment. *JAMA* 259(23):3406–3407.

Mayo-Smith MT (1997). Pharmacologic management of alcohol withdrawal: a meta-analysis and evidence-based practice guidelines. *JAMA* 278:144–151.

McArthur JC, McDermott MP, McClernon D, St Hillaire C, Conant K, Marder K, Schifitto G, Selnes OA, Sacktor N, Stern Y, Albert SM, Kieburtz K, deMarcaida JA, Cohen B, Epstein LG (2004) McArthur JC, McDermott MP, McClernon D, St Hillaire C, Conant K, Marder K, Schifitto G, Selnes OA, Sacktor N, Stern Y, Albert SM, Kieburtz K, deMarcaida JA, Cohen B, Epstein LG (2004). Attenuated central nervous system infection in advanced HIV/AIDS with combination antiretroviral therapy. *Arch Neurol* 61: 1687–1696.

McCann UD, Ricuarte GA (2000). Drug abuse and dependence: hazards and consequences of heroin, cocaine, amphetamines. *Curr Opin Psychiatry* 13:321–325.

McCann UD, Slate SO, and Ricuarte GA (1996). Adverse reactions with 3,4-methylenedioxymethamphetamine (MDMA, ecstasy). *Drug Saf* 15:107–116.

McKinnon K, Cournos F, Sudgen R, Guido JR, Herman R (1996). The relative contributions of psychiatric symptoms and AIDS knowledge to HIV risk behaviors among people with severe mental illness. *J Clin Psychiatry* 57:506–513.

Meehan RA, Brush JA (2001). An overview of AIDS dementia complex. *Am J Alzheimer Dis Other Demen* 16:225–229.

Miguez-Burbano MJ, Burbano X, Ashkin D, Pitchenik A, Allan R, Pineda L, Rodriguez N, Shor-Posner G (2003). Impact of tobacco use on the development of opportunistic respiratory infections in HIV seropositive patients on antiretroviral therapy. *Addict Biol* 8:39–43.

Morrison MF, Petitto JM, Ten Have T, Gettes DR, Chiappini MS, Weber AL, Brinker-Spence P, Bauer RM, Douglas SD, Evans DL (2002). Depressive and anxiety disorders in women with HIV infection. *Am J Psychiatry* 159 (5):789–796.

Mulder CL, Emmelkamp PM, Antoni MH, Mulder JW, Sandfort TG, de Vries MJ (1994). Cognitive-behavioral and experiential group psychotherapy for HIV-infected homosexual men: a comparative study. *Psychosom Med* 56 (5):423–431.

Nath A, Schiess N, Venkatesan A, Rumbaugh J, Sacktor N, McArthur J (2008). Evolution of HIV dementia with HIV infection. *Int Rev Psychiatry* 20:25–31.

New York State Department of Health AIDS Institute Guidelines, 2000–2009. Retrieved April 19, 2009, from http://www.hivguidelines.org/GuideLine. aspx?GuideLineID=53

Niaura R, Shadel WG, Morrow K, Tashima K, Flanigan T, Abrams DB (2000). Human immunodeficiency virus infection, AIDS, and smoking cessation: The time is now. *Clin Infect Dis* 31:808–812.

Nightingale SD, Koster FT, Mertz GJ, Loss SD (1995). Clarithromycin-induced mania in two patients with AIDS. *Clin Infect Dis* 20(6):1563–1564.

NIH Consensus Development Conference (1998). Effective medical treatment of opiate addiction. *JAMA* 280:1936–1943.

O'Dowd MA, Natali C, Orr D, McKegney FP (1991). Characteristics of patients attending an HIV-related psychiatric clinic. *Hosp Community Psychiatry* 42 (6):615–619.

Pages KP, Ries RK (1998). Use of anticonvulsants in benzodiazepine withdrawal. *Am J Addict* 7:198–204.

Parisi A, DiPerri G, Stroselli M, Nappi G, Minoli L, Rondanelli EG (1989). Usefulness of computerized electroencephalography in diagnosing, staging, and monitoring AIDS-dementia complex. *AIDS* 3:209–223.

Petry NM (1999). Alcohol use in HIV patients: what we don't know may hurt us. *Int J STD AIDS* 10:561–570.

Pickles RW, Spelman DW (1996). Suspected ethambutol-induced mania. *Med J Aust* 164(7):445–446.

Pollack MH, Otto MW, Bernstein JG, Rosenbaum JF (2004). Anxious patients. In TA Stern, GL Fricchione, NH Cassem, MS Jellinek, and JF Rosenbaum (eds.), *Massachusetts General Hospital Handbook of General Hospital Psychiatry*, fifth edition. Philadelphia: Mosby.

Price RW, Spudich S (2008). Antiretroviral therapy and central nervous system HIV type 1 infection. *J Infect Dis* 15(Suppl. 3):S294–S306.

Rabkin JG, McElhiney M, Rabkin R, Ferrando SJ (2004b). Modafinil treatment for fatigue in HIV+ patients: a pilot study. *J Clin Psychiatry* 65(12):1688–1695.

Reichenberg A, Gorman JM, Dieterich DT (2005). Interferon-induced depression and cognitive impairment in hepatitis C virus patients: a 72-week prospective study. *AIDS* 19:S174–S178.

Reynolds A, Kammogne G, Kadiu I, Gendelman HF (2008). HIV and the central nervous system. In MA Cohen and JM Gorman (eds.), *Comprehensive Textbook of AIDS Psychiatry* (pp. 207–253). New York: Oxford University Press.

Ricart F, Cohen MA, Alfonso CA, Hoffman RG, Quiñones N, Cohen A, Indyk, D (2002). Understanding the psychodynamics of non-adherence to medical treatment in persons with HIV infection. *Gen Hosp Psychiatry* 24:176–180.

Ryan EL, Morgello S, Isaacs K, Naseer M, Gerits P, for the Manhattan HIV Brain Bank (2004). Neuropsychiatric impact of hepatitis C on advanced HIV. *Neurology* 62(6):957–962.

Scalori A, Pozzi M, Bellia V, Apale P, Santamaria G, Bordoni T, Redaelli A, Avolio A, Parravicini P, Pioltelli P, Roffi L (2005). Interferon-induced depression: prevalence and management. *Dig Liver Dis* 37(2):102–107.

Schurman RA, Kramer PD, Mitchell JB (1985). The hidden mental health network. Treatment of mental illness by nonpsychiatrist physicians. *Arch Gen Psychiatry* 42(1):89–94.

Sevigny JJ, Albert SM, McDermott MP, Schifitto G, McArthur JC, Sacktor N, Conant K, Selnes OA, Stern Y, McClernon DR, Palumbo D, Kieburtz K, Riggs G, Cohen B, Marder K, Epstein LG (2007). An evaluation of neurocognitive status and markers of immune activation as predictors of time to death in advanced HIV infection. *Arch Neurol* 64:97–102.

Sewell MC, Goggin KJ, Rabkin JG, Ferrando J, McElhiney MC, Evans S (2000). Anxiety syndromes and symptoms among men with AIDS: a longitudinal controlled study. *Psychosomatics* 41(4):294–300.

Shen JM, Blank A, Selwyn PA (2005). Predictors of mortality for patients with advanced disease in an HIV palliative care program. *J Acquir Immune Defic Syndr* 40:445–447.

Sherman AC, Leszcz M, Mosier J, Burlingame GM, Cleary T, Ulman KH, Simonton S, Latif U, Strauss B, Hazelton L (2004). Group interventions for patients with cancer and HIV disease: Part II. Effects on immune, endocrine, and disease outcomes at different phases of illness. *Int J Group Psychother* 54 (2):203–233.

Shiboski CH, Neuhaus JM, Greenspan D, Greenspan JS (1999). Effect of receptive oral sex and smoking on the incidence of hairy leukoplakia in HIV-positive gay men. *J Acquir Immune Defic Syndr* 21:236–242.

Sikkema KJ, Hansen NB, Kochman A, Tate DC, Difranceisco W (2004). Outcomes from a randomized controlled trial of a group intervention for HIV positive men and women coping with AIDS-related loss and bereavement. *Death Stud* 28(3):187–209.

Sikkema KJ, Hansen NB, Meade CS, Kochman A, Lee RS (2005). Improvements in health-related quality of life following a group intervention for coping with AIDS-bereavement among HIV-infected men and women. *Qual Life Res* 14 (4):991–1005.

Silberstein CH, O'Dowd MA, Schoenbaum EE, Friedland GH, Chartock P, Feiner C, McKegney FP (1993). Association of baseline neuropsychological function and progression of illness over 4 years in HIV-seropositive individuals. *Psychosomatics* 34:502–505.

Sledjeski EM, Delahanty DL, Bogart LM (2005). Incidence and impact of post-traumatic stress disorder and comorbid depression on adherence to HAART and CD4+ counts in people living with HIV. *AIDS Patient Care STDS* 19 (11):728–736.

Smith MY, Egert J, Winkel G, Jacobson J (2002). The impact of PTSD on pain experience in persons with HIV/AIDS. *Pain* 98(1-2):9–17.

Spitzer RL, Kroenke K, Williams JB (1999). Validation and utility of a self-report version of PRIME-MD: the PHQ primary care study. Primary Care Evaluation of Mental Disorders. Patient Health Questionnaire. *JAMA* 282:1737–1744.

Szerlip MA, DeSalvo KB, Szerlip HM (2005). Predictors of HIV-infection in older adults. *J Aging Health* 17:293–304.

Thienhaus OJ, Khosla N (1984). Meningeal cryptococcosis misdiagnosed as a manic episode. *Am J Psychiatry* 141:1459–1460.

Tozzi V, Balestra P, Bellagamba R, Corpolongo A, Salvatori MF, Visco-Comandini U, et al. (2007). Persistence of neuropsychologic deficits despite long-term highly active antiretroviral therapy in patients with HIV-related neurocognitive impairment: prevalence and risk factors. *J Acquir Immune Defic Syndr* 45:174–82.

Treisman G, Fishman M, Schwartz J, Hutton H, Lyketsos C (1998). Mood disorders in HIV infection. *Depress Anxiety* 7(4):178–187.

Tsao JCI, Dobalian A, Naliboff BD (2004). Panic disorder and pain in a national sample of persons living with HIV. *Pain* 109:172–180.

Urbina A, Jones K (2004). Crystal methamphetamine, its analogues, and HIV infection: medical and psychiatric aspects. *Clin Infect Dis* 38:890–894.

U.S. FDA Public Health Advisory on Chantix (2008). Retrieved April 19, 2009, from http://www.fda.gov/bbs/topics/NEWS/2008/NEW01788.html

Uthman OA, Abdulmalik JO (2008). Adjunctive therapies for AIDS dementia complex. *Cochrane Database Syst Rev* 3:CD006496.

Venable PA, McKirnan DJ, Buchbinder SP, et al. (2004). Alcohol use and high-risk behavior among men who have sex with men: the effects of consumption level and partner type. *Health Psychol* 23:525–532.

Wells KB, Golding JM, Burnam MA (1988). Psychiatric disorder in a sample of the general population with and without chronic medical conditions. *Am J Psychiatry* 145(8):976–981.

Wells KB, Golding JM, Burnam MA (1989). Chronic medical conditions in a sample of the general population with anxiety, affective, and substance use disorders. *Am J Psychiatry* 146(11):1440–1446.

Woody GE, Donnell D, Seage GR (1999). Non-injection substance use correlates with risky sex among men having sex with men: Data from HIVNET. *Drug Alcohol Depend* 53:197–205.

7

Psychopharmacologic Treatment Issues in AIDS Psychiatry

Kelly L. Cozza, Harold W. Goforth, and Sharon M. Batista

Persons with HIV and AIDS are often prescribed a plethora of medications, all of which require special attention and are based on well-defined principles. In the first part of this chapter, Drug Interaction Principles, we provide a short but essential review of these principles in order to prepare the reader to critically weigh the potential for drug interactions between psychotropics and antiretroviral therapy (ART) and those between ART and other medications. In the second part, Psychotropics and HIV, a brief review of the available literature on the effectiveness of psychotropics in treating patients with HIV is provided, followed by an overview of issues relating to drug interactions for each psychotropic or class of psychotropic. The third part of the chapter, Antiretrovirals, provides an introductory overview of currently available antiretrovirals and of medications prescribed in treating HIV/ AIDS. Readers are referred to an excellent review of pharmacological treatment for persons with addictions and HIV/AIDS, by Wynn and colleagues (2005), and to Chapters 2, 6, 8, and 10 of this handbook for more information on treating substance abuse and dependence.

Brief Review of Drug Interaction Principles

Understanding drug–drug interactions in the care of HIV patients is essential. For a full explanation of psychotropic pharmacology and drug interactions, the reader is referred to additional texts on the subject (Cohen and Gorman, 2008; Schatzberg and Nemeroff, 2009; Wynn et al., 2009).

Pharmacodynamic interactions are those that occur at the intended receptor site of a medication and involve absorption, distribution, metabolism, and excretion. ART drugs may be affected by timing with food or buffers, which is relatively predictable. Metabolic interactions are a bit more complex, as they are affected by metabolic inhibition, induction, and pharmacogenetics (the particular metabolic enzymes that a patient is born with). Metabolic interactions may occur in either phase I or II metabolic enzymes and also may include the cell membrane transporter enzymes (also known as p-glycoproteins). For a complete explanation of pharmacokinetic interactions, the reader is referred to the text by Wynn et al. (2009).

Figure 7.1 represents serum levels of drug A when a potent inhibitor of drug A's metabolic enzyme (usually in the gut wall or the liver) is present. Inhibition of metabolism is immediate and generally causes the serum level of the parent drug to increase. If that parent drug (e.g., a tricyclic antidepressant) has a narrow margin of safety, then toxicity may result. Inhibition slows the metabolism of a drug dependent on the inhibited enzyme. Inhibition may occur at cytochrome P450 enzymes in the liver and gut wall (phase I metabolism) or during phase II metabolism (glucuronidation [UGTs], sulfation [SULTs], methylation, etc.) in the liver. P450 enzymes that metabolize medications include cytochromes 3A4, 2D6, 1A2, 2C9,

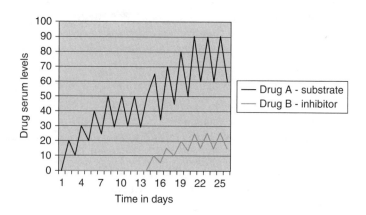

FIGURE 7.1 Drug–drug interaction—inhibition. Drug A develops steady-state concentrations after 4 half-lives ($t_{1/2}$). Its peak levels are 50 and trough levels 30 at steady state. Drug B is introduced sometime later after drug A is in steady-state concentrations. Drug B develops its own steady state after 4 halflives. Drug B, however, is a competitive inhibitor of the enzyme(s) that drug A uses for its metabolism. Drug A develops a new steady state, with peak levels at 90 and trough levels at 60. Adapted with permission from Cozza KL, Armstrong SC, and Oesterheld JR. *Concise Guide to Drug Interaction Principles for Medical Practice: Cytochrome P450s, UGTs, P-Glycoproteins*, second edition. Copyright (2003), American Psychiatric Press, Inc.

2C19, 2E1, and 2B6, among others. ART and psychotropics most commonly affect 3A4, 2D6, and glucuronidation reactions.

Figure 7.2 represents drug A when a potent inducer of drug A's metabolic enzymes is introduced. Induction of metabolism increases the number of sites available for metabolism. This process is not immediate and can take up to 2 weeks to occur. When more enzymes are available, more drug is metabolized, and the net effect is a lowering of available parent drug or a more rapid metabolism. An inducer may cause the level of a drug dependent on that enzyme to drop below the level needed for clinical effectiveness.

Table 7.1 presents common inhibitors and inducers of 3A4 and 2D6, as well as medications with narrow therapeutic windows that are dependent on those enzymes for metabolism.

Interactions may also occur with phase II enzymes (e.g., glucuronidation via uridine 5' diphosphate glucuronosyltransferase [UGTs] and sulfation). UGT enzymes are the most numerous and clinically important phase II enzymes. They are found in the endoplasmic reticulum and the nuclear membrane of kidney, brain, and placental cells (Radominska-Pandya et al., 2002). Many drugs are metabolized first by phase I metabolism (P450 and others) and then by glucuronidation, but some drugs are directly conjugated by UGTs, such as lorazepam, temazepam, and oxazepam. Drugs primarily metabolized by UGTs include lamotrigine, valproate, nonsteroidal anti-inflammatory drugs,

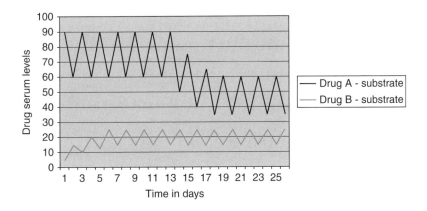

FIGURE 7.2 Drug–drug interaction—induction. Drug A is in steady state, having been introduced sometime before this graph, with peak levels of 90 and trough levels of 60. Drug B is started on day 1 and develops steady state after 4 half lives. After 2 weeks, levels of drug A decrease, as drug B has gradually induced the enzyme(s) involved in metabolizing drug A. Drug A now has a steady state, with peak levels at 60 and trough levels at 35. Adapted with permission from Cozza KL, Armstrong SC, and Oesterheld JR. *Concise Guide to Drug Interaction Principles for Medical Practice: Cytochrome P450s, UGTs, P-Glycoproteins,* second edition. Copyright (2003), American Psychiatric Press, Inc.

TABLE 7.1 Common Substrates, Inhibitors, and Inducers of Cytochrome P450
Enzymes 2D6 and 3A4

P450 Enzyme	Common Substrates*	Common Inhibitors	Common Inducers
2D6	Antiarrhythmics	**Bupropion**	Pan-inducers,[†] possibly
	Metaclopramide	Fluoxetine	
	Metoprolol	Paroxetine	
	Tramadol	Quinidine	
	Tricyclic antidepressants	Ritonavir	
	Typical antipsychotics		
3A4	Antitarrythmics	**Atanazanavir**	**Carbamazepine**
	Beta-blockers	Cimetidine	Efavirenz
	Carbamazepine	**Clarithromycin**	**Etravirine**
	Calcium channel blockers	Delavirdine	Nevirapine
	Cyclosporine	Diltiazem	Oxcarbazepine
	Methadone	Efavirenz	**Pan-inducers**[†]
	Oral contraceptives	**Erythromycin**	**Ritonavir**
	Protease inhibitors	**Grapefruit juice**	**St. John's wort**
	Statins	Indinivir	
	Triazolobenzodiazepines[‡]	**Itraconazole**	
	Zolpidem	**Ketoconazole**	
		Nefazodone	
		Ritonavir	
		Tipranavir	

All drugs in **bold** type are potent in their inhibition or induction.
*A substrate is a drug that must utilize the enzyme for metabolism. If this enzyme is altered by inhibition or induction, substrate serum levels will be affected.
[†]Carbamazepine, phenobarbital, phenytoin, and rifamycins, and ritonavir.
[‡]Alprazolam, midazolam, and triazolam.

zidovudine, and most opioids. Most glucuronide metabolites are inactive, so inhibition or induction of these enzymes produces no clinically relevant effects. A few drugs are known to produce active metabolites via glucuronidation, such as morphine to morphine-6-glucuronide, a metabolite of morphine that is about 20 times more potent as an analgesic compound than morphine. Inhibition of glucuronidation may reduce morphine's effectiveness (Court, 2009).

Membrane transporters may also be inhibited or induced via drug interactions. The membrane-bound transporters are sometimes called *phase 0* or *phase III* of the metabolic system. They were first called *p-glycoproteins*. Transporters are present in the blood–brain barrier, placenta, intestine, hepatocytes, renal tubule cells, and many other sites. They regulate the transfer of drugs into and out of organs and other target cells. Transporters play a large role in penetration of drugs into the brain and help explain how HIV can find "sanctuary" in some organ sites. A full explanation of the importance of transporters may be found in a chapter by Oesterheld (2009b). Transported activity is listed in the tables presented with the drug classes discussed in the next sections (see Tables 7.2–7.9).

PSYCHOTROPICS AND HIV

In some clinical settings, more than 50% of HIV patients seeking medical care have a comorbid psychiatric disorder or substance use disorder (Treisman et al., 2001). It is imperative that psychiatrists who treat HIV-infected patients become part of the multidisciplinary treatment team and assist in medication management. An understanding of the drug–drug interactions between ART and psychotropics, including narcotics, can help prevent morbidity, support adherence, and improve quality of life (Yun et al., 2005).

Antidepressants

Treatment of HIV itself can improve depressive symptoms, and ART has been associated with a decrease in severity of depression (Brechtl et al., 2001). Treatment of depression in patients with HIV in many ways mirrors the treatment of non-HIV-infected patients. However, patients with HIV are more susceptible to drug–drug interactions and may be more sensitive to side effects, making treatment similar to that for the geriatric population (Goldstein and Goodnick, 1998). Treatment is important not just for emotional well-being but also for physical well-being, since comorbid mood disorders increase the risk of nonadherence to medical care (DiMatteo et al., 2000; Horberg et al., 2008). Although not supported by multiple, well-controlled clinical trials nor systematically studied, most psychotropics have been found to be clinically effective. Many clinicians advocate, therefore, that the selection of an antidepressant be based on its side-effect profile, comorbid symptomatology, and the potential for drug–drug interactions. An overview of antidepressant metabolism, special clinical considerations, and potential drug interactions is provided in Table 7.2 at the end of this section.

Selective serotonin reuptake inhibitors

Selective serotonin reuptake inhibitors (SSRIs) are usually first-line medication choices for treating and managing depression, depression and anxiety, and panic disorder in the medically ill. In addition to their general effectiveness in treating depression, HIV-associated neurocognitive disorders (HAND) may benefit from SSRIs by both treating depression and providing neurocognitive protection from toxic by-products of HIV replication and neuroinflammation (Ances et al., 2008). SSRIs are mostly metabolized at cytochromes 2D6 and 3A4, which are both potently inhibited by ritonavir and fluoxetine. Patients taking fluoxetine with the protease inhibitor ritonavir may develop serotonin syndrome, a constellation of symptoms including mental status changes, diarrhea, and myoclonus (DeSilva et al., 2001). Theoretically, the same may be true with other SSRIs, but there have been no clinical reports of this to date.

Citalopram and escitalopram. Citalopram and escitalopram are the most selective antidepressants for the serotonin receptor and have few reported drug–drug interactions. They are metabolized by CYP 2C19, 2D6, and 3A4 and are substrates of transporters. They are mild inhibitors of CYP 2D6 and transporters. They have an advantageous side-effect profile compared with that of many other antidepressants. Citalopram and escitalopram are very commonly used in treating HIV patients, although they have not been studied well in this population.

Laguno and colleagues (2004) studied interferon-alpha-induced depression in 113 patients with chronic hepatitis C and HIV who were not suffering from major depression prior to interferon-alpha therapy. Forty percent (N = 45) of the patients had developed depressive symptoms, and 20 were treated with citalopram. The authors reported that 95% of the citalopram-treated patients responded to treatment and there were no reported drug–drug interactions or adverse events. Another small (N = 20) open-label, flexible-dose study also had favorable results (Currier et al., 2004). HIV patients suffer the same common side effects as noninfected patients, including dry mouth, somnolence, carbohydrate craving, and sexual dysfunction. Less common side effects seen in HIV patients include diplopia (Dorell et al., 2005).

Fluoxetine. Since fluoxetine is the oldest SSRI, there are considerable data to support its use in HIV patients, both for depressive symptoms and for decreasing cocaine cravings (Levine et al., 1990; Batki et al., 1993; Cazzullo et al., 1998). Early data comparing efficacy to imipramine showed comparable results and greater tolerability (Rabkin et al., 1994b). In 1997, Ferrando and colleagues performed a small, 6-week open-label trial using fluoxetine, sertraline, and paroxetine. All of the medications improved depressive symptoms but the power was not great enough to detect any difference among the SSRIs. Interestingly, there was a statistically significant improvement (up to 80%) in somatic symptoms. This is an important point, since presenting somatic symptoms such as weight loss, fatigue, decreased libido, gastrointestinal upset, musculoskeletal complaints and even cardiopulmonary symptoms may be attributed to the HIV illness instead of depression. The most common side effects reported and the reasons for discontinuation included agitation, anxiety, and insomnia (Ferrando et al., 1997). Fluoxetine was also found to be synergistic with psychotherapy with significant improvement in symptoms when fluoxetine was combined with psychotherapy compared with psychotherapy alone (Zisook et al., 1998).

The first large double-blind, placebo-controlled trial involving an SSRI compared fluoxetine to placebo (Rabkin et al., 1999) and found fluoxetine to be more effective than placebo, despite a large placebo effect. Fluoxetine, because of its long half-life and active metabolite, may be useful in patients who have difficulty remembering to take their medication on a daily basis. Fluoxetine's propensity for P450-mediated drug interactions and its active metabolite's long half life are of clinical importance as they may limit its usefulness in some HIV patients.

Fluvoxamine. Fluvoxamine has not been well tolerated in patients with HIV and is not recommended for routine use. The only published study had a 63% discontinuation rate due to insomnia, gastrointestinal disturbance, anorexia, behavioral changes, and sedation (Grassi et al., 1995). Fluvoxamine is also extensively metabolized by the liver through multiple pathways and inhibits many of the enzymes responsible for metabolizing antiretrovirals and antimicrobials in general.

Paroxetine. Elliot and colleagues (1998) showed equivalent efficacy in a randomized, placebo-controlled trial comparing paroxetine and imipramine. Paroxetine was better tolerated, but there was a significant attrition rate from both medications and placebo, and the sample size was small. Paroxetine may be useful in patients with insomnia since it is one of the more sedating SSRIs. In addition, there are in vitro data to suggest that paroxetine may also have antiviral activity and may work synergistically with ART (Kristiansen and Hansen, 2000). Paroxetine's significant withdrawal syndrome, which includes autonomic instability and influenza-like symptoms, may be problematic for nonadherent patients and for neonates of mothers taking paroxetine (Thormhalen, 2006). Paroxetine is a very potent inhibitor of cytochrome 2D6 and will increase serum levels of medications dependent on 2D6 for metabolism, such as metoprolol.

Sertraline. Sertraline has an advantageous side-effect profile compared with that of many other antidepressants, and it is very safe in overdose (Hansen et al., 2005). The first study of sertraline in HIV patients with depression was a small, open-label trial conducted in 1994. The results were quite impressive, showing a 70% response rate with a dropout rate of 18%. Sertraline has also been shown to have a strong safety profile in patients with HIV, with no appreciable effect on CD4 count or natural killer cell count (Rabkin et al., 1994c).

Serotonin and norepinephrine reuptake inhibitors (venlafaxine, duloxetine)

Serotonin and norepinephrine reuptake inhibitors (SNRIs) may have a role in treating HIV depression as they have demonstrated effectiveness for somatic symptoms (Barkin and Barkin, 2005) such as pain and urinary incontinence. They have not, however, been systematically studied in the setting of HIV. They both utilize cytochromes 3A4 and 2D6, and patients on potential pan-inhibitors such as ritonavir may be at risk of increased serum levels and hence worsened side effects when coadministered. In addition, all protease inhibitors are inhibitors of metabolism at 3A4 and may potentially raise serum levels of SNRIs.

Venlafaxine is an inhibitor of 2D6 and may increase serum levels of medications dependent on 2D6 for metabolism. Levin and colleagues (2001) studied the interaction of indinivir and venlafaxine in healthy volunteers and found that coadministration did not significantly affect serum levels of venlafaxine, but venlafaxine did modestly decrease the area under the concentration curve (AUC) and maximum plasma concentration (C_{max}) of plasma indinivir, for unclear reasons. Although this was a small study in healthy volunteers, any decrease in the plasma concentration of a protease inhibitor may place a patient at risk for treatment failure and viral resistance. Venlafaxine should be used with caution in combination with protease inhibitors until further studied.

Desvenlafaxine is metabolized via glucuronidation (uridine diphosphate–glucuronosyltransferase enzymes [UGTs]) and cytochrome 3A4 and is a mild inhibitor of 2D6. It is possible that potent inhibitors of 3A4, such as all protease inhibitors, and inducers of glucuronidation, such as ritonavir, may affect serum levels of desvenlafaxine, but there are no data to support this.

Tricyclic antidepressants

While many clinicians avoid use of tricyclic antidepressants (TCAs) for fear of anticholinergic side effects, tachycardia, hypotension, and toxicity in overdose, this class remains effective, especially when monitired (Rabkin and Harrison 1990, Rabkin et al., 1994a; Razali and Hasanah, 1999). It is possible to use TCA side effects to clinical advantage, especially in patients who have diarrhea, weight loss, insomnia, or a comorbid pain disorder. Despite the potential for toxicity due to drug–drug interactions, therapeutic drug monitoring (TDM) and clinical observation allow for safer use in combination with HIV medications. All tricyclics utilize cytochrome 2D6 as well as 3A4 and others for metabolism. Potent pan-inhibitors such as ritonavir may lead to tricyclic toxicity (Bertz et al., 1996; Abbott Laboratories, 2007), but the risk is reduced if TDM is used.

Atypical antidepressants

Nefazodone. Potential drug–drug interactions are a concern with nefazodone, as it is a potent inhibitor of cytochrome 3A4, the primary metabolic enzyme for all protease inhibitors and many other medications. Coadministration with medications with a narrow margin of safety that are dependent on CYP 3A4 may lead to toxicity of those coadministered drugs. Generic formulations of nefazodone remain on the U.S. market.

Mirtazepine. Mirtazapine may have a niche in the treatment of AIDS wasting syndrome, as it can reduce nausea through $5HT_3$ blockade and promote weight gain and improved sleep through its antihistaminergic effects (Elliot and Roy-Byrne, 2000).

Trazodone. Trazodone may be an attractive adjunct antidepressant for HIV patients with depression and anxiety, especially when the clinician is fearful of prescribing potentially addictive benzodiazepines. One study found that trazodone was slightly more effective than the benzodiazepine clorazepate for HIV patients with adjustment disorder. Although this study failed to achieve statistical significance, it highlights trazodone's properties of sedation and its ability to reduce anxiety without the abuse or dependence risks of benzodiazepines (De Wit et al., 1999). In a single-dose, blinded, four-way crossover study of healthy volunteers, Greenblatt and colleagues (2003) found that ritonavir significantly increased trazodone plasma concentration, which in turn increased sedation and fatigue and impaired performance on the digit-symbol substitution test. Induction of cytochrome 3A4 by pan-inducers may also lead to a preferential accumulation of a trazodone metabolite, mCPP, which has been linked to increased anxiety and panic-like reactions (Zuardi, 1990; Rotzinger et al., 1998).

Bupropion. A 6-week open-label trial of bupropion in 20 HIV-positive patients with major depression showed relatively good efficacy, with 60% of patients responding, whereas 25% of patients dropped out because of intolerable side effects. No changes in the CD4 count or drug toxicity were noted (Currier et al., 2003). Caution should also be used when treating patients with central nervous system (CNS) pathology, such as opportunistic infections or metastases, or patients at risk for alcohol or benzodiazepine withdrawal because of bupropion's propensity to lower the seizure threshold.

Use of bupropion may also be limited because of the potential for drug interactions with antiretrovirals. Bupropion is primarily metabolized by the minor P450 enzyme 2B6 (Hesse et al., 2001). Nelfinavir, ritonavir, and efavirenz are all inhibitors of this enzyme. Since bupropion has the potential to lower the seizure threshold at high doses, there is a potential for bupropion to become toxic when coadministered with 2B6 inhibitors. HIV patients with a previous history of seizures or who are severely immunocompromised and at risk for secondary seizures are not candidates for these combinations. However, a recent case series (Park-Wyllie and Antoniou, 2003) in which concomitant use of these agents occurred for as long as 2 years found no recorded episodes of seizures. Although encouraging, no pharmacokinetic data were available and none of the patients were on high-dose ritonavir. Thus further pharmacokinetic study is needed. Careful monitoring when using lower doses of bupropion (preferably of the longer-acting formulation) and careful informed consent and monitoring for potential seizures would be prudent with this medication.

Reboxetine

Reboxetine is the first medication in a new class of antidepressants termed norepinephrine reuptake inhibitors (NARI). Currently unavailable in the United States, the NARI data from Europe suggest efficacy in patients without medical comorbidity. There is also one small, open-label study from Brazil that suggests good efficacy in patients with HIV (Carvalhal et al., 2003). It is not yet clear whether this drug will gain U.S. Food and Drug Administration (FDA) approval, but it may have a role in treating HIV patients since it is not metabolized by P450 enzymes and may have a lower potential for drug–drug interactions.

An overview of antidepressant metabolism, special clinical considerations, and potential drug interactions is provided in Table 7.2.

TABLE 7.2 Psychotropic Medications and Special Considerations for HIV: Antidepressants

Antidepressant	Metabolic Site(s)	Inhibits	Clinical Pearls and Potential Drug–Drug Interaction with ART
SSRIs			All may cause sexual dysfunction, carbohydrate craving, apathy, withdrawal syndrome, serotonin syndrome
Citalopram (Celexa)	CYP 2C19, 2D6, 3A4 Transporter ABCB1	CYP2D6[c] ABCB1	Low potential for pharmacokinetic interactions
Escitalopram (Lexapro)	CYP 2C19, 2D6, 3A4	CYP2D6[c]	Low potential for pharmacokinetic interactions

	Transporter ABCB1	ABCB1	Protease inhibitors[1]
Fluoxetine (Prozac)	CYP2C9, 2C19, 2D6, 3A4	CYP2D6[a], 2C19[a], 2B6[b], 2C9[b], 3A4[b], 1A2[c]	Very long–acting active metabolite Protease inhibitors[1]
	Transporter ABCB1	ABCB1	Advantage in nonadherent populations
Fluvoxamine (Luvox)	CYP1A2, 2D6	CYP1A2[a], 2C19[a], 2B6[b], 2C9[b], 3A4[b], 2D6[b]	Great potential for multiple drug interactions
	Transporter ABCB1	ABCB1	Requires BID dosing Tenofovir[4]
Paroxetine (Paxil)	CYP2D6, 3A4	CYP2D6[a], 2B6[a], 3Ab[c], 2C19[c], 1A2[c], 2C9[c]	Sedating Most severe withdrawal syndrome, especially in neonates
Sertraline (Zoloft)	CYP2B6, 2C9, 2C19, 2D6, 3A4 UGT2B7, UGT1A1	CYP2D6[d], 2B6[c], 2C9[c], 2C19[c], 3A4[c], 1A2[c]	Low potential for pharmacokinetic interactions
	Transporter ABCB1	ABCB1	Protease inhibitors[1]

Atypical Antidepressants

Buproprion (Wellbutrin/ Zyban)	CYP2B6, 2D6, 1A2, 2C9, 2E1, 3A4, 2A6 Glucuronidation	CYP2D6[b]	Not recommended with seizure patients Advantage for nicotine cessation therapy Stimulating antidepressant Protease inhibitors[1] Tenofovir[4]
Desvenlafaxine (Pristiq)	UGTs, CYP3A4	CYP2D6[c]	Protease inhibitors[1,2]
Duloxetine (Cymbalta)	CYP 1A2, 2D6	CYP2D6[b]	Approved for neuropathic pain Tenofovir[4]
Mirtazepine (Remeron)	CYP1A2, 2D6, 3A4 glucuronidation	None known	Advantages in sleep, appetite, nausea, failure to thrive Tenofovir[4]
Nefazodone (Serzone)	CYP3A4, 2D6	CYP3A4[a]	Not recommended in HIV disease Protease inhibitors[1,2,3]
Trazodone (Deseryl)	CYP3A4	None known	Advantages in sleep, anxiety Protease inhibitors[2]

(*continued*)

TABLE 7.2 (Continued)

Antidepressant	Metabolic Site(s)	Inhibits	Clinical Pearls and Potential Drug–Drug Interaction with ART
Venlafaxine (Effexor)	CYP2D6, 2C19, 3A4	CYP2D6[c]	Potential effects for neuropathic pain Protease inhibitors[1]
Tricyclics			All protease inhibitors may increase TCA serum levels to toxicity[1] Use therapeutic drug monitoring (TDM/serum levels)
Amitriptyline (Elavil)	CYP1A2, 2C19, 2D6, 3A4 UGT1A4	CYP1A2[c], 2C19[c], 2D6[c]	Very anticholinergic Advantages in patients with sleep issues, diarrhea, weight loss Delirium risk Protease inhibitors[1,2] Tenofovir[4]
Clomipramine (Anafranil)	CYP 1A2, 2C19, 2D6, 3A4	CYP2D6[c], 1A2[c], 2C19[c]	Effective in obsessive compulsive disorder Protease inhibitors[1,2] Tenofovir[4]
Desipramine (Norpramin)	CYP2D6	CYP2D6[c], 2C19[c]	Least anticholinergic of the tricyclics More stimulating than other TCAs Protease inhibitors[1]
Doxepin (Adapin, Sinequan)	CYP1A2, 2D6, 2C19, 3A4 UGT1A3, UGT1A4	CYP1A2[c], 2C19[c], 2D6[c]	Advantages in patients with sleep, pain, GERD, allergies Protease inhibitors[1,2] Efavirenz Tenofovir[4]
Imipramine (Tofranil)	CYP1A2, 2C19, 2D6, 3A4 UGT1A3, UGT1A4	CYP2C19[c], 2D6[c]	Very anticholinergic Protease inhibitors[1,2] Tenofovir[4]
Nortriptyline (Pamelor)	CYP2D6	CYP2D6[c], 2C19[c]	Advantages in patients with sleep or pain complaints Metabolite of amitryptiline and better tolerated with fewer side effects Therapeutic window (50–150 ng/dL) provides for best TDM Protease inhibitors[1]

| Protriptyline (Vivactil) | CYP2D6 (perhaps) | Unknown | Protease inhibitors[1] |
| Trimipramine (Surmontil) | CYP2C19, 2D6, 3A4 | Unknown | Potential advantages in insomnia Protease inhibitors[1,2] |

Note: Primary route of metabolism listed first. ABCB = ATP binding cassette B transporter; ART = antiretroviral therapy; CYP = cytochrome; GERD = gastroesophageal reflux disease; UGT = uridine 5′-diphosphate glucuronosyltransferase.
Bold type indicates **potent** inhibition or induction at that site.
[a] Potent inhibition.
[b] Moderate inhibition.
[c] Mild inhibition.
[d] Sertraline is a MILD inhibitor at doses below 150 mg. It may become a POTENT inhibitor at doses >150 mg/day.
[1] The most likely of the protease inhibitors to cause increased drug levels is ritonavir because of pan-inhibition, potentially worsening antidepressant side effects or toxicity.
[2] The most likely of the protease inhibitors to cause increased drug levels are ritonavir, atazanavir, and indinavir because of potent CYP3A4 inhibition, which may worsen antidepressant side effects or toxicity.
[3] Nefazodone's potent CYP3A4 inhibition will likely cause an increase in protease inhibitor levels.
[4] Potential interaction due to inhibition of CYP 1A2 by tenofovir, potentially worsening antidepressant side effects or toxicity.
Source: Adapted from Wynn GH, Sandson N, Muniz J (2009). Psychiatry. In GH Wynn, JR Oesterheld, KL Cozza KL, and SC Armstrong (eds.), *Clinical Guide to Drug Interaction Principles for Medical Practice.* Washington, DC: American Psychiatric Press, used with permission.

Stimulants

Although the above data suggest that most of the currently available anti-depressant medications have good clinical efficacy with respect to mood state, many patients may require rapidly effective interventions for acute stabilization. Others may continue to experience fatigue and generalized low energy, especially those with advanced HIV or AIDS (Wagner et al., 1997). There are subpopulations with severe medical illness who may benefit from the use of psychostimulants (Satel and Nelson, 1989). In addition to their use for fatigue and depression in the medically ill, stimulants may be necessary in patients with comorbid attention-deficit hyperactivity disorders.

Dextroamphetamine

Dextroamphetamine has been reported as being effective for fatigue and depression in HIV since the late 1980s. Early case reports touted its quick onset of action and positive effects on concentration and cognition (Fernandez et al., 1988). In 1997, Wagner and colleagues conducted a small open-label trial of dextroamphetamine with a 75% response rate according to intention-to-treat analysis. Results were seen as quickly as 2 to 3 days after starting treatment. Only two patients discontinued the study because of adverse effects with "overstimulation" as the most common adverse side effect. The same group later found that 73% of patients with HIV, depression, and fatigue responded, and there was no evidence of tolerance, abuse, or dependence (Wagner and Rabkin, 2000).

Methylphenidate

There are few high-quality data to analyze the efficacy of methylphenidate in HIV patients. Methylphenidate was used in an open-label trial with dextroamphetamine, and both medications demonstrated significant improvement (Holmes et al., 1989) in depression. When compared with desipramine, methylphenidate showed equal efficacy; however, the study was not powered to detect significant differences. Interestingly, methylphenidate did not produce antidepressant effects any faster than desipramine but was very well tolerated in this study (Fernandez et al., 1995). Methylphenidate is mainly metabolized extracellularly via de-esterification into an inactive metabolite. Less than 2% of metabolism involves oxidation or conjugation (Royal College of Psychiatrists, 2009). Clinically, methylphenidate is well tolerated by HIV patients, even those with severe medical complications, and is flexibly dosed (patch, long-, mid-, and short-release formulations). Many persons with HIV/AIDS have comorbid diagnoses of attention-deficit disorder (ADD) or attention-deficit-hyperactivity disorder (ADHD), and/or severe depression indistinguishable from delirium or dementia. Methylphenidate products, particularly the patch and all-day formulations, offer the most effectiveness with the least complications or potential for abuse.

Non–amphetamine-based stimulants (atomoxetine, modafinil)

To date, there is no trial documenting the effects of atomoxetine in patients with HIV. One open-label trial by Rabkin and colleagues (2004) showed promising results using modafinil to treat fatigue in HIV. In this study, patients also had affective improvement, but there was no placebo to compare the magnitude of the effect. There was no significant effect on CD4 count or viral load, and the treatment was well tolerated.

Mood stabilizers and anticonvulsants

Lithium has the fewest pharmacokinetics interactions with ART, although side effects may limit its use in patients with HIV. Ritonavir may induce the metabolism of lamotrigine and valproic acid, lowering serum levels (Back, 2006). Most older antiepileptics are pan-inducers of multiple P450 enzymes. Phenytoin, phenobarbital, carbamazepine, and oxcarbazepine induce metabolism at 3A4 (Armstrong and Cozza, 2000, Kato et al., 2000) and thus may reduce the serum levels of protease inhibitors and non-nucleoside reverse transcriptase inhibitors (NNRTIs), resulting in the lowering of serum levels and viral resistance. The newer antiepileptics that are not inducers of 3A4 (e.g., levetiracetam or gabapentin) may be better first choices for patients on ART who require seizure treatment.

Careful attention to viral load, disease progression, and therapeutic drug monitoring of antiepileptics is prudent whenever prescribing antiretrovirals with anticonvulsants. Lithium, either alone or in combination with other antiepileptic mood stabilizers, is an effective treatment for bipolar disorder–spectrum symptoms. Lithium has also been used with some success for antidepressant augmentation in the general population (Stein and Bernadt, 1993). There have been no studies to support its use in depressed patients with HIV.

Lithium's common side effects, which include fatigue and slowed cognition, weight gain, and skin changes, may pose significant burdens to medically ill patients. Symptoms of lithium toxicity (nausea, vomiting, diarrhea, confusion) may mimic symptoms common in AIDS. Lithium use also requires adequate electrolyte balance, which may be difficult to obtain in patients with AIDS who have diarrhea, nausea and vomiting, and general debility. Patients with HIV-associated nephropathy may also be poor candidates for lithium treatment (Harvey et al., 2002; Cohen and Alfonso, 2004). Starting lithium after there has been significant neurological damage as evidence by MRI findings predicts poor tolerability.

Anticonvulsants

In addition to the mood-stabilizing effects of anticonvulsants, some have also shown efficacy in the treatment of HIV neuropathy. Carbamazepine and phenytoin have been studied in treatment of trigeminal neuralgia and diabetic peripheral neuropathy, but not HIV-associated neuropathy. Carbamezapine's potential for leukopenia, anticholinergic effects, and metabolic enzyme induction limit its use in patients with HIV. Gabapentin was studied initially in an open-label trial of 19 HIV-positive patients. Pain was significantly improved, independent of whether neurotoxic antiretroviral therapy was used (La Spina et al., 2001). Hahn and colleagues (2004) studied gabapentin in 26 patients and concluded that it was effective, compared to placebo, in controlling neuropathic pain. It was very well tolerated at up to 3600 mg/day, with somnolence being the most common side effect.

Lamotrigine was shown to be superior to placebo in a small, randomized trial, but adverse events did limit its use in a small number of patients (Simpson et al., 2000). Of the adverse reactions, rash was the most common and potentially the most serious. No patients developed Stevens–Johnson

syndrome, and all dermatological manifestations resolved with discontinuation of the study drug. A larger trial by the same group showed that
lamotrigine was effective in treating pain among patients receiving neurotoxic antiretroviral therapy. However, there was no change, compared to
placebo, for patients who were not receiving neurotoxic antiretroviral
therapy. The authors postulated that different mechanisms of neuropathy
in these patients might account for the lack of therapeutic response
(Simpson et al., 2003).

There have been reports of valproic acid–induced hepatotoxicity with
coadministration of P450 inducers such as nevirapine (Cozza et al., 2000).
Ritonavir, efavirenz, and lopinavir may also have complicated drug–drug
interactions with valproic acid. There is some debate in the literature about
valproate acid potentially increasing viral replication (Maggi and Halman,
2001; Romanelli and Pomeroy, 2003), which may limit its usefulness even
more.

For an overview of drug interactions and other considerations with mood
stabilizers and anticonvulsant medications see Table 7.3.

Antipsychotics

Most antipsychotics are partially metabolized at cytochrome 2D6 (ziprasi-
done and pimozide being notable exceptions). Those that are would be
susceptible to inhibition by ritonavir, which has been reported to lead to
worsened side effects, including extrapyramidal symptoms (Kelly et al.,
2002) and possibly tardive dyskinesia.

It is important to remember that HIV-infected patients may be more
susceptible to extrapyramidal symptoms and may even have abnormal
movements prior to therapy with dopamine antagonists, given that HIV
can attack the basal ganglia (Nath et al., 1987, Lera and Zirulnik, 1999).
Patients with HIV seem to be exquisitely vulnerable to side effects of high-
potency conventional neuroleptics (Ramachandran et al., 1997). Molindone
has been used with HIV patients with few side effects (Fernandez and Levy,
1993). Pimozide, generally used in the treatment of tic disorders, has risks for
arrhythmias, seizures, and blood disorders. Pimozide is metabolized primarily at cytochrome 3A4 and thus must never be coadministered with
protease inhibitors or NNRTIs (Abbott Laboratories, 2007).

HIV patients may also be at greater risk for side effects with the newer
neruoleptics than the general population. Although some clinicians have
reported good response with few side effects with neuroleptics such as
risperidone in the years prior to protease inhibitor therapy (Singh et al.,
1997), it is important to remember that risperidone may have a greater
propensity to cause extrapyramidal side effects than most other atypicals
neuroleptics. In addition, risperidone is metabolized at cytochrome 2D6 and

TABLE 7.3 Psychotropic Medications and Special Considerations for HIV: Mood Stabilizers and Anticonvulsants

Mood Stabilizer	Metabolic Site(s)	Inhibits/Induces	Clinical Pearls and Potential Drug–Drug Interactions with ART
Carbamazepine (CBZ, Tegretol)	CYP 3A4, 2B6, 2C8, 2E1, 2C9, 1A2 UGT2B7 Transporter ABCB1	Inhibits CYP2C19 (possibly) Induces CYP3A4, 1A2, 2B6, 2C8, 2C9, UGT1A4	Data for use in pain disorders including trigeminal neuralgia Potential for diminished white blood cell count Delavirdine[f] Efavirenz[e,f] Etravirine[e] Nevirapine[e] Protease inhibitors[b,c] Zidovudine[d]
Gabapentin (Neurontin)	Excreted in urine unchanged	None known	Strong evidence for use in neuropathic pain Poor mood stabilization No drug–drug interactions known
Lamotrigine (Lamictal)	UGT 1A4 Also excreted in urine unchanged	Induces UGT1A4[a]	Strong mood stabilizing properties Increased risk of Stevens–Johnson Syndrome (SJS) if not titrated slowly Use with caution with abacavir which may also cause SJS.
Levitiracetam (Keppra)	1/3 by noncytochromal hydrolysis	None	Can be used as monotherapy for seizure prophylaxis and treatment No drug–drug interactions known May alter mood

(continued)

TABLE 7.3 (Continued)

Mood Stabilizer	Metabolic Site(s)	Inhibits/Induces	Clinical Pearls and Potential Drug–Drug Interactions with ART
Lithium	Renal	None	Use with caution in patients concurrently taking NSAIDs, ACE inhibitors, angiotensin receptor antagonists, and diurectics Therapeutic drug monitoring required (serum levels) Narrow margin of safety May cause slowed/poor cognition
Oxcarbazepine (Trileptal)	Noncytochromal metabolism, CYP3A4 Transporter ABCB1	Inhibits CYP2C19[a] Induces CYP3A4[a], 3A5[a], UGTs[a]	Data for mood stabilization less strong than for carbamazepine Hyponatremia relatively common Delavirdine[f] Efavirenz[e,f] Etravirine[e] Nevirapine[e] Protease Inhibitors[e] Zidovudine[d]
Tiagabine (Gabitril)	CYP3A4, UGTs	None known	Delavirdine[f] Efavirenz[e,f] Etravirine[e]

Drug	Pharmacokinetics	Enzyme effects	Notes
Topiramate (Topamax)	70% excreted unchanged in urine Phase I and II UGTs Transporter ABCB1	Inhibits 2C19[a]	Nevirapine[e] Protease inhibitors[b] Works via multiple mechanisms Effective for migraine prophylaxis Risk of cognitive impairment and drug-induced mood disorder depression Protease inhibitors[e]
Valproic acid (VPA, Depakote, Depakene)	CYP 2C9, 2C19, 2A6 UGT 1A6, UGT 1A9 UGT 2B7, β-oxidation	Induces 3A4[a], UGTs[a] Inhibits UGT 1A4, UGT1A9, UGT2B7, UGT 2B15, CYP2D6, 2C9, Epoxide hydroxylase Induces perhaps CYP3A4, ABCB1	Strong mood-stabilizing properties Effective for migraine prophylaxis Hepatotoxicity, especially with CYP inducers such as nevirapine, efavirenz, and ritonavir Hepatotoxic metabolite is not measured in standard lab tests Use with caution in those with hepatitis C/HIV coinfection Weight gain Hair loss

(continued)

TABLE 7.3 (Continued)

Mood Stabilizer	Metabolic Site(s)	Inhibits/Induces	Clinical Pearls and Potential Drug–Drug Interactions with ART
Vigabatrin (Sabril)	Excreted in urine unchanged	None known	None known
Zonisamide (Zonegran)	CYP3A4 Acetylation, Sulfonation	None known	Delavirdine[f] Efavirenz[e,f] Etravirine[e] Nevirapine[e] Protease inhibitors[b]

Note: Primary route of metabolism listed first. ABCB = ATP binding cassette B transporter; CYP = cytochrome; UGT = uridine 5′-diphosphate glucuronosyltransferase.

Bold type indicates **potent** inhibition or induction at that site.

[a] Moderate.

[b] The most likely of the protease inhibitors to cause increased anticonvulsant/mood stabilizer serum levels are ritonavir, atazanavir, and indinavir because of CYP 3A4 inhibition.

[c] This anticonvulsant/mood stabilizer's potent induction of metabolism at CYP3A4 will likely reduce protease inhibitor levels and increase risk of viral resistance to ART

[d] May decrease zidovudine levels because of induction of UGTs and increase risk of viral resistance to ART

[e] Induction of CYP3A4 metabolism may reduce anticonvulsant/mood stabilizer levels and reduce effectiveness.

[f] A potent inhibitor of CYP3A4 metabolism and may increase serum levels of anticonvulsants/mood stabilizers dependent on this enzyme, leading to increased side effects and toxicity.

Source: Adapted from Wynn GH, Sandson N, Muniz J (2009). Psychiatry. In GH Wynn, JR Oesterheld, KL Cozza, and SC Armstrong (eds.), *Clinical Guide to Drug Interaction Principles for Medical Practice.* Washington DC: American Psychiatric Press, used with permission.

3A4 and may be prone to metabolic inhibition (and hence worsened side effects, including movement disorders) by 3A4 inhibitors such as protease inhibitors, especially the pan-inhibitor ritonovir (Jover et al., 2002, Kelly et al., 2002).

Antipsychotics dependent on 1A2, such as many of the newer or novel antipsychotics, may be susceptible to reduced serum levels and hence less effectiveness when coadministered with the mixed inhibitor–inducers ritonavir or ritonavir/lopinavir (Penzak et al., 2002).

For an overview of drug interactions and other considerations with antipsychotic medications see Table 7.4.

TABLE 7.4 Psychotropic Medications and Special Considerations for HIV: Classic and Novel Antipsychotics

Antipsychotics	Metabolic Site(s)	Inhibits/ Induces	Clinical Pearls and Potential Drug–Drug Interaction with ART
Classic Antipsychotics			Since these are older drugs, there are fewer data about specific metabolic sites and drug interactions Risk for extrapyramidal symptoms (EPS) and tardive dyskinesia
Chlorpromazine (Thorazine)	CYP2D6, 1A2, 3A4 UGT1A4, UGT1A3	Inhibits CYP2D6[a]	Very anticholinergic Very sedating Ritonavir[i]
Fluphenazine (Prolixin)	CYP2D6, 1A2	Inhibits CYP2D6[a], 1A2	High-potency neuroleptic Higher risk for EPS Tenofovir[d] Ritonavir[i]
Haloperidol (Haldol)	CYP 2D6, 3A4, 1A2	Inhibits CYP2D6[a]	High-potency neuroleptic Higher risk for EPS Ritonavir[i] Tenofovir[d]
Mesoridazine (Serentil)	CYP2D6, 1A2	Unknown	Uncommonly used Very sedating Ritonavir[i] Tenofovir[d]
Molindone (Moban)	CYP2D6 and phase II	None known	Medium-potency antipsychotic Less risk for EPS Generally well tolerated Ritonavir[i]
Thioridazine (Mellaril)	CYP2D6, 1A2, 2C19, FMO3	Inhibits CYP2D6[c]	Very anticholinergic Very sedating Risk of retinitis pigmentosa at higher doses Ritonavir[i] Tenofovir[d]

(continued)

TABLE 7.4 (Continued)

Antipsychotics	Metabolic Site(s)	Inhibits/ Induces	Clinical Pearls and Potential Drug–Drug Interaction with ART
Perphenazine (Trilafon)	CYP2D6, 3A4, 1A2, 2C19	Inhibits CYP 2D6[a], 1A2	High-potency neuroleptic Higher risk for EPS Protease inhibitors[e] Ritonavir[i] Tenofovir[d]
Pimozide (Orap)	CYP3A4, 1A2	Inhibits CYP2D6[a], 3A4	High-potency neuroleptic Arrhythmia risk Higher risk for EPS Not recommended in HIV patients since delavirdine, efqavirenz and protease inhibitors may cause arrhythmia when coadministered with CYP3A4-dependent pimozide Efavirenz[f,g] Etravirine[h] Nevirapine[g] Protease inhibitors[e] Tenofovir[d]

Novel Antipsychotics

Antipsychotics	Metabolic Site(s)	Inhibits/ Induces	Clinical Pearls and Potential Drug–Drug Interaction with ART
Aripiprazole (Abilify)	CYP2D6, 3A4	None known	Risk of metabolic syndrome—weight gain, hypertriglyceridemia, diabetes mellitus Akathesia most common side effect Ritonavir[i]
Clozapine (Clozaril)	CYPCYP1A2, 3A4, 2D6, 2C9, 2C19, UGT 1A3 UGT 1A4 FMO3	Inhibits 2D6[c]	Risk of agranulocytosis; requires frequent CBCs to screen for adverse events Risk of metabolic syndrome, rhabdomyolysis, myocarditis, pericarditis, sialorhea, Should be used only by experienced provider Ritonavir[i] Tenofovir[d]
Olanzapine (Zyprexa)	UGT 1A4 CYP 1A2, 2D6, FMO3	None	High risk of metabolic syndrome—weight gain, hypertriglyceridemia, diabetes mellitus Sedating Advantages in sleep, appetite, nausea, failure to thrive Tenofovir[d]

Quetiapine (Seroquel)	CYP3A4 Sulfoxidation Oxidation Transporter ABCB1	None	High risk of metabolic effects— weight gain, hypertriglyceridemia, diabetes mellitus Low risk of EPS Very sedating Delavirdine[f] Efavirenz [f,g] Etravirine[h] Nevirapine[g] Protease inhibitors[e]
Risperidone (Risperdal)	CYP 2D6, 3A4	Inhibits 2D6,[b]	Highest risk for EPS avoid in HIV/AIDS Risk of metabolic syndrome— weight gain, hypertriglyceri- demia, diabetes mellitus Ritonavir[i]
Ziprasidone (Geodon)	Aldehyde oxidase (mostly) CYP3A4, 1A2 (minimal)	None	Risk of metabolic syndrome— weight gain, hypertriglyceri- demia, diabetes mellitus

Note: Primary route of metabolism listed first. ABCB = ATP binding cassette B transporter; CYP = cytochrome, FMO3 = flavin monooxygenase; UGT = uridine 5′-diphosphate glucuronosyltransferase.
Bold type indicates **potent** inhibition or induction at that site.
[a] Potent.
[b] Moderate.
[c] Mild.
[d] Tenofovir may reduce serum levels and effectiveness because of induction of metabolism at CYP 1A2.
[e] The most likely of the protease inhibitors to cause increased antipsychotic levels and increased risk of side effects and toxicity are ritonavir, atazanavir, and indinavir because of potent CYP 3A4 inhibition.
[f] NNRTIs delavirdine and efavirenz are potent inhibitors of CYP3A4 and may increase serum levels of antipsychotics that are primarily metabolized at CYP 3A4, worsening side effects/ sedation.
[g] Efavirenz and nevirapine are moderate inducers of CYP3A4 and may reduce serum levels of antipsychotics dependent upon CYP 3A4, reducing effectiveness.
[h] Etravirine is a potent inducer of CYP3A4 and may reduce serum levels of antipsychotics dependent upon CYP 3A4, reducing effectiveness.
[i] Rironavir is a potent pan-inhibitor of many CYP enzymes and may increase serum levels and antipsychotic side effects/toxicity.
Source: Adapted from Wynn GH, Sandson N, Muniz J (2009). Psychiatry. In GH Wynn, JR Oesterheld, KL Cozza, and SC Armstrong (eds.), *Clinical Guide to Drug Interaction Principles for Medical Practice*. Washington DC: American Psychiatric Press, used with permission.

Anxiolytics

Benzodiazepines

The only benzodiazepine that has been studied specifically in HIV-positive patients is lorazepam. Breitbart and colleagues (1996) compared lorazepam to the neuroleptics haloperidol and chlorpromazine in treating delirium, and benzodiazepine use was shown to be ineffective. In fact, adverse side effects caused an early termination of this treatment arm. There are no clinical trials evaluating the commonly used agents diazepam, clonazepam, alprazolam, midazolam, or temezepam in HIV-infected patients, but literature on their use in other medically ill populations suggests that they are efficacious if used wisely (Fernandez and Levy, 1991).

HIV-infected patients may be very sensitive to the effects of benzodiazepines, leading to confusion, cognitive impairment, disinhibition, and frank delirium (Uldall and Berghuis, 1997). Long-acting formulations with active metabolites should be avoided to limit the possibility of disinhibition, amnesia, and delirium.

The triazolobenzodiazepines alprazolam, triazolam, and midazolam are all dependent on 3A4 for metabolism. All protease inhibitors inhibit the metabolism of these medications. Merry and colleagues (1997) reported a case of prolonged sedation for bronchoscopy with a protease inhibitor and midazolam combination. Ritonavir's interaction with alprazolam and triazolam has proven to be more complex. Short-term use of ritonavir has been shown to potently inhibit metabolism of these drugs, resulting in enhanced sedation and impairment (Greenblatt et al., 2000). After using ritonavir for more than a few days, the clearance of the benzodiazepines increases, resulting in reduced effect due to a slight net 3A4 induction by ritonavir.

Nonbenzodiazepine anxiolytics

Buspirone has the potential for confusion related to its dopaminergic effects, and drug–drug interactions, particularly with protease inhibitors and efavirenz, limit its use. Thus, some clinicians advocate using buspirone in patients not taking ART who may have substance abuse problems (Fernandez and Levy, 1994). Buspirone is metabolized at 3A4. Clay and Adams (2003) reported a case of pseudo-parkinsonism in a 54-year-old HIV-positive patient after ritonavir was added to his high-dose buspirone (70 mg/day).

For an overview of drug interactions and other considerations with these medications and other sedative-hypnotics see Table 7.5.

Substance Abuse Medications

This section includes a brief overview of pharmacological issues in the use of prescription medications for treating substance abuse and dependence. For in-depth information on pharmacological issues concerning nonprescription use of drugs of abuse, readers are referred to publications by Wynn et al.

TABLE 7.5 Psychotropic Medications and Special Considerations for HIV: Sedative-Hypnotics

Sedative-Hypnotic	Metabolic Site(s)	Inhibits/Induces	Clinical Pearls and Potential Drug–Drug Interactions with ART
Benzodiazepines			
Triazolobenzodiazepines			
Alprazolam (Xanax) Midazolam (Versed) Triazolam (Halcion)	CYP3A4 Glucuronidation	None known	Higher risk of abuse and may need to increase dose over time Susceptible to drug interactions May cause amnesia, cognitive impairment, delirium, discoordination Protease inhibitors[a] Delavirdine[d] Efavirenz[d,e] Entravirine[f] Nevirapine[e]
Clonazepam (Klonopin)	3A4 Acetylation	None known	Long half-life Potential cognitive impairment, especially in advanced hepatic disease or AIDS Antiepileptic properties Good muscle relaxant properties Protease inhibitors[a] Delavirdine[d] Efavirenz[d,e] Entravirine[f] Nevirapine[e]

(continued)

TABLE 7.5 (Continued)

Sedative-Hypnotic	Metabolic Site(s)	Inhibits/Induces	Clinical Pearls and Potential Drug–Drug Interactions with ART
Diazepam (Valium)	CYP2C19, 3A4, 2B6, 2C9, Glucuronidation	None known	Long half-life Potential cognitive impairment, especially in advanced hepatic disease or AIDS Antiepileptic properties Good muscle relaxant properties Ritonavir may increase serum levels via CYP pan-inhibition
Flunitrazepam (Rohypnol)	CYP2C19, 3A4	Inhibits UGT 1A1, UGT 1A3, UGT 2B7	Used only in treatment of narcolepsy Stringent prescribing guidelines; should be restricted to experienced providers Ritonavir may initially increase serum levels, then reduce serum levels via CYP pan-inhibition Zidovudine[b]
Lorazepam (Ativan)	UGT 2B7, Glucuronidation	None known	Mid length half-life No active metabolites Useful in patients with liver disease, but requires lower dosing
Oxazapem (Serax)	Soxazepam—UGT 2B15 Roxazepam—UGT 1A9, UGT 2B7	None known	None known Mid length half-life No active metabolites Useful in patients with liver disease, but requires lower dosing
Temazepam (Restoril)	UGT 2B7, Glucuronidation 2C19, 3A4	None known	None known Mid-length half-life No active metabolites Approved only for sleep

Non-benzodiazepines			
Barbiturates	CYP2C9, 2C19, 2E1	Pan-inducer	Narrow margin of safety
			Risk of tachyphylaxis
			Highly lethal in overdose
			Coadministration with ART may reduce ART effectiveness
Buspirone (Buspar)	CYP3A4	None known	Non-addictive—potential advantage in substance use disorders
			Delayed response time of 2 weeks or more
			Protease inhibitors[a]
			Delavirdine[d]
			Efavirenz[d,e]
			Entravirine[f]
			Nevirapine[e]
Diphenhydramine (Benadryl)	CYP2D6	2D6	Highly anticholinergic; high risk for cognitive effects
Zaleplon (Sonata)	CYP3A4, 1A2, 2D6 aldehyde oxidase,	None known	Very short half-life
			Effective only for sleep-onset insomnia
			Protease inhibitors[a]
			Delavirdine[a,d]
			Efavirenz[a,d,e]
			Nevirapine[e]
			Tenofovir[c]
Zolpidem (Ambien)	CYP3A4, 1A2, 2C9, 2C19, 2D6	None known	Effective for sleep-onset and maintenance insomnias
			Inhibition of metabolic enzymes, may increase serum levels
			Protease inhibitors, [a]
			Delavirdine[d]
			Efavirenz[a,d,e]
			Etravirine[f]
			Nevirapine[e]
			Tenofovir[c]

(continued)

TABLE 7.5 (Continued)

Sedative-Hypnotic	Metabolic Site(s)	Inhibits/Induces	Clinical Pearls and Potential Drug–Drug Interactions with ART
Zopiclone (Zimovane)	CYP3A4, 2C9	None known	Effective for sleep-onset and maintenance insomnias Metallic taste Protease inhibitors[a] Delavirdine[d] Efavirenz[a,d,e] Etravirine[f] Nevirapine[e]
Eszopiclone (Lunesta)	CYP3A4, 2C9	None known	Best evidence for effective sleep-onset and maintenance insomnias Metallic taste Inhibition of 3A4 and 2C9 may increase serum levels Protease inhibitors[a] Delavirdine[d] Efavirenz[d,e] Nevirapine[e]

Note: Primary route of metabolism listed first. CYP = cytochrome, UGT = uridine 5'-diphosphate glucuronosyltransferase. **Bold** type indicates **potent** inhibition or induction at that cytochrome or UGT.

[a]The most likely of the protease inhibitors to cause increased drug levels of sedative-hypnotics dependent upon CYP 3A4 are ritonavir, atazanavir, and indinavir.

[b]Flunitrazepam may increase zidovudine levels because of inhibition of UGT 2B7.

[c]Potential interaction due to induction of CYP 1A2 by tenofovir.

[d]NNRTIs delavirdine and efavirenz are potent inhibitors of CYP3A4 and may increase serum levels of sedative-hypnotics that are primarily metabolized at CYP 3A4, worsening side effects/sedation.

[e]Efavirenz and nevirapine are moderate inducers of CYP3A4 and may reduce serum levels of sedative-hypnotics dependent upon CYP 3A4, reducing effectiveness.

[f]Etravirine is a potent inducer of CYP3A4 and may reduce serum levels of sedative-hypnotics dependent upon CYP 3A4, reducing effectiveness.

Source: Adapted from Wynn GH, Sandson N, Muniz J (2009). Psychiatry. In GH Wynn, JR Oesterheld, KL Cozza, and SC Armstrong SC (eds.), *Clinical Guide to Drug Interaction Principles for Medical Practice.* Washington DC: American Psychiatric Press, used with permission.

(2005), Armstrong and Cozza (2003a, 2003b), Oesterheld et al. (2004), Sandson et al. (2005), and McDowell et al. (2000).

Methadone

In a review of 28 clinical studies, methadone therapy has been shown to decrease the risk of transmission of HIV through the reduction of injection drug use and of sharing of injection drug paraphernalia (Gowing et al., 2006). It has been associated with an increase in the likelihood of using antiretroviral therapy (Wood et al., 2005). Methadone has been shown to decrease the number of reports of multiple sex partners and the practice of exchanging drugs for money (Stark et al., 1996). Methadone may also decrease the risk for heroin overdose (Brugal et al., 2005).

Methadone is metabolized primarily by the CYP3A4, so when beginning medications that inhibit 3A4 metabolism, careful monitoring of this narcotic is required to prevent toxicity. Similarly, if 3A4 is induced, then previously stable methadone levels can diminish and induce narcotic withdrawal reactions. Importantly, antiretrovirals can serve as both inhibitors and inducers of this enzyme, requiring continued careful monitoring for ongoing reactions (Iribarne et al., 1998; Altice et al., 1999; Geletko and Erickson 2000; Boffito et al., 2002, Hendrix et al., 2004; Boehringer Ingelheim Pharmaceuticals, 2008). Coadministration of methadone with potent CYP3A4 inhibitors such as atazanavir, delavirdine, efavirenz, indinivir, ritonavir, clarithromycin, erythromycin, and even grapefruit juice may cause opiate toxicity. Coadministration of methadone with potent CYP3A4 inducers such as ritonavir, entravirine, St. John's wort, or the pan-inducers rifampin, carbamazepine, phenobarbital, or phenytoin may lead to opiate withdrawal (see Table 7.1 for a review of CYP 3A4 inhibitors and inducers of metabolism). Patients with HIV who are on methadone maintenance for chronic pain or as part of addiction treatment will also occasionally need acute pain management. Increased or new pain should be treated as a separate problem, with additional opioids including methadone administered carefully, monitoring for drug interactions. Methadone maintenance therapy cannot be thought of as analgesia, but rather as agonist therapy for relapse and withdrawal prevention. Methadone for relapse prevention will target opioid tolerance needs and prevent withdrawal but will not provide analgesia for pain. Clinicians may have to advocate for increased methadone replacement dosing for these patients to achieve previously stable pain relief and symptom control.

Buprenorphine

Buprenorphine has been shown to be very effective worldwide in the opioid-dependent population, but its efficacy in preventing HIV risk behavior and transmission has not been well studied. A 12-week trial combining buprenorphine, bupropion, and psychotherapy showed some benefit over standard treatment with methadone in HIV-positive patients with opioid and cocaine dependency. The small sample size and short duration of treatment coupled with no data on long-term follow-up make it difficult to generalize this treatment approach (Avants et al., 1998). A more recent randomized trial has demonstrated a decrease in HIV risk behaviors, but there was no significant improvement in its ability to suppress heroin use over that with methadone treatment (Mattick et al., 2003). Another consideration when using buprenorphine is drug–drug interactions, since buprenorphine, like methadone, is metabolized via cytochrome 3A4 and is susceptible to interactions with all protease inhibitors and efavirenz.

Naltrexone

Currently there are no trials studying naltrexone use exclusively in HIV-positive patients. Since adherence and pill burden are issues in HIV care, the newly developed long-acting depot formulation of naltrexone may be promising (Hulse et al., 2004).

Disulfiram

Although there are no studies of disulfiram treatment in HIV patients, a drug safety trial has shown no negative immunomodulatory effects and concluded that the use of disulfiram should not enhance disease progression (Hording et al., 1990). The potential for hepatotoxicity, particularly in HIV patients also infected with hepatitis B and C, has not been formally studied and requires monitoring (Forns et al., 1994). Continuous alcohol ingestion may carry a greater risk of morbidity than disulfiram use; further study in HIV patients is needed (Kulig and Beresford, 2005).

REVIEW OF ANTIRETROVIRAL THERAPY (ART)

At the time of publication, ART includes protease inhibitors (PIs), nucleotide analogue reverse transcriptase inhibitors (NRTIs), non-nucleoside reverse transcriptase inhibitors (NNRTIs), CCR5 inhibitors, invirase inhibitors, and fusion inhibitors. These medications have helped transform HIV/AIDS from being a fatal disease to becoming a more manageable chronic illness. To select adequate psychopharmacological therapies and provide helpful consultation to HIV specialists, one needs an understanding of the components of ART, including drug interactions and special idiosyncrasies. Presented here is a brief review of the ART medications.

Protease inhibitors

Protease inhibitors, like all HIV therapies, have significant side effects that warrant monitoring in combination with patient education. The side effects common to the entire class include gastrointestinal disruption, dysfunction of lipid and glucose metabolism, sexual dysfunction, and hepatic toxicity.

Protease inhibitors are primarily metabolized at 3A4 with some minor involvement by 2D6 for ritonavir and 2C19 for nelfinavir. Enzymatic inhibition by protease inhibitors also occurs primarily at 3A4. Of all the protease inhibitors, ritonavir causes the most varied and potent inhibition (a pan-inhibitor) and requires the most monitoring when used in combination with other medications.

See Table 7.6 for a review of metabolism and special clinical considerations for each protease inhibitor.

Nucleoside reverse transcriptase inhibitors

The NRTIs in general do not interact with the P450 system. NRTIs have several significant side effects, including mitochondrial toxicity, ototoxicity, and hematopoietic toxicity. The most common severe manifestations of mitochondrial toxicity include neuropathy, myopathy, lactic acidosis, hepatic steatosis, pancreatitis, and lipodystrophy (Moyle, 2000). Hematopoietic toxicity can negatively affect any of the three major cell lines, causing anemia, neutropenia, or thrombocytopenia. Notable side effects outside of those applicable to the entire class include a potentially fatal hypersensitivity reaction in up to 5% of patients on abacavir (Clay, 2002). Definitive therapy consists of permanent discontinuation of abacavir, as rechallenge has been associated with significant worsening of symptoms.

See Table 7.7 for a review of metabolism and special clinical considerations for the NRTIs.

Non-nucleoside reverse transcriptase inhibitors

Though different in chemical structure, non-nucleoside reverse transcriptase inhibitors (NNRTIs) are similar in mechanism of action, side effects, and in some aspects of metabolism (see Table 7.8). Most frequently, rash, elevation of liver-associated enzymes, and lipodystrophy are the side effects associated with the NNRTIs. Unlike abacavir, the rash associated with NNRTIs is usually mild in nature and does not always require discontinuation. The elevation of liver-associated enzymes is most often asymptomatic and usually requires no intervention outside of periodic monitoring. Lipodystrophy frequently causes discontinuation of therapy and does not always resolve after discontinuation of therapy (Dieterich et al., 2004).

TABLE 7.6 Protease Inhibitors (PIs)

Drug	Metabolic Site(s)/ Transporter Activity	Inhibition[a]	Induction[a]	Common Side Effects, Toxicities, and Clinical Considerations	Some Potential Medication Interactions
All protease inhibitors	3A4 Transporters	3A4	Varies	Bleeding risk Gastrointestinal disturbance Headaches Hepatitis Lipodystrophy Sexual dysfunction	All 3A4-dependent medications with narrow safety margins, such as: Antiarrhythmics Ergots Lovastatin Pimozide Simvastatin Triazolobenzodiazepines[2] Warfarin Grapefruit juice raises PI serum levels Pan-inducers[1] and St. John's wort decrease PI serum levels
Amprenavir (Agenerase) Fosamprenavir (Lexiva)	3A4 Transporters	3A4[b]	3A4 (possibly) Transporters (possibly)	Lactic acidosis Perioral and peripheral paresthesias Stevens–Johnson syndrome Discontinue vitamin D (high content in formulation) Do not take with high-fat meals	Propafenone

Drug	Substrate	Inhibits	Induces	Adverse effects	Interactions
Atazanavir (Reyataz)	3A4 Transporters (possibly)	3A4, 1A2, 2C9, UGT1A1	None known	Direct (unconjugated) hyperbilirubinemia Lactic acidosis Prolonged P-R interval Take with food/high-fat meal	Irinotecan Proton pump inhibitors
Indinavir (Crixivan)	3A4 Transporters	3A4	None known	Altered taste Chelitis Dry eyes, skin, mouth Hyperbilirubinemia Nephrolithiasis Neutropenia Paronychia Rash Leukocytoclastic vasculitis Do not take with high-fat meals	
Lopinavir/ ritonavir (Kaletra)	3A4 Transporters	Lopinavir: 3A4[b], 2D6 Ritonavir: 3A4, 2D6, 2C9, 2C19, 2B6 Transporters (acute)	Lopinavir: Glucuronidation Ritonavir: 3A4, 1A2[b], 2C9[b], 2C19 Transporters (chronic)	Diarrhea Pancreatitis Altered taste Take with food	Same as ritonavir Propafenone
Nelfinavir (Viracept)	3A4, 2C19 Transporters	3A4[c], 1A2, 2B6[b], Transporters	2C9 (possibly)	Diarrhea (worst of PIs) Nephrolithiasis	

(continued)

TABLE 7.6 (Continued)

Drug	Metabolic Site(s)/ Transporter Activity	Inhibition[a]	Induction[a]	Common Side Effects, Toxicities, and Clinical Considerations	Some Potential Medication Interactions
Ritonavir (Norvir)	**3A4**, **2D6** Transporters	**3A4**, **2D6**, **2C9**, **2C19**, 2B6 Transporters (acute)	**3A4**, 1A2[b], 2C9[b], 2C19 Transporters (chronic)	Pancreatitis Altered taste	Clozapine Estradiol Meperidine Methadone Propafenone
Saquinavir (Invirase, Fortovase)	3A4 Transporters	3A4[c] Transporters	None known	Altered taste Take with food	
Tipravavir (Aptivus)	3A4 Transporters	3A4	None known	Intracranial hemorrhage Hepatotoxicity Rash Sulfa-based drug Must be taken with ritonavir "boost"	NSAIDs SSRIs (possible bleeding) Vitamin E (bleeding)

NSAID = nonsteroidal anti-inflammatory drug; SSRI = selective serotonin reuptake inhibitor; UGT = uridine 5′-diphosphate glucuronosyltransferase.
[1] Pan-inducers are drugs that induce many if not all cytochrome P450 enzymes and include barbiturates, carbamazepine, ethanol, phenytoin, and rifmycins.
[2] Alprazolam (Xanax), midazolam (Versed), triazolam (Halcion).
[a] **Bold** type indicates potent inhibition or induction.
[b] Moderate inhibition or induction.
[c] Mild inhibition or induction.

Source: Wise JE, Cozza KL (2009). Infectious diseases. In GH Wynn, JR Oesterheld, KL Cozza, and SC Armstrong (eds.), Clinical Manual of Drug Interaction Principles for Medical Practice (pp. 284–288). Washington, DC: American Psychiatric Press, used with permission.

TABLE 7.7 Nucleoside Reverse Transcriptase Inhibitors (NRTIs)

Drug	Metabolic Site(s)/ Transporter Activity	Inhibition	Induction	Common side Effects, Toxicities, and Clinical Considerations	Some Potential Interactions
All NRTIs			None known	Hepatomegaly with steatosis Lactic acidosis Lipodystrophy Myopathy Pancreatitis Peripheral neuropathy	
Abacavir (Ziagen)	Alcohol dehydrogenase, Glucuronyl transferase	None known	Unknown	Hypersensitivity reaction Take with or without food	Alcohol
Didanosine (ddl, Videx, Videx EC)	Purine nucleoside phosphorylase	Unknown	None known	Optic neuritis Retinal depigmentation Pancreatitis Peripheral neuropathy Take on empty stomach Do not crush or chew EC tablets	Allopurinol Dapsone[1] Delavirdine Ganciclovir Itraconazole[1] Ketoconazole[1] Methadone Quinolones[2] Ribavirin Stavudine Tenofovir Tetracyclines[2] Trimethoprim/ sulfamethoxazole
Emtricitabine (Emtriva)	Full recovery in urine and feces	None known	None known	Discontinuation with hepatitis B virus; may exacerbate hepatitis	

(continued)

TABLE 7.7 (Continued)

Drug	Metabolic Site(s)/ Transporter Activity	Inhibition	Induction	Common side Effects, Toxicities, and Clinical Considerations	Some Potential Interactions
Lamivudine (3TC, Epivir)	Minimal metabolism Renal transporters	None known	None known	Generally well tolerated	Ribavirin Trimethoprim/ sulfameth-oxazole Zalcitabine[3]
Stavudine (d4T, Zerit)	Not yet known	None known	None known	Peripheral neuropathy (increased risk with didanosine)	Didanosine Ribavirin Trimethoprim/ sulfamethoxazole Zidovudine[4]
Tenofovir disoproxil fumarate (Viread)	Renal transporters	1A2	None known	Nausea	Atazanavir Didanosine[5]
Zalcitabine (ddC, Hivid)	Renal transporters	Unknown	None known	Pancreatitis Peripheral neuropathy Stomatitis	Antacids[6] Didanosine Doxorubicin

Zidovudine (AZT, Retrovir)	UGT2B7 Transporters	Unknown	Anemia Granulocytopenia Headache Gastrointestinal cytopenia	Lamivudine Metoclopramide[6] Ribavirin Stavudine Atovaquone[7] Fluconazole[7] Ganciclovir[8] Methadone Rifampin[9] Ritonavir[9] Valproic acid[7]

[1] Drug that requires an acidic pH for absorption and thus should not be coadministered with didanosine, which is buffered with an antacid.

[2] Antibiotic that would be chelated by didanosine's buffered formulation.

[3] Lamivudine and zalcitabine may inhibit each other's intracellular phosphorylation, worsening toxicity, and should not be coadministered.

[4] Zidovudine may inhibit the intracellular phosphorylation of stavudine, worsening toxicity, so these two drugs should not be coadministered.

[5] Take tenofovir 2 hours before or 1 hour after didanosine.

[6] Decrease absorption of zalcitabine.

[7] Increase zidovudine levels and toxicity.

[8] Increase hematologic toxicity.

[9] Decrease zidovudine levels.

Source: Wise JE, Cozza KL (2009). Infectious diseases. In GH Wynn, JR Oesterheld, KL Cozza, and SC Armstrong (eds.), *Clinical Manual of Drug Interaction Principles for Medical Practice* (pp. 284–288). Washington, DC: American Psychiatric Press, used with permission.

All NNRTIs are primarily metabolized at 3A4, with minor contribution by 2B6 for efavirenz and nevirapine and 2C9 and 2C19 for entravirine (Tibotec, 2008). Cytochromes 2D6, 2C9, and 2C19 play a small role in delavirdine's metabolism. Efavirenz, nevirapine, and entravirine are multi-enzyme inhibitors, whereas nevirapine has not shown any enzymatic inhibition. Efavirenz and delavirdine both inhibit 3A4 potently with mild in vitro inhibition of 2C9, 2D6, and 2C19. In addition, efavirenz weakly inhibits 1A2 (Smith et al., 2001; von Moltke et al., 2001).

Delavirdine and entravirine induce metabolism at 3A4 (Seminari et al., 2008, Tibotec, 2008). Although efavirenz initially inhibits 3A4 in vitro, clinical evidence shows that, over time, efavirenz becomes a potent inducer of metabolism at 3A4 (Clarke et al., 2001; Mouly et al., 2002). This initial inhibition followed by long-term induction necessitates close monitoring of any coadministered medication using 3A4 for metabolism.

A summary of NNRTIs, including metabolism and clinical considerations, is given in Table 7.8.

Cell membrane fusion inhibitors

Enfuvirtide is a synthetic peptide derived from viral membrane protein. It requires subcutaneous injection. The most noted side effect is a local injection-site reaction, often leading to subcutaneous nodules, most of which resolve on their own and do not interfere with continuation for most patients. Rotation of injection sites is recommended, but the need for injections may decrease adherence (Maggi et al., 2004). Studies thus far have shown no P450 interactions (Zhang et al., 2004).

CCR5 antagonists

Maraviroc's mechanism is to prevent HIV from entering target cells, thus preventing the initiation of HIV's replication cycle. Maraviroc is a substrate of 3A4 and P-gp transporters and has potential interactions with protease inhibitors. Serum levels of maraviroc may be increased in patients also taking atazanavir, ritonavir-boosted lopinavir, and ritonavir-boosted saquinavir (Muirhead et al., 2004). Potent inducers of 3A4 may lower serum levels of maraviroc, necessitating higher doses of miraviroc.

Integrase inhibitor

Raltegravir is an HIV integrase strand transfer inhibitor that prevents HIV from inserting HIV DNA into host DNA. Side effects include gastrointestinal symptoms and headaches, with less impact on lipids than many other anti-retrovirals (Grinsztejn et al., 2007). Raltegravir does not affect or use the

TABLE 7.8 Non-Nucleoside Reverse Transcriptase Inhibitors (NNRTIs)

Drug	Metabolic Site(s)/ Transporter Activity	Inhibition[a]	Induction[a]	Common side Effects, Toxicities, and Clinical Considerations	Some Potential Medication Interactions
All NNRTIs				Rash	
Delavirdine (Rescriptor)	3A4, 2D6, 2C9, 2C19	**3A4**, 2C9, 2D6, 2C19	None known	Asymptomatic elevation of liver-associated enzymes	Atorvastatin Calcium channel blockers Ergots Lovastatin Phenobarbital Phenytoin Pimozide Rifampin St. John's wort Triazolobenzodiazepines
Etravirine (Intelence)	Methyl hydroxylation 3A4, 2C19, 2C9 glucuronidation	2C9[c], 2C19[c]	**3A4,** glucuronidation	Rash (severe) Peripheral neuropathy	NNRTs Oral contraceptives Pan-inducers Protease inhibitors St. John's wort Triazolobenzodiazepines

(continued)

TABLE 7.8 (Continued)

Drug	Metabolic Site(s)/ Transporter Activity	Inhibition[a]	Induction[a]	Common side Effects, Toxicities, and Clinical Considerations	Some Potential Medication Interactions
Efavirenz (Sustiva)	3A4, 2B6	**3A4**, 2C9, 2C19, 2D6, 1A2	3A4[b], 2B6[c]	CNS symptoms: Confusion Depression Euphoria Insomnia Vivid dreams Agitation Altered cognition Amnesia Hallucinations Stupor	Atorvastatin Carbamazepine Ergots Lovastatin Pimozide Phenobarbital Phenytoin Rifampin St. John's wort
Nevirapine (Viramune)	3A4, 2B6	None known	3A4[b], 2B6[b]	Hepatotoxicity	Antiarrhythmics Beta-blockers Cyclosporine Protease inhibitors St. John's wort Tacrolimus

[1] Alprazolam (Xanax), midazolam (Versed), triazolam (Halcion).
[a]**Bold** type indicates potent inhibition or induction.
[b]Moderate induction.
[c]Mild inhibition or induction.
Source: Wise JE, Cozza KL (2009). Infectious diseases. In GH Wynn, JR Oesterheld, KL Cozza, and SC Armstrong (eds.), *Clinical Manual of Drug Interaction Principles for Medical Practice* (pp. 284–288). Washington, DC: American Psychiatric Press, used with permission.

P450 system. Raltegravir is mainly metabolized by UGT1A1 via glucuronidation (Isentress, 2007). Potent inducers of glucuronidation/UGT1A1, such as rifampin and tipranavir/ritonavir, reduce plasma concentrations of raltegravir. Potent inhibitors of glucuronidation, such as atazanavir, may increase serum levels of raltegravir and potentially worsen side effects and toxicity.

For a summary of CCR5 antagonsits, fusion inhibitors, and integrase inhibitors see Table 7.9.

TABLE 7.9 CCR5 Antagonists, Fusion Inhibitors, Integrase Inhibitors

Drug	Metabolic Site(s)/ Transporter Activity	P450 and Transporter Inhibition/ Induction	Common Side Effects, Toxicities, and Clinical Considerations	Some Potential Medication Interactions
CCR5 Antagonist				
Maraviroc (Selzentry)	3A4 Transporters	None	Allergic reactions (systemic) Hepatotoxicity Rash	Clarithromycin Efavirenz Inhibitors of 3A4, e.g., grape fruit juice Inducers of 3A4, e.g., St. John's wort Protease inhibitors Rifampin
Fusion Inhibitor				
Enfuvirtide (Fuzeon)	Peptidases in liver and kidneys	None	Subcutaneous nodules	None known
Integrase Inhibitor				
Raltegravir (Isentress)	UGT1A1	None	Gastrointestinal Headache	Inhibitors of glucuronidation, e.g., atazanavir Inducers of glucuronidation, e.g., rifampin

UGT = uridine 5′-diphosphate glucuronosyltransferase.
Source: Wise JE, Cozza KL (2009). Infectious diseases. In GH Wynn, JR Oesterheld, KL Cozza, and SC Armstrong (eds.), *Clinical Manual of Drug Interaction Principles for Medical Practice* (pp. 284–288). Washington, DC: American Psychiatric Press, used with permission.

Selected nonpsychotropics and interactions with ART

Ergots

Ergots are metabolized at 3A4, and coadministration with 3A4-inhibiting ART medications may lead to frank ergotism. Vila et al. (2001) reported that after 5 days of coadministration of an ergot-containing antimigraine drug with newly administered ritonavir, a patient developed pain, claudication, paresthesia, coldness, and cyanosis of both lower limbs. This is one of many reported cases of serious ergotism associated with ritonavir.

Glucocorticoids

Some ritonavir interactions may take longer to become apparent. There are case reports of patients taking ritonavir who developed Cushing's syndrome after many months of inhaled fluticasone because of ritonavir's inhibition of 3A4 metabolism of the corticosteroid (Clevenbergh et al., 2002; Gupta and Dube, 2002). Although metabolic inhibition of 3A4 was immediate, the pharmacodynamic effects of the higher concentrations of substrate became apparent over time. Other glucocorticoids such as prednisilone may also have elevated serum levels when coadministered with ritonavir (Abbott Laboratories, 2007; Roche Pharmaceuticals, 2003/2004). Dexamethasone is a 3A4 inducer and may decrease saquinavir and other protease inhibitor levels.

Oral contraceptives

Oral contraceptives (OCPs) are dependent on 3A4, 2C9, glucuronidation, and sulfation for metabolism. Most protease inhibitors and efavirenz inhibit 3A4 and place patients at risk for increased side effects (headache, breast tenderness, weight gain) (Bristol-Myers Squibb, 2008). Ritonavir, being both an inhibitor and inducer of 3A4, has been found to reduce the AUC and C_{max} of ethinyl estradiol (EE) (Ouellet et al., 1998; Piscitelli et al., 2000), placing patients at risk for breakthrough bleeding and pregnancy. Lopinavir, which induces glucuronidation, and the 3A4-inducing NNRTIs etravirine, efavirenz, and nevirapine may also do the same. Women of childbearing age taking OCPs who are placed on ART need to be warned to use barrier methods of contraception. Higher-dose preparations of OCPs may also be an option, but these recommendations have not been thoroughly studied with ART (Oesterheld, 2009a).

Statins

Slowed or inhibited metabolism of the statins can lead to toxicity (muscle breakdown and rhabdomyolysis). Only pravastatin and rosuvastatin have minimal or non-P450 metabolic pathways. All other statins are dependent on 3A4 for their metabolism. All protease inhibitors, efavirenz, and delavirdine inhibit 3A4. Entravirine, favirenz and nevirapine induce 3A4 metabolism. Protease inhibitors given with simvastatin in healthy volunteers raised simvastatin levels 30-fold (Fichtenbaum et al., 2002).

In a retrospective cohort study of 3448 persons receiving protease inhibitors, one of every five persons on a protease inhibitor and on a statin (N = 200) was on a contraindicated combination (Hulgan et al., 2005). In a review of 2110 claims of persons on ART from a database of private insurance holders (MarketScan, 1999–2000; Hellinger and Encinosa, 2005), 2% had "inappropriate statin drug combination" (IDC), and those with an IDC had a higher number of claims and 39% higher costs than those without an IDC. Those on an IDC were 17 times more likely to have myopathy, polyneuropathy, or myositis. One-half of those cases with an IDC involved simvastatin. Those patients on simvastatin and protease inhibitors had claims for muscle damage. Efavirenz-induced metabolism of simvastatin, atorvastatin, and even pravastatin lowered effectiveness (patients developed an increase in low-density lipoprotein with a simvastatin-efavirenz combination) (Gerber et al., 2005).

CONCLUSIONS

The prescribing of psychotropics or any other class of medications to HIV-positive patients taking ART is a complicated undertaking. An understanding of the potential drug–drug interactions is essential and is helpful to the multidisciplinary team. Knowing that the potential exists for an interaction allows for either more careful monitoring (as in the case of tricyclic antidepressants) or the choice of alternative treatments or precautions (such as barrier contraceptive methods).

Protease inhibitors are the most difficult antiretrovirals in terms of drug–drug interactions. All protease inhibitors are metabolized by cytochrome 3A4 and are susceptible to inhibition and, more importantly, induction (i.e., lowered serum levels leading to viral resistance to ART). All protease inhibitors are inhibitors of 3A4 metabolism and can increase levels of medications dependent on 3A4 (this is especially important for drugs with potential toxicity or narrow margins of safety). Ritonavir is a pan-inhibitor of multiple enzymes and an inducer of 3A4. This induction can lower serum levels of OCPs, immunosuppressants, and other medications. Efavirenz is also a mixed inhibitor and inducer of 3A4, and nevirapine is an inducer of 3A4. Understanding the role of cytochrome P450, phase II enzymes (such as UGTs), and transporters in psychopharmacology of patients with HIV/AIDS will enhance efficacy, adherence, and patient health. Information about

TABLE 7.10 Basic Clinical Pearls

- START VERY LOW and GO VERY SLOW: HIV/AIDS psychopharmacology is similar to geriatric psychopharmacology, particularly in advanced AIDS.
- Persons with HIV/AIDS are exquisitely vulnerable to extrapyramidal, anticholinergic, and sedating side effects of all medications.
- Become familiar with medications that are cytochrome P450 3A4 inhibitors and inducers since these medications can alter ART, leading to toxicity or ineffectiveness of ART (consider memorizing Table 7.1).
- Recognize that ART, particularly the protease inhibitors (PIs) and some non-nucleoside reverse transcriptase inhibitors (NNRTIs), may profoundly alter the metabolism of medications dependent upon CYP 3A4, such as methadone, sedative-hypnotics, antipsychotics, cardiac medications, statins, and others, which may lead to toxicity or ineffectiveness of some non-ART medications that the patient may be taking.
- Review all medications being taken (including over-the-counter [OTC] and herbal substances) at every visit, keeping a medication log updated.
- Teach patients to use labeled pill boxes, and have them bring them to visits to monitor adherence (and catch newly prescribed medications you were unaware of).
- Educate HIV/AIDS patients and their caretakers about drug interactions and invite them to check with you (and every prescribing provider) before adding any new medication or drug.

these medications, from dosing to interactions, changes regularly. Some helpful Web sites providing updated information on these medications include the following:

http://www.hopkins-hivguide.org/
http://www.hiv-druginteractions.org/
http://www.tthhivclinic.com/interact_tables.html

A summary of basic principles in using psychotropics and other medications in persons with HIV or AIDS is provided in Table 7.10.

ACKNOWLEDGMENTS

The opinions and assertions contained herein are the private views of the individual authors and are not to be construed as official or as reflecting the views of the Department of the Army or the Department of Defense of the United States of America.

REFERENCES

Abbott Laboratories (2007). Norvir prescribing information.
Altice FL, Friedland GH, Cooney EL. (1999). Nevirapine induced opiate withdrawal among injection drug users with HIV infection receiving methadone. *AIDS* 13(8):957–962.

Ances BM, Letendre SL, Alexander T, Ellis RJ (2008). Role of psychiatric medications as adjunct therapy in the treatment of HIV associated neurocognitive disorders. *Int Rev Psychiatry* 20(1):89–93.

Armstrong SC, Cozza KL (2000). Consultation-liaison psychiatry drug–drug interactions update. *Psychosomatics* 41(6):541–543.

Armstrong SC, Cozza KL (2003a) Pharmacokinetic drug interactions of morphine, codeine, and their derivatives: theory and clinical reality, part I. *Psychosomatics* 44:167–171.

Armstrong SC, Cozza KL (2003b) Pharmacokinetic drug interactions of morphine, codeine, and their derivatives: theory and clinical reality, part II. *Psychosomatics* 44:515–520.

Avants SK, Margolin A, DePhilippis D, Kosten TR (1998). A comprehensive pharmacologic–psychosocial treatment program for HIV-seropositive cocaine- and opioid-dependent patients. Preliminary findings. *J Subst Abuse Treat* 15(3):261–265.

Back D (2006). HIV drug interactions. Retrieved June 19, 2006, from www.HIV-druginteractions.org

Barkin RL, Barkin S (2005). The role of venlafaxine and duloxetine in the treatment of depression with decremental changes in somatic symptoms of pain, chronic pain, and the pharmacokinetics and clinical considerations of duloxetine pharmacotherapy. *Am J Ther* 12(5):431–438.

Batki SL, Manfredi LB, Jacob P 3rd, Jones RT (1993). Fluoxetine for cocaine dependence in methadone maintenance: quantitative plasma and urine cocaine/benzoylecgonine concentrations. *J Clin Psychopharmacol* 13(4):243–250.

Bertz RJ, Cao G, Cavanaugh JH (1996). Effect of ritonavir on the pharmacokinetics of desipramine. Abstract no. B.1201. Presented at the 11th International Conference on AIDS, Vancouver, Canada.

Boehringer Ingelheim Pharmaceuticals (2008). Nevirapine prescribing information.

Boffito M, Rossati A, Reynolds HE, Hoggard PG, Back DJ, Di Perri G (2002). Undefined duration of opiate withdrawal induced by efavirenz in drug users with HIV infection and undergoing chronic methadone treatment. *AIDS Res Hum Retroviruses* 18(5):341–342.

Brechtl JR, Breitbart W, Galietta M, Krivo S, Rosenfeld B (2001). The use of highly active antiretroviral therapy (HAART) in patients with advanced HIV infection: impact on medical, palliative care, and quality of life outcomes. *J Pain Symptom Manage* 21(1):41–51.

Breitbart W, Marlotta R, Platt MM, Weisman H, Derevenco M, Grau C, Corbera K, Raymond S, Lund S, Jacobson P (1996). A double-blind trial of haloperidol, chlorpromazine, and lorazepam in the treatment of delirium in hospitalized AIDS pstients. *Am J Psychiatry* 153(2):231–237.

Bristol-Myers Squibb Pharmaceuticals (2008). Sustiva prescribing information.

Brugal MT, Domingo-Salvany A, Puig R, Barrio G, Garcia de Olalla P, de la Fuente L (2005). Evaluating the impact of methadone maintenance programmes on mortality due to overdose and AIDS in a cohort of heroin users in Spain. *Addiction* 100(7):981–989.

Carvalhal AS, de Abreu PB, Spode A, Correa J, Kapczinski F (2003). An open trial of reboxetine in HIV-seropositive outpatients with major depressive disorder. *J Clin Psychiatry* 64(4):421–424.

Cazzullo CL, Bessone E, Bertrando P, Pedrazzoli L, Cusini M (1998). Treatment of depression in HIV-infected patients. *J Psychiatry Neurosci* 23(5):293–297.

Clarke SM, Mulcahy FM, Tjia J, Reynolds HE, Gibbons SE, Barry MG, Back DJ. (2001). The pharmacokinetics of methadone in HIV-positive patients receiving the non-nucleoside reverse transcriptase inhibitor efavirenz. *Br J Clin Pharmacol* 51(3):213–217.

Clay PG (2002). The abacavir hypersensitivity reaction: a review. *Clin Ther* 24(10):1502–1514.

Clay PG, Adams MM (2003). Pseudo-Parkinson disease secondary to ritonavir-buspirone interaction. *Ann Pharmacother* 37(2):202–205.

Clevenbergh P, Corcostegui M, Gerard D, Hieronimus S, Mondain V, Chichmanian RM, Sadoul JL, Dellamonica P (2002). Iatrogenic Cushing's syndrome in an HIV-infected patient treated with inhaled corticosteroids (fluticasone propionate) and low dose ritonavir enhanced PI containing regimen. *J Infect* 44(3):194–195.

Cohen MA, Alfonso CA (2004). AIDS psychiatry: psychiatric and palliative care, and pain management. In GP Wormser (ed.), *AIDS and Other Manifestations of HIV Infection* (pp. 537–576). New York: Elsevier.

Cohen MA, Gorman JM (eds.) (2008). *Comprehensive Textbook of AIDS Psychiatry*. New York: Oxford University Press.

Court M (2009). Metabolism in depth: phase II. In GH Wynn, JR Oesterheld, KL Cozza, and Armstrong SC (eds.), *Clinical Manual of Drug Interaction Principles for Medical Practice* (pp 23–41). Washington, DC: American Psychiatric Press.

Cozza KL, Swanton EJ, Humphreys CW (2000). Hepatotoxicity with combination of valproic acid, ritonavir, and nevirapine: a case report. *Psychosomatics* 41(5):452–453.

Currier MB, Molina G, Kato M (2003). A prospective trial of sustained-release bupropion for depression in HIV-seropositive and AIDS patients. *Psychosomatics* 44(2):120–125.

Currier MB, Molina G, Kato M (2004). Citalopram treatment of major depressive disorder in Hispanic HIV and AIDS patients: a prospective study. *Psychosomatics* 45(3):210–216.

DeSilva KE, Le Flore DB, Marston BJ, Rimland D (2001). Serotonin syndrome in HIV-infected individuals receiving antiretroviral therapy and fluoxetine. *AIDS* 15(10):1281–1285.

De Wit S, Cremers L, Hirsch D, Zulian C, Clumeck N, Kormoss N (1999). Efficacy and safety of trazodone versus clorazepate in the treatment of HIV-positive subjects with adjustment disorders: a pilot study. *J Int Med Res* 27(5):223–232.

Dieterich DT, Robinson PA, Love J, Stern JO (2004). Drug-induced liver injury associated with the use of nonnucleoside reverse-transcriptase inhibitors. *Clin Infect Dis* 38(Suppl. 2):S80–S89.

DiMatteo MR, Lepper HS, Croghan TW (2000). Depression is a risk factor for noncompliance with medical treatment: meta-analysis of the effects of anxiety and depression on patient adherence. *Arch Intern Med* 160(14):2101–2107.

Dorell K , Cohen MA, Huprikar SS, Gorman JM, Jones M (2005). Citalopram-induced diplopia. *Psychosomatics* 46:91–93.

Elliott AJ, Roy-Byrne PP (2000). Mirtazapine for depression in patients with human immunodeficiency virus. *J Clin Psychopharmacol* 20(2):265–267.

Elliott AJ, Uldall KK, Bergam K, Russo J, Claypoole K, Roy-Byrne PP (1998). Randomized, placebo-controlled trial of paroxetine versus imipramine in depressed HIV-positive outpatients. *Am J Psychiatry* 155(3):367–372.

Fernandez F, Levy JK (1991). Benzodiazepines in the medically ill. In PP Roy-Byrne and D Cowlet (eds.), *Benzodiazepines in Clinical Practice: Risks and Benefits* (pp. 179–200). Washington, DC: American Psychiatric Press.

Fernandez F, Levy JK (1993). The use of molindone in the treatment of psychotic and delirious patients infected with the human immunodeficiency virus. Case reports. *Gen Hosp Psychiatry* 15(1):31–35.

Fernandez F, Levy JK (1994). Psychopharmacology in HIV spectrum disorders. *Psychiatr Clin North Am* 17(1):135–148.

Fernandez F, Levy JK, Galizzi H (1988). Response of HIV-related depression to psychostimulants: case reports. *Hosp Community Psychiatry* 39(6): 628–631.

Fernandez F, Levy JK, Samley HR, Pirozzolo FJ, Lachar D, Crowley J, Adams S, Ross B, Ruiz P (1995). Effects of methylphenidate in HIV-related depression: a comparative trial with desipramine. *Int J Psychiatry Med* 25(1):53–67.

Ferrando SJ, Goldman JD, Charness WE (1997). Selective serotonin reuptake inhibitor treatment of depression in symptomatic HIV infection and AIDS. Improvements in affective and somatic symptoms. *Gen Hosp Psychiatry* 19(2):89–97.

Fichtenbaum CJ, Gerber JG, Rosenkranz SL, Segal Y, Aberg JA, Blaschke T, Alston B, Fang F, Kosel B, Aweeka F (2002). Pharmacokinetic interactions between protease inhibitors and statins in HIV seronegative volunteers: ACTG study a5047. *AIDS* 16(4):569–577.

Forns X, Caballeria J, Bruguera M, Salmeron J.M, Vilella A, Mas A, Pares A, Rodes L (1994). Disulfiram-induced hepatitis. Report of four cases and review of the literature. *J Hepatol* 21(5):853–857.

Geletko SM, Erickson AD (2000). Decreased methadone effect after ritonavir initiation. *Pharmacotherapy* 20(1):93–94.

Gerber JG, Rosenkranz SL, Fichtenbaum CJ, Vega JM, Yang A, Alston BL, Brobst SW, Segal Y, Aberg JA (2005). Effect of efavirenz on the pharmacokinetics of simvastatin, atorvastatin, and pravastatin: results of AIDS clinical trials group 5108 study. *J Acquir Immune Defic Syndr* 39(3):307–312.

Goldstein BJ, Goodnick PJ (1998). Selective serotonin reuptake inhibitors in the treatment of affective disorders—III. Tolerability, safety and pharmacoeconomics. *J Psychopharmacol* 12(3 Suppl. B):S55–S87.

Gowing LR, Farrell M, Bornemann R, Sullivan LE, Ali RL (2006). Brief report: methadone treatment of injecting opioid users for prevention of HIV infection. *J Gen Intern Med* 21(2):193–195.

Grassi B, Gambini O, Garghentini G, Lazzarin A, Scarone S (1997). Efficacy of paroxetine for the treatment of depression in the context of HIV infection. *Pharmacopsychiatry* 30(2):70–71.

Grassi B, Gambini O, Scarone S (1995). Notes on the use of fluvoxamine as treatment of depression in HIV-1-infected subjects. *Pharmacopsychiatry* 28(3):93–94.

Greenblatt DJ, von Moltke LL, Harmatz JS, Durol AL, Daily JP, Graf JA, Mertzanis P, Hoffman JL, Shader RI (2000). Alprazolam–ritonavir interaction: implications for product labeling. *Clin Pharmacol Ther* 67(4):335–341.

Greenblatt DJ, von Moltke LL, Harmatz JS, Fogelman SM, Chen G, Graf JA, Mertzanis P, Byron S, Culm KE, Granda BW, Daily JP, Shader RI (2003). Short-term exposure to low-dose ritonavir impairs clearance and enhances adverse effects of trazodone. *J Clin Pharmacol* 43(4):414–422.

Grinsztejn B, Nguyen BY, Katlama C, et al. (2007). Safety and efficacy of the HIV-1 integrase inhibitor raltegravir (MK-0518) in treatment-experienced patients with multidrug-resistant virus: a phase II randomised controlled trial. *Lancet* 369:1261–1269.

Gupta SK, Dube MP (2002). Exogenous Cushing syndrome mimicking human immunodeficiency virus lipodystrophy. *Clin Infect Dis* 35(6): E69–E71.

Hachad H, Ragueneau-Majlessi I, Levy RH (2002). New antiepileptic drugs: review on drug interactions. *Ther Drug Monit* 24(1):91–103.

Hahn K, Arendt G, Braun JS, von Giesen HJ, Husstedt IW, Maschke M, Straube ME, Schiekle E. (2004). A placebo-controlled trial of gabapentin for painful HIV-associated sensory neuropathies. *J Neurol* 251(10): 1260–1266.

Hansen RA, Gartlehner G, Lohr KN, Gaynes BN, Carey TS (2005). Efficacy and safety of second-generation antidepressants in the treatment of major depressive disorder. *Ann Intern Med* 143(6):415–426.

Harvey BH, Meyer CL, Gallichio VS, Manji HK (2002). Lithium salts in AIDS and AIDS-related dementia. *Psychopharmacol Bull* 36(1):5–26.

Hellinger FJ, Encinosa WE (2005). Inappropriate drug combinations among privately insured patients with HIV disease. *Med Care* 43(9 Suppl.): III53–III62.

Hendrix CW, Wakeford J, Wire MB, Lou Y, Bigelow GE, Martinez E, Christopher J, Fuchs EJ, Snidow JW (2004). Pharmacokinetics and pharmacodynamics of methadone enantiomers after coadministration with amprenavir in opioid-dependent subjects. *Pharmacotherapy* 24(9):1110–1121.

Hesse LM, von Moltke LL, Shader RI, Greenblatt DJ (2001). Ritonavir, efavirenz, and nelfinavir inhibit cyp2b6 activity in vitro: potential drug interactions with bupropion. *Drug Metab Dispos* 29(2): 100–102.

Holmes VF, Fernandez F, Levy JK (1989). Psychostimulant response in AIDS-related complex patients. *J Clin Psychiatry* 50(1):5–8.

Horberg MA, Silverberg MJ, Hurley LB, Towner WJ, Klein DB, Bersoff-Matcha S, Weinberg WG, Antoniskis D, Mogyoros M, Dodge WT, Dobrinich R, Quesenberry CP, Kovach DA (2008). Effects of depression and selective serotonin reuptake inhibitor use on adherence to highly active antiretroviral therapy and on clinical outcomes in HIV-infected patients. *J Acquir Immune Defic Syndr* 47(3):384–90.

Hording M, Gotzsche PC, Bygbjerg IC, Christensen LD, Faber V (1990). Lack of immunomodulating effect of disulfiram on HIV positive patients. *Int J Immunopharmacol* 12(2):145–147.

Hulgan T, Sterling TR, Daugherty J, Arbogast PG, Raffanti S, Ray W (2005). Prescribing of contraindicated protease inhibitor and statin combinations among HIV-infected persons. *J Acquir Immune Defic Syndr* 38 (3):277–282.

Hulse GK, Arnold-Reed DE, O'Neil G, Chan CT, Hansson RC (2004). Achieving long-term continuous blood naltrexone and 6-beta-naltrexol coverage following sequential naltrexone implants. *Addict Biol* 9(1):67–72.

Iribarne C, Berthou F, Carlhant D, Dreano Y, Picart D, Lohezic F, Riche C (1998). Inhibition of methadone and buprenorphine N-dealkylations by three HIV-1 protease inhibitors. *Drug Metab Dispos* 26(3):257–260.

Isentress (package insert) (2007) Whitehouse Station, NJ, Merck & Co.

Jover F, Cuadrado JM, Andreu L, Merino J (2002) Reversible coma caused by risperidone–ritonavir interaction. *Clin Neuropharmacol* 25(5):251–253.

Kato Y, Fujii T, Mizoguchi N, Takata N, Ueda K, Feldman MD, Kayser SR (2000). Potential interaction between ritonavir and carbamazepine. *Pharmacotherapy* 20(7):851–854.

Kelly DV, Beique LC, Bowmer MI (2002). Extrapyramidal symptoms with ritonavir/indinavir plus risperidone. *Ann Pharmacother* 36(5):827–830.

Kristiansen JE, Hansen JB (2000). Inhibition of HIV replication by neuroleptic agents and their potential use in HIV infected patients with AIDS related dementia. *Int J Antimicrob Agents* 14(3):209–213.

Kulig CC, Beresford T P (2005). Hepatitis C in alcohol dependence: drinking versus disulfiram. *J Addict Dis* 24(2):77–89.

Laguno M, Blanch J, Murillas J, Blanco JL, Leon A, Lonca M, Larrousse M. Biglia A, Martinez E, Garcia F, Miro JM, de Pablo J, Gatell JM, Mallolas J (2004). Depressive symptoms after initiation of interferon therapy in human immunodeficiency virus–infected patients with chronic hepatitis C. *Antivir Ther* 9(6):905–909.

La Spina I, Porazzi D, Maggiolo F, Bottura P, Suter F (2001). Gabapentin in painful HIV-related neuropathy: a report of 19 patients, preliminary observations. *Eur J Neurol* 8(1):71–75.

Lera G, Zirulnik J (1999). Pilot study with clozapine in patients with HIV-associated psychosis and drug-induced parkinsonism. *Mov Disord* 14(1):128–131.

Levin GM, Nelson LA, DeVane CL, Preston SL, Eisele G, Carson SW (2001). A pharmacokinetic drug–drug interaction study of venlafaxine and indinavir. *Psychopharmacol Bull* 35(2):62–71.

Levine S, Anderson D, Bystritsky A, Baron D (1990). A report of eight HIV-seropositive patients with major depression responding to fluoxetine. *J Acquir Immune Defic Syndr* 3(11):1074–1077.

Maggi JD, Halman MH (2001). The effect of divalproex sodium on viral load: a retrospective review of HIV-positive patients with manic syndromes. *Can J Psychiatry* 46(4):359–362.

Maggi P, Ladisa N, Cinori E, et al. (2004). Cutaneous injection site reactions to long-term therapy with enfuvirtide. *J Antimicrob Chemother* 53:678–681.

Marketscan (1999–2000). http://www.medstatmarketscan.com/. Ann Arbor, MI: Thomson Medstat.

Mattick RP, Ali R, White JM, O'Brien S, Wolk S, Danz C (2003). Buprenorphine versus methadone maintenance therapy: a randomized double-blind trial with 405 opioid-dependent patients. *Addiction* 98(4): 441–452.

McDowell JA, Chittick GE, Stevens CP, Edwards KD, Stein DS (2000) Pharmacokinetic interaction of abacavir (1592U89) and ethanol in human immunodeficiency virus–infected adults. *Antimicrob Agents Chemother*; 44(6):1686–90.

Merry C, Mulcahy F, Barry M, Gibbons S, Back D (1997). Saquinavir interaction with midazolam: pharmacokinetic considerations when prescribing protease inhibitors for patients with HIV disease. *AIDS* 11(2):268–269.

Mouly S, Lown KS, Kornhauser D, Joseph JL, Fiske WD, Benedek IH, Watkins PB (2002). Hepatic but not intestinal CYP3A4 displays dose-dependent induction by efavirenz in humans. *Clin Pharmacol Ther* 72(1):1–9.

Moyle G (2000). Clinical manifestations and management of antiretroviral nucleoside analog-related mitochondrial toxicity. *Clin Ther* 22(8):911–936; discussion 898.

Muirhead G, Ridgway C, Leahy D, et al. (2004). A study to investigate the combined coadministration of P450 CYP3A4 inhibitors and inducers on the pharmacokinetics of the novel CCR5 inhibitor UK-427,857. *Seventh International Congress on Drug Therapy in HIV Infection*, Glasgow, abstract P284.

Nath A, Jankovic J, Pettigrew LC (1987). Movement disorders and AIDS. *Neurology* 37(1):37–41.

Oesterheld JR (2009a). Gynecology: oral contraceptives. In GH Wynn, JR Oesterheld, KL Cozza, SC Armstrong (eds.), *Clinical Manual of Drug Interaction Principles for Medical Practice* (pp. 191–210). Washington, DC: American Psychiatric Press.

Oesterheld JR (2009b). Transporters. In GH Wynn, JR Oesterheld, KL Cozza, SC Armstrong (eds.), *Clinical Manual of Drug Interaction Principles for Medical Practice* (pp. 42–70). Washington, DC: American Psychiatric Press.

Oesterheld JR, Armstrong SC, Cozza KL (2004). Ecstasy: pharmacodynamic and pharmacokinetic interactions. *Psychosomatics* 45:84–87.

Ouellet D, Hsu A, Qian J, Locke CS, Eason CJ, Cavanaugh JH, Leonard JM, Granneman GR (1998). Effect of ritonavir on the pharmacokinetics of ethinyl oestradiol in healthy female volunteers. *Br J Clin Pharmacol* 46(2):111–116.

Park-Wyllie LY, Antoniou T (2003). Concurrent use of bupropion with CYP2B6 inhibitors, nelfinavir, ritonavir and efavirenz: a case series. *AIDS* 17 (4):638–640.

Penzak SR, Hon YY, Lawhorn WD, Shirley KL, Spratlin V, Jann MW (2002). Influence of ritonavir on olanzapine pharmacokinetics in healthy volunteers. *J Clin Psychopharmacol* 22(4):366–370.

Piscitelli SC, Kress DR, Bertz RJ, Pau A, Davey R (2000). The effect of ritonavir on the pharmacokinetics of meperidine and normeperidine. *Pharmacotherapy* 20(5):549–553.

Rabkin JG, McElhiney MC, Rabkin R, Ferrando SJ (2004). Modafinil treatment for fatigue in HIV+ patients: a pilot study. *J Clin Psychiatry* 65(12):1688–1695.

Rabkin JG, Harrison WM (1990). Effect of imipramine on depression and immune status in a sample of men with HIV infection. *Am J Psychiatry* 147(4):495–497.

Rabkin JG, Rabkin R, Harrison W, Wagner G (1994a). Effect of imipramine on mood and enumerative measures of immune status in depressed patients with HIV illness. *Am J Psychiatry* 151(4):516–523.

Rabkin JG, Rabkin R, Wagner G (1994b). Effects of fluoxetine on mood and immune status in depressed patients with HIV illness. *J Clin Psychiatry* 55(3):92–97.

Rabkin JG, Wagner G, Rabkin R (1994c). Effects of sertraline on mood and immune status in patients with major depression and HIV illness: an open trial. *J Clin Psychiatry* 55(10):433–439.

Rabkin JG, Wagner GJ, Rabkin R (1999). Fluoxetine treatment for depression in patients with HIV and AIDS: a randomized, placebo-controlled trial. *Am J Psychiatry* 156(1):101–107.

Radominska-Pandya A, Pokrovskaya ID, Xu J, Little JM, Jude AR, Kurten RC, Czernik PJ (2002). Nuclear UDP-glucuronosyltransferases: identification of UGT2B7 and UGT1A6 in human liver nuclear membranes. *Arch Biochem Biophys* 399:37–48.

Ramachandran G, Glickman L, Levenson J, Rao C (1997). Incidence of extrapyramidal syndromes in AIDS patients and a comparison group of medically ill patients. *J Neuropsychiatry Clin Neurosci* 9(4):579–583.

Razali SM, Hasanah CI (1999). Cost-effectiveness of cyclic antidepressants in a developing country. *Aust N Z J Psychiatry* 33(2):283–284.

Roche Pharmaceuticals (2003/2004). Fortovase/invirase prescribing information.

Romanelli F, Pomeroy C (2003). Concurrent use of antiretrovirals and anticonvulsants in human immunodeficiency virus (HIV) seropositive patients. *Curr Pharm Des* 9(18):1433–1439.

Rotzinger S, Fang J, Coutts RT, Baker GB (1998). Human CYP2D6 and metabolism of m-chlorophenylpiperazine. *Biol Psychiatry* 44(11):1185–1191.

Royal College of Psychiatrists (2009). Metabolism of methylphenidate. Retrieved September 18, 2009, from http://www.rcpsych.ac.uk/training/cpd/adhd/therapy/methylphenidate/pharmacokinetics/metabolism.aspx

Sandson NB, Armstrong SC, Cozza KL (2005). An overview of psychotropic drug–drug interactions. *Psychosomatics* 46:464–494.

Satel SL, Nelson JC (1989). Stimulants in the treatment of depression: a critical overview. *J Clin Psychiatry* 50(7):241–249.

Schatzberg AF, Nemeroff CB (eds.) (2009) *The American Psychiatric Publishing Textbook of Psychopharmacology*, fourth edition. Arlington, VA: American Psychiatric Publishing.

Seminari E, Castagna A, Lazzarin A (2008). Etravirine for the treatment of HIV infection. *Expert Rev Anti Infect Ther* 6(4):427–433.

Simpson DM, McArthur JC, Olney R, Clifford D, So Y, Ross D, Baird BJ, Barrett P, Hammer AE (2003). Lamotrigine for HIV-associated painful sensory neuropathies: a placebo-controlled trial. *Neurology* 60(9):1508–1514.

Simpson DM, Olney R, McArthur JC, Khan A, Godbold J, Ebel-Frommer K (2000). A placebo-controlled trial of lamotrigine for painful HIV-associated neuropathy. *Neurology* 54(11):2115–2119.

Singh AN, Golledge H, Catalan J (1997). Treatment of HIV-related psychotic disorders with risperidone: a series of 21 cases. *J Psychosom Res* 42(5): 489–493.

Smith PF, DiCenzo R, Morse GD (2001). Clinical pharmacokinetics of nonnucleoside reverse transcriptase inhibitors. *Clin Pharmacokinet* 40(12): 893–905.

Stark K, Muller R, Bienzle U, Guggenmoos-Holzmann I (1996). Methadone maintenance treatment and HIV risk-taking behaviour among injecting drug users in Berlin. *J Epidemiol Community Health* 50(5):534–537.

Stein G, Bernadt M (1993). Lithium augmentation therapy in tricyclic-resistant depression. A controlled trial using lithium in low and normal doses. *Br J Psychiatry* 162:634–640.

Thormhalen M (2006). Paroxetine use during pregnancy: is it safe? *Ann Pharmacother* 40(10):1834–1837.

Tibotec (2008). Intelence (entravirine) prescribing information.

Treisman GJ, Angelino AF, Hutton HE (2001). Psychiatric issues in the management of patients with HIV infection. *JAMA* 286(22):2857–2864.

Uldall KK, Berghuis JP (1997). Delirium in AIDS patients: recognition and medication factors. *AIDS Patient Care STDS* 11(6):435–441.

Vila A, Mykeitiuk A, Bonvehi P, Temporiti E, Uruena A, Herrera F (2001). *Scand J Infect Dis* 33(10):788–789.

von Moltke LL, Greenblatt DJ, Granda BW, Giancarlo GM, Duan SX, Daily JP, Hamatz JS, Shader RI (2001). Inhibition of human cytochrome p450 isoforms by nonnucleoside reverse transcriptase inhibitors. *J Clin Pharmacol* 41(1):85–91.

Wagner GJ, Rabkin R (2000). Effects of dextroamphetamine on depression and fatigue in men with HIV: a double-blind, placebo-controlled trial. *J Clin Psychiatry* 61(6):436–440.

Wagner GJ, Rabkin JG, Rabkin R (1997). Dextroamphetamine as a treatment for depression and low energy in AIDS patients: a pilot study. *J Psychosom Res* 42(4):407–411.

Wise JE, Cozza KL (2009) Infectious diseases. In GH Wynn, JR Oesterheld, KL Cozza, and SC Armstrong (eds.), *Clinical Manual of Drug Interaction*

Principles for Medical Practice. Washington, DC: American Psychiatric Press.

Wood E, Hogg RS, Kerr T, Palepu A, Zhang R, Montaner JS (2005). Impact of accessing methadone on the time to initiating HIV treatment among antiretroviral-naive HIV-infected injection drug users. *AIDS* 19(8):837–839.

Wynn GH, Cozza KL, Zapor MJ, Wortmann GW, Armstrong SC (2005). Antiretrovirals. Part III: antiretrovirals and drugs of abuse. *Psychosomatics* 46:79–87.

Wynn GH, Oesterheld JR, Cozza KL, Armstrong SC (2009). *Clinical Manual of Drug Interaction Principles*. Washington, DC: American Psychiatric Press.

Yun LW, Maravi M, Kobayashi JS, Barton PL, Davidson AJ (2005). Antidepressant treatment improves adherence to antiretroviral therapy among depressed HIV-infected patients. *J Acquir Immune Defic Syndr* 38(4): 432–438.

Zhang X, Lalezari JP, Badley AD, Dorr A, Kolis SJ, Kinchelow T, Patel IH (2004). Assessment of drug–drug interaction potential of enfuvirtide in human immunodeficiency virus type 1–infected patients. *Clin Pharmacol Ther* 75(6):558–568.

Zisook S, Peterkin J, Goggin KJ, Sledge P, Atkinson JH, Grant I (1998). Treatment of major depression in HIV-seropositive men. HIV Neurobehavioral Research Center Group. *J Clin Psychiatry* 59(5):217–224.

Zuardi AW (1990). 5-HT-related drugs and human experimental anxiety. *Neurosci Biobehav Rev* 14(4):507–510.

8

PSYCHOTHERAPEUTIC TREATMENT OF PSYCHIATRIC DISORDERS

Jocelyn Soffer and Mary Ann Cohen

Persons living with HIV and AIDS face a complex array of stresses and challenges, as discussed throughout this book, which may overwhelm psychological functioning. This leads to considerable distress and suffering (Cohen et al., 2002), manifests in a multitude of psychiatric symptoms, and increases nonadherence to risk reduction and medical care. The aim of psychotherapeutic care for persons with HIV is to mitigate such distress through a combination of psychosocial interventions. Goals of such therapies may include enhancing adaptive coping strategies, facilitating adjustment to living with HIV, increasing social supports, and improving a patient's sense of purpose, self-esteem, and overall well-being. Goals may also include improving adherence to risk reduction and medical care, as well as preventing HIV transmission.

Psychological distress in persons with HIV infection is associated with decreased quality of life, disease progression, and mortality (Leserman, 2008). Considering the biopsychosocial model, emotional distress in HIV can be viewed as resulting from a combination of medical, psychological, and social factors related to the illness (see Table 8.1).

In some studies, improved social support and active coping styles in response to illness and stress have correlated with improved immunological parameters. Studies have also linked depressed mood and stressful life events to worsened immunological status, including decreased CD4 cell counts. Nonetheless, randomized controlled data demonstrating the ability of behavioral and social interventions to improve immune status remain conflicted; further evidence-based research is needed. While improving immunological status is a potential benefit of psychosocial treatment for people with HIV

TABLE 8.1 Biopsychosocial Model of Emotional Distress in Persons with HIV

1. **Medical**—e.g., multimorbid medical illness, physical symptoms, pain, and compromised energy level
2. **Psychological**—e.g., multimorbid psychiatric disorders; responses to diagnosis of HIV and loss of health; coping with HIV-stigma, rejection, bereavement, and loss; conflicts about disclosure, dependency, and meaning of life
3. **Social**—e.g., negotiation of social and intimate relationships and disclosure; stigma, and rejection by family, friends, and community; job loss, financial stress, and housing difficulties

infection, it is relieving the suffering inherent to psychiatric illness and improving patients' quality of life that remain the primary goals.

A variety of psychosocial interventions are available to persons with HIV, from individual to group-based formats. Such treatments span a spectrum of psychotherapeutic approaches, including supportive, psychodynamic, interpersonal, and cognitive-behavioral. This chapter will consider the benefits of such psychosocial interventions by summarizing the current state of research and findings for each of these treatment approaches, addressing both individual and group settings.

SUPPORTIVE PSYCHOTHERAPY

Most psychological interventions for persons with HIV focus on supporting and counseling to enhance adjustment to living with HIV. Supportive therapy primarily aims to reduce symptoms and ameliorate distress, by bolstering a patient's defenses and strengths, rather than seeking to change character structure or address deeper intra-psychic conflicts. Supportive therapy may take the form of individual or group treatment. While many psychiatrists and other mental health clinicians find supportive psychotherapy to be a useful modality in the care of persons with HIV and AIDS, there is little formalized research to provide an evidence base for its efficacy.

Group supportive treatments typically take the form of a "support group." Support groups provide a remarkable forum for persons with HIV and AIDS and have been described as a valuable modality for coping with general stresses of the illness and its treatments as well as HIV stigma. A summary of the functions of heterogeneous support groups can be found in Table 8.2.

Support groups often focus on particular issues, including bereavement support, parenting concerns, or trauma work. The benefits of such groups in reducing psychological distress and improving immunological parameters in HIV patients have been confirmed by several studies. Sikkema and

TABLE 8.2 Functions of HIV Support Groups

- Provide a safe environment to discuss concerns about HIV, its stigma, and its treatments
- Provide support from both members and leaders
- Confidential
- Nonjudgmental
- Compassionate
- Caring
- Participants are "all in the same boat"
- Acceptance and sense of family

colleagues (2004a) demonstrated the efficacy of a bereavement coping intervention for both general health-related quality of life and health issues specific to HIV, compared to a community standard of care, although findings were stronger in the group of women than in the men. Goodkin and colleagues (1998) reported on a randomized, controlled trial of a bereavement support group intervention, finding decreased levels of psychological distress and grief in the intervention group. There was also an improvement of immunological factors; the clinical relevance was supported by a decrease in health care use 6 months after the intervention. Because bereavement is an example of a severe life stressor, this conclusion may also hold for stressor-management interventions generally.

Other support groups may be tailored to specific patient populations, such as on the basis of gender, sexual orientation, or stage of illness. Evidence for the utility of such supportive interventions lies mostly in the subjective reports of patients, with many citing positive experiences and increased feelings of well-being and social support. Controlled trials for such interventions, both individual and group, however, remain sparse. One randomized study comparing a weekly supportive-expressive group intervention with an educational control condition found that distress and depressive symptoms decreased similarly in both groups (Weiss et al., 2003).

HIV-positive individuals often have a history of childhood physical and sexual trauma (Cohen, 1999; Sikkema et., 2004b). Feelings of mistrust, isolation, and anxiety in abuse victims frequently result in emotional and physical detachment from others and avoidance of intimacy, which can be targeted through a supportive group therapy approach (Sikkema et al., 2004b). Sikkema and colleagues (2004b) reported improvement in mood and symptoms of trauma in patients who participated in a trauma-focused coping group intervention. Working through exposure and trauma must be done carefully and with adequate support in order for patients to experience the treatment as safe and to avoid worsening of symptoms in a population with psychological vulnerability and multiple stresses. A helpful focus can be on skills building, use of coping tools, and practical application to everyday life.

The adjunctive use of medication should be considered in patients with significant depressive symptoms, given that some studies have shown it to be more effective at reducing symptoms than supportive psychotherapy. In a randomized study, fluoxetine plus group psychotherapy was found to be more effective than group psychotherapy alone in HIV-positive men with major depression (Zisook et al., 1998).

PSYCHODYNAMIC PSYCHOTHERAPY

Psychodynamic psychotherapy, which involves exploration of a patient's defenses, resistance, and intra-psychic conflicts, with a focus on unconscious mental life, transference issues, and a developmental perspective (Gabbard, 2007), is another modality that may be used to alleviate psychological distress in persons with HIV. Controlled studies of psychodynamically oriented psychotherapy are difficult to design, with correspondingly limited research. There is, however, considerable literature on the utility of psychodynamic therapy for patients struggling to maintain or regain a stable sense of self while coping with the challenges of HIV. The enhanced understanding of the conflicts and struggles of the HIV-positive patient afforded by such techniques has been described by multiple authors (Rogers, 1989; Weiss, 1997; Cohen, 1999; Cohen et al., 2001; Ricart et al., 2002; Cohen and Alfonso, 2004). Even early on in the epidemic of HIV, psychodynamic factors were identified as important to recognize and address in treatment, in ways that could both ameliorate suffering and decrease the transmission of the virus (Rogers, 1989).

This modality of treatment may be especially suited for patients with a trauma history, as physical illness, changes in the body, and relationship stresses can awaken conflicts triggered by early trauma and neglect. As described earlier, a history of childhood emotional, physical, and sexual trauma as well as neglect is associated with risk behaviors and is prevalent in persons with HIV (Lodico and DiClemente, 1994; Lenderking et al., 1997; Thompson et al., 1997; Wingood and DiClemente, 1997; Goodman and Fallot, 1998). Early childhood trauma-induced posttraumatic stress disorder (PTSD) is also prevalent in persons with HIV and has been reported to be as high as 40% (Cohen et al., 2002) and is associated with nonadherence to risk reduction and HIV medical care and antiretroviral medication (Cohen et al., 2001; Ricart et al., 2002). Psychodynamic psychotherapy can help persons with HIV and PTSD to heal and experience a decrease in distress as they work though such issues. Addressing childhood trauma in psychodynamic psychotherapy can not only improve psychiatric symptoms but also decrease risk behaviors and increase adherence to treatment (Ricart et al., 2002).

Other major themes that may surface and be addressed in psychodynamic work include fears about mortality, with the erosion of defensive denial as illness progresses, and conflicts surrounding sexuality. Severe illness and increased awareness of mortality can serve as catalysts for change, leading to motivation for reflective work, conflict resolution, and healing (Cohen, 1999). Exploration of the unique role and meaning of being HIV positive for each patient can facilitate acceptance and master and an increased sense of a functional and cohesive self (Weiss, 1997).

INTERPERSONAL PSYCHOTHERAPY

Interpersonal therapy was initially developed by Gerald Klerman, MD, and Myrna Weissman, PhD, as a focused and time-limited psychotherapy for the treatment of depression, with attention to the interpersonal and social context in which symptoms occur, rather than on intrapsychic conflicts and defense mechanisms. The aim of the therapy is to help patients link depressive symptoms to specific interpersonal stresses and facilitate resolution of those stresses. The therapy targets one of four areas: unresolved grief (following the death of a loved one), role transitions (difficulty adjusting to changed life circumstances), interpersonal role disputes (conflicts with a significant other), or interpersonal deficits (impoverished social networks) (Blanco and Weissman, 2007). This therapy has been adapted for patients with HIV with initial promising results.

One large randomized study found better outcomes with a 16-week interpersonal psychotherapy intervention for patients with HIV and depressive symptoms than outcomes both with supportive psychotherapy and with cognitive behavioral therapy (Markowitch et al., 1995, 1998). A recent telephone-delivered interpersonal therapy intervention in a rural area of the United States demonstrated a decrease in depressive symptoms and overall psychiatric distress, compared to the usual care control condition (Ransom et al., 2008). Interpersonal therapy has been suggested to be particularly appropriate for patients with HIV given its emphasis on life events and role transitions. More research of this modality is warranted.

COGNITIVE-BEHAVIORAL THERAPY

The largest body of evidence for effective psychological treatment of psychiatric symptoms and emotional distress in patients with HIV exists in the cognitive-behavioral realm. Originally developed by Aaron Beck for depression, cognitive-behavioral therapy (CBT) has now been demonstrated to have efficacy for many psychiatric conditions. Cognitive behavioral approaches vary in emphasis but share the common underlying features of being problem focused, goal directed, and time limited (Grant et al., 2007). The aim of CBT is to decrease symptoms by changing cognitions ("cognitive restructuring") and behaviors that are associated with dysfunction or distress. There are typically educational components to help the patient acquire skills and knowledge that can increase functioning. There is also an emphasis on a collaborative approach between patient and therapist, with an active role for the latter. A wide body of literature demonstrates the efficacy of CBT for patients with HIV, especially in conjunction with emphasis on stress management techniques, although more robust data exist for group than individual interventions.

In the first randomized trial comparing individual CBT with other psychotherapeutic approaches in patients with HIV, depressive symptoms decreased in all groups. In this 16-week intervention, CBT was found to be less effective than interpersonal therapy, and similarly effective to supportive psychotherapy (Markowitz et al., 1998). The authors make the point that functional scores improved in all groups, suggesting that some symptoms previously ascribed to HIV had been due to untreated depression, and that depressive symptoms should never be seen as "normal" in patients with HIV.

Cognitive-behavioral approaches can also be useful for decreasing substance use or increasing adherence to treatment in persons with HIV. One small study combined motivational interviewing with individual CBT sessions and found effective reduction of substance use (Parsons et al., 2005). Other studies have employed a contingency management (CM) individual intervention with positive results (Schroeder et al., 2006). This approach uses behavioral reinforcement techniques, such as tangible rewards (e.g., vouchers) for refraining from negative behaviors (e.g., drug use) or demonstrating positive behaviors.

The bulk of the literature on CBT for patients with HIV pertains to group rather than individual settings. A 16-week cognitive-behavioral group psychotherapy intervention for HIV-infected patients found improvement on measures of depression and anxiety, with effects that persisted at 3-month follow-up (Blanch et al., 2002). While most studies of CBT interventions have been positive, those comparing the specific efficacy to that of other types of psychotherapeutic modalities have yielded mixed results. Some have demonstrated CBT to be superior to other modalities, such as peer support/ counseling (for example, in a pilot study of Chinese patients examining psychological distress and quality of life [Molassiotis et al., 2002]). Other studies have found CBT techniques to be approximately as effective as other group psychotherapy modalities, such as experiential group psychotherapy (Mulder et al., 1995) or social support groups (Kelly et al., 1993).

Researchers have examined whether CBT methods might help reduce risk behaviors in HIV-positive populations, with largely mixed results. One study found that a cognitive-behavioral intervention in persons with substance use had limited advantages over a two-session standard drug counseling and testing protocol developed by the National Institute on Drug Abuse (NIDA) (Herschberger et al., 2003). Studies using contingency management interventions, as described above, have demonstrated more success at decreasing sexual risk behaviors (Shoptaw et al., 2005).

Intervention styles aiming to reduce emotional distress through psychoeducation and coping styles training have also been used. Chesney and colleagues (2003) compared the effects of a theory-based coping effectiveness training (CET) intervention with an active informational control and a wait-list control on psychological distress and positive mood. The CET participants showed significantly greater decreases in perceived stress and burnout as well as decreases in anxiety, with treatment differences for positive morale maintained at 12 months. Coping models have also been described that include examination of cognitive appraisals, emotional coping patterns, and behavior patterns, with improved immunological parameters in persons with HIV (Temoshok et al., 2008).

CBT has also been combined with stress management, relaxation techniques, and expressive-supportive therapeutic strategies, with significant improvement in depressive symptoms that were maintained at 1-year follow-up (Laperriere et al., 2005). A number of studies have examined the effects of a cognitive-behavioral stress management (CBSM) intervention on various immunological, psychological, and endocrine factors. The idea behind such research is that through stress reduction, interventions might correct functioning of the hypothalamic–pituitary–adrenal axis, known to be dysregulated in many patients with HIV infection (Cole, 2008).

In one series of such studies, the treatment protocol consisted of 10 weekly group sessions consisting of relaxation techniques (including muscle relaxation, guided imagery, meditation, and breathing exercises) and stress management (identifying automatic thoughts, using cognitive restructuring, increasing coping skills and assertiveness, and enhancing strategies for anger management and use of social supports) (Antoni et al., 2005). Patients were instructed to practice relaxation exercises twice daily between sessions and were assigned cognitive homework exercises. Compared to a wait-list control group, the CBSM group showed significantly lower depressed affect, anxiety, anger, and confusion.

Interestingly, multiple endocrine and immunological changes were also associated with these effects. The treatment group had lower levels of urinary cortisol, with decreases in depressed mood paralleling cortisol decreases in urine and decreased urinary norepinephrine (NE) output and anxiety decreases correlating with NE reduction (Antoni et al., 2000b). Immunological benefits were seen in the CBSM group as well (Antoni et al., 2000a). Other studies have similarly demonstrated improved immunological and endocrine parameters as well as mood improvements in HIV and cancer patients (Leszcz et al., 2004; Sherman et al., 2004). As summarized in a research review, "Irrespective of the treatment modality, it seems that interventions that are successful in improving psychological adjustment are more likely to have salutary effects on neuroendocrine regulation and immune status" (Carrico et al., 2008).

SPIRITUALLY FOCUSED CARE

Attention to the spiritual well-being of the medically ill has recently added a different dimension to the psychological treatment of these patients. A spiritual approach can help mitigate emotional distress and decrease the impact of depressive symptoms on health-related quality of life and illness morbidity (McClain et al., 2003; Newlin et al., 2003). While few studies in the literature specifically address spiritual care in the patients with HIV, one can draw on work using this approach with other medically ill populations. Dickerman and colleagues (2008) have written a multifaceted chapter on the palliative and spiritual care of persons with HIV, some of which is reviewed below.

Meaning-centered and spiritually focused interventions

Rousseau (2000) has developed an approach to the treatment of spiritual suffering that encompasses a blend of several basic psychotherapeutic principles, shown in Table 8.3.

This approach to spiritual suffering emphasizes religious expression that may be extremely helpful to some patients, but not comfortable for all patients or clinicians.

Breitbart and colleagues have applied the work of Frankl and his concepts of meaning-based psychotherapy (Frankl, 1955) to address spiritual suffering. This approach may benefit patients seeking guidance in dealing with issues of sustaining meaning, hope, and understanding in the face of their illness, while avoiding overt religious emphasis. "Meaning-centered group psychotherapy"

TABLE 8.3 Psychotherapeutic Principles in Spiritually Focused Treatment

1. Controlling physical symptoms
2. Providing a supportive presence
3. Encouraging life review to assist in recognizing purpose, value, and meaning
4. Exploring guilt, remorse, forgiveness, and reconciliation
5. Facilitating religious expression
6. Reframing goals
7. Encouraging meditative practices
8. Focusing on healing rather than cure

(Greenstein and Breitbart, 2000) uses a mixture of didactics, discussion, and experiential exercises that can also be used in individual therapy.

Treatment of demoralization and dignity therapy

Chochinov (2002) has developed a short-term dignity therapy for palliative patients to bolster the dying patient's will to live, decrease overall level of distress, and combat what has been termed the "syndrome of demoralization." The dignity model establishes the concept of "generativity" as a central dignity theme; as such, the sessions are taped, transcribed, edited, and then returned within days to the patient. The creation of a tangible product that will live beyond the patient and the immediacy of the returned transcript help to foster the patient's sense of purpose, meaning, and worth. Such transcripts can be left for family members or loved ones as part of a personal legacy that the patient has actively participated in creating.

OTHER GROUP FORMATS

Couple therapy

The psychological well-being of the HIV patient will inevitably affect the relationships and social systems in which he or she is involved. Both members of a couple face significant challenges in managing the relationship, with changing role dynamics and uncertainty about the future. Marshall Forstein (2008) has written extensively on the complexities that arise in work with couples affected by HIV; some key issues are summarized in this section.

Coping with HIV illness can challenge basic conceptions of sexuality and identity—fundamental aspects of the self that work to maintain psychological and physiological homeostasis. It can awaken fears of abandonment, existential anxiety about death, feelings of failure, and unacceptable rage leading to reaction formation, all of which can, consciously or unconsciously, affect relationship behaviors and patterns. Some people may emotionally distance themselves to protect their partner or themselves, while others may seek additional intimacy and closeness. Guilt and blame are common themes that emerge in work with both serodiscordant and seroconcordant couples. The sexual nature of HIV transmission also creates practical issues; mixed-status couples will need to negotiate satisfying and safe sexual practices. The AIDS-infected person can lose interest in sexual relations or feel unattractive because of the progressive nature of the illness.

Evaluation of the HIV-concordant or HIV-discordant couple should thus include not only review of a complete medical and psychiatric history but also assessment of psychological structures and defenses. One must also be

Table 8.4 Questions to Consider During Evaluation and Treatment of HIV-Seroconcordant and HIV-Serodiscordant Couples

- Is the major focus of the couple's decision to come for therapy to stay together or to find ways of separating? Is the goal the same for both members of the relationship?
- What is the customary nature of unions within the cultural background of each member?
- What is the current medical status of each partner? If there has been a major episode of illness, how have the individual and the couple coped?
- What does each member of the couple know about the other's sexual or intravenous drug use history, or both?
- To whom else has the HIV-positive person disclosed their status, and what was the response?
- What is the nature of support in the couple's social and familial network?
- How has the HIV-positive person's illness changed expectations about role identity in the relationship, and how has the couple reacted to and managed such changes?
- What are the individual coping strengths and how does the couple use the strengths of each to support the stability of the relationship?

sensitive to the cultural and individual factors that govern beliefs about and expectations for what the illness means and what the future is likely to bring. Table 8.4 contains examples of questions that may guide a clinician toward understanding of the meaning of the behavior, anxieties, fears, and coping mechanisms involved in a couple's relationship, in addition to the more concrete questions usually covered in a psychiatric evaluation.

Developing a trusting, nonjudgmental relationship with providers allows the couple to reflect on a dynamic individual and relationship process that is often unpredictable for providers and patients alike. Therapists can help couples manage these emotional complexities and the psychological impact of HIV infection.

Studies evaluating the efficacy of psychiatric interventions in this domain have largely been limited to the ability of couple therapy to reduce unprotected sex within serodiscordant couples. Some research has demonstrated benefit in promoting safe sexual practices by providing intervention sessions jointly to both members of a couple, with increased HIV testing and condom use. A six-session relationship-based intervention provided to women and their sexual partners significantly reduced the number of unprotected sexual acts at 12 months post-intervention compared with a control group (El Bassel et al., 2005). A recent study based on a psychosocial educational model incorporated four 2-hour sessions focused on communication, stress appraisal, adaptive coping strategies, and building social support in persons with HIV and their partners and found increased adaptive coping (Fife et al., 2008). A manual is now available for this treatment approach.

Clinical work with HIV-discordant couples may elicit strong counter-transference feelings in the therapist, as people do not always act in a way that an outside observer would deem "rational." Therapists may experience frustration and anxiety when witnessing continued risk-taking behavior within discordant couples. Cultural norms of gender roles, autonomy, and beliefs that differ from the therapist's own views may elicit countertransference that, if unexamined, can affect the therapy process. Powerful emotional reactions may also occur when HIV-affected couples discuss issues related to child rearing. Supervision can be very helpful to the clinician in understanding and facing ambivalent feelings that may arise.

As more HIV-infected people are treated with and maintain adherence to antiretrovirals, there is a shift in identification with a chronic to that with a lethal illness. Many are searching for ways to move forward in changing careers, having children, and re-entering the social world. Therapeutic strategies should address the complex factors and underlying strengths and vulnerabilities brought out in couples trying to remain alive and connected in the face of a terrible illness. Couples may find that issues of intimacy, fears of transmission, adherence, and the many emotional aspects of coping with an unpredictable chronic disease will fluctuate at different periods in the normal course of development. Health-care providers should maintain a dynamic view of the medical and mental health concerns of individuals and those of couples over time.

Family therapy

Medically ill parents who care for their children while simultaneously coping with ongoing physical symptoms face particular challenges and are especially vulnerable to psychosocial stressors that may affect their health. These parents often struggle with social and financial difficulties that have a great impact on their children's well-being. If the children themselves are HIV positive, maintaining healthy family dynamics can be especially difficult. Issues around disclosure, emotional reactions to the HIV diagnosis, fear of death, role adjustments, loss and bereavement, and social stigma are all examples of challenges to families with HIV. Pressure to reduce risky behaviors also commonly presents as a struggle.

Multiple studies have reported increased adherence, improved well-being, and improved health measures in families receiving family group support (Kmita et al., 2002; Lyon et al., 2003; Mitrani et al., 2003; Rotheram-Borus et al., 2003; McKay et al., 2004). These interventions have been conducted in various settings, including outpatient clinic and therapeutic camp (Kmita et al., 2002), using different modalities, such as a peer approach with "treatment buddies" (Lyon et al., 2003), and using different facilitators, including school staff and community-based agency representatives to deliver family-based preventive intervention (McCay et al., 2004). Family-focused grief therapy (FFGT) represents a family approach to bereavement that aims to enhance family functioning while supporting the expression of grief (Kissane et al., 2006). This approach promotes open communication of thoughts and feelings and teaches effective problem solving to reduce conflict and increase tolerance of different opinions. The improved functioning of the family as a unit helps advance adaptive mourning.

One study of a family-based intervention helped parents with HIV and their adolescent children to cope with the HIV diagnosis, promote positive health behaviors, support healthy family dynamics, and reduce risk behaviors, even as parents were dying (Rotheram-Borus et al., 2001). The intervention was delivered in 24 modules over 12 Saturdays and was found to reduce emotional distress, decrease problem behaviors, and improve developmental outcomes of the children in up to 6- year follow-up measures (Roheram-Borus et al., 2004). Additionally, follow-up studies found that grandchildren in the intervention condition displayed fewer behavioral symptoms, had more positive home environments, and scored higher on measures of cognitive development, suggesting the intergenerational benefits of family intervention (Rotheram-Borus et al., 2006). For further discussion of treatment of children and adolescents with HIV, please refer to Chapter 3, HIV through the Life Cycle.

Summary

The mental health needs of persons with HIV vary widely, depending on many factors including the stage of illness, current and past life circumstances, and prior psychological functioning. A variety of psychosocial interventions are available to persons with HIV, from individual to group-based formats, spanning a spectrum of psychotherapeutic approaches including supportive, psychodynamic, interpersonal, and cognitive-behavioral, as well as specific group formats such as couples and families. Benefits of psychosocial treatment include decreasing emotional distress, improving adaptive coping skills, improving adherence, decreasing risk behaviors, and facilitating overall improved physical and mental health, along with improved immunological parameters. Each interventional approach and treatment setting offers different merits and must be carefully selected to best suit the particular needs of the individual, couple, or family presenting for treatment.

References

Antoni MH, Cruess DG, Cruess S, Lutgendorf S, Kumar M, Ironson G, Klimas N, Fletcher MA, Schneiderman N (2000a). Cognitive-behavioral stress management intervention effects on anxiety, 24-hr urinary norepinephrine output, and

T-cytotoxic/suppressor cells over time among symptomatic HIV-infected gay men. *J Consult Clin Psychol* 68(1):31–45.

Antoni MH, Cruess DG, Klimas N, Carrico AW, Maher K, Cruess S, Lechner SC, Kumar M, Lutgendorf S, Ironson G, Fletcher MA, Schneiderman N (2005). Increases in a marker of immune system reconstitution are predated by decreases in 24-h urinary cortisol output and depressed mood during a 10-week stress management intervention in symptomatic HIV-infected men. *J Pscyhosom Res* 58:3–13.

Antoni MH, Cruess S, Cruess DG, Kumar M, Lutgendorf S, Ironson G, Dettmer E, Williams J, Klimas N, Fletcher MA, Schneiderman N (2000b). Cognitive-behavioral stress management reduces distress and 24-hour urinary free cortisol output among symptomatic HIV-infected gay men. ó*Ann Behav Med* 22(1):29–37.

Blanch J, Rousaud A, Hautzinger M, Martínez E, Peri J-M, Andrés S, Cirera E, Gatell JM, Gastó C (2002). Assessment of the efficacy of a cognitive-behavioural group psychotherapy programme for HIV-infected patients referred to a con-sultation-liaison psychiatry department. *Psychother Psychosom* 71:77–84.

Blanco C, Weissman MM (2007). Interpersonal psychotherapy. In GO Gabbard, JS Beck, and J Holmes (eds.), *Oxford Textbook of Psychotherapy* (pp. 27–34). New York: Oxford University Press.

Carrico AW, Antoni MH (2008). Effects of psychological interventions on neuroendocrine hormone regulation and immune status in HIV-positive persons: a review of randomized controlled trials. *Psychosom Med* 70 (5):575–584.

Chesney MA, Chamber DB, Taylor JM, Johnson LM, Folkman S (2003). Coping effectiveness training for men living with HIV: results from a randomized clinical trial testing a group-based intervention. *Psychosom Med* 65(6):1038–1046.

Chochinov HM (2002). Dignity-conserving care: a new model for palliative care: helping the patient feel valued. *JAMA* 287(17):2253–2260.

Cohen MA (1999). Psychodynamic psychotherapy in an AIDS nursing home. *J Am Acad Psychoanal* 27(1):121–133.

Cohen MA, Alfonso CA, Hoffman RG, Milau V, Carrera G (2001). The impact of PTSD on treatment adherence in persons with HIV infection. *Gen Hosp Psychiatry* 23:294–296.

Cohen MA, Alfonso CA (2004). AIDS psychiatry: psychiatric and palliative care, and pain management. In GP Wormser (ed.), *AIDS and Other Manifestations of HIV Infection*, fourth edition. (pp. 537–576). New York: Elsevier.

Cohen MA, Gorman JM (2008). *Comprehensive Textbook of AIDS Psychiatry*. New York: Oxford University Press.

Cohen, MA, Hoffman, RG, Cromwell C, Schmeidler J, Ebrahim F, Carrera G, Endorf F, Alfonso CA, Jacobson JM (2002). The prevalence of distress in persons with human immunodeficiency virus infection. *Psychosomatics* 43:10–15.

Cole SW (2008). Psychosocial influences on HIV-1 disease progression: neural, endocrine, and virologic mechanisms. *Psychosom Med* 70(5):562–568.

Dickerman AL, Breitbart W, Chochinov HM (2008). Palliative and spiritual care of persons with HIV and AIDS. In MA Cohen and JM Gorman (eds.), *Comprehensive Textbook of AIDS Psychiatry* (pp. 417–437). New York: Oxford University Press.

El-Bassel N, Witte S, Gilbert L, Wu E, Chang M, Hill J, Steinglass P (2005). Long-term effects of an HIV/STI sexual risk reduction intervention for heterosexual couples. *AIDS Behav* 9(1):1–13.

Fife BL, Scott LL, Fineberg NS, Zwickl BE (2008). Promoting adaptive coping by persons with HIV disease: evaluation of a patient/partner intervention model. *Psychosom Med* 70(5):562–568.

Forstein M (2008). Young adulthood and serodiscordant couples. In MA Cohen and JM Gorman (eds.), *Comprehensive Textbook of AIDS Psychiatry* (pp. 341–355). New York: Oxford University Press.

Frankl VF (1955). *The Doctor and the Soul.* New York: Random House.

Gabbard G (2007). Major modalities: psychoanalytic/psychodynamic. In GO Gabbard, JS Beck, and J Holmes (eds.), *Oxford Textbook of Psychotherapy* (pp. 3–14). New York: Oxford University Press.

Goodkin K, Feaster DJ, Asthana D, et al. (1998). A bereavement support group intervention is longitudinally associated with salutary effects on CD4 cell count and on number of physician visits. *Clin Diagn Lab Immunol* 5:382–391.

Goodman LA, Fallot RD (1998). HIV risk-behavior in poor urban women with serious mental disorders: association with childhood physical, and sexual abuse. *Am J Orthopsychiatry* 68:73–83.

Grant P, Young PR, DeRubeis RJ (2007). Cognitive and behavioral therapies. In GO Gabbard, JS Beck, and J Holmes (eds.), *Oxford Textbook of Psychotherapy* (pp. 15–26). New York: Oxford University Press.

Greenstein M, Breitbart W (2000). Cancer and the experience of meaning: a group psychotherapy program for people with cancer. *Am J Psychother* 54:486–500.

Hershberger SL, Wood MM, Fisher DG (2003). A cognitive-behavioral intervention to reduce HIV risk behaviors in crack and injection drug users. *AIDS Behav* 7(3):229–243.

Kelly JA, Murphy DA, Bahr GR, Kalichman SC, Morgan MG, Stevenson LY, Koob JJ, Brasfield TL, Bernstein BM (1993). Outcomes of cognitive-behavioral and support group brief therapies for depressed, HIV-infected persons. *Am J Psychiatry* 150(11):1679–1686.

Kissane DW, McKenzie M, Bloch S, Moskowitz C, McKenzie DP, O'Neill I (2006). Family focused grief therapy: a randomized, controlled trial in palliative care and bereavement. *Am J Psychiatry* 163(7):1208–1218.

Kmita G, Baranska M, Niemiec T (2002). Psychosocial intervention in the process of empowering families with children living with HIV/AIDS—a descriptive study. *AIDS Care* 14(2):279–284.

Laperriere A, Ironson GH, Antoni MH, Pomm H, Jones D, Ishii M, Lydston D, Lawrence P, Grossman A, Brondolo E, Cassells A, Tobin JN, Schneiderman N, Weiss SM (2005). Decreased depression up to one year following CBSM+ intervention in depressed women with AIDS: the smart/EST women's project. *J Health Psychol* 10(2):223–231.

Lenderking WR, Wold D, Mayer KH, et al. (1997). Childhood sexual abuse among homosexual men. Prevalence and association with unsafe sex. *J Gen Intern Med* 12:250–253.

Leserman J (2008). Role of depression, stress, and trauma in HIV disease progression. *Psychosom Med* 70(5):539–545.

Leszcz M, Sherman A, Mosier J, Burlingame GM, Cleary T, Ulman KH, Simonthon S, Latif U, Strauss B, Hazelton L (2004). Group interventions for patients with cancer and HIV disease: part IV. Clinical and policy recommendations. *Int J Group Psychother* 54(4):539–556; discussion, 557–562, 563–568, 569–574.

Lodico MA, DiClemente RJ (1994). The association between childhood abuse, and prevalence of HIV-related risk behaviors. *Clin Pediatr* 33:498–502.

Lyon ME, Trexler C, Akpan-Townsend C, Pao M, Selden K, Fletcher J, Addlestone IC, D'Angelo LJ (2003). A family group approach to increasing adherence to therapy in HIV-infected youths: results of a pilot project. *AIDS Patient Care STDS* 17(6):299–308.

Markowitz JC, Klerman GL, Clougherty KF, Spielman LA, Jacobsberg LB, Fishman B, Frances AJ, Kocsis JH, Perry SW (1995). Individual psychotherapies for depressed HIV-positive patients. *Am J Psychiatry* 152:1504–1509.

Markowitz JC, Kocsis JH, Fishman B, et al. (1998). Treatment of depressive symptoms in human immunodeficiency virus–positive patients. *Arch Gen Psychiatry* 55:452–457.

McClain CS, Rosenfeld B, Breitbart W (2003). Effect of spiritual well-being on end-of-life despair in terminally ill cancer patients. *Lancet* 361:1603–1607.

McKay MM, Chasse KT, Paikoff R, McKinney LD, Baptiste D, Coleman D, Madison S, Bell CC (2004). Family-level impact of the CHAMP Family Program: a community collaborative effort to support urban families and reduce youth HIV risk exposure. *Fam Process* 43(1):79–93.

Mitrani VB, Prado G, Feaster DJ, Robinson-Batista C, and Szapocznik J (2003). Relational factors and family treatment engagement among low-income, HIV-positive African American mothers. *Fam Process* 42(1):31–45.

Molassiotis A, Callaghan P, Twinn SF, Lam SW, Chung WY, Li CK (2002). A pilot study of the effects of cognitive-behavioral group therapy and peer support/counseling in decreasing psychological distress and improving quality of life in Chinese patients with symptomatic HIV disease. *AIDS Patient Care STDS* 16(2):83–96.

Mulder CL, Antoni MH, Emmelkamp PM, Veugelers PJ, Sandfort TG, van de Vijver FA, de Vries MJ (1995). Psychosocial group intervention and the rate of decline of immunological parameters in asymptomatic HIV-infected homosexual men. *Psychother Psychosom* 63(3-4):185–192.

Newlin K, Melkus GD, Chyun D, Jefferson V (2003). The relationship of spirituality and health outcomes in Black women with type 2 diabetes. *Ethnic Dis* 13:61–68.

Parsons JT, Rosof E, Punzalan JC, Di Maria L (2005). Integration of motivational interviewing and cognitive behavioral therapy to improve HIV medication adherence and reduce substance use among HIV-positive men and women: results of a pilot project. *AIDS Patient Care STDS* 19(1):31–39.

Ransom D, Heckman TG, Anderson T, Garske J, Holroyd K, Basta T (2008). Telephone delivered, interpersonal psychotherapy for HIV-infected rural persons with depression: a pilot trial. *Psychiatr Serv* 59(8):871–877.

Ricart F, Cohen MA, Alfonso CA, Hoffman RG, Quiñones N, Cohen A, Indyk D (2002). Understanding the psychodynamics of non-adherence to medical treatment in persons with HIV infection. *Gen Hosp Psychiatry* 24(3):176–180.

Rogers RR (1989). Beyond morality: the need for psychodynamic understanding and treatment of responses to the AIDS crisis. *Psychiatr J Univ Ott* 14(3):456–459.

Rotheram-Borus MJ, Lee MB, Gwadz M, Draimin B (2001). An intervention for parents with AIDS and their adolescent children. *Am J Public Health* 91(8):1294–1302.

Rotheram-Borus MJ, Lee M, Leonard N, Lin YY, Franzke L, Turner E, Lightfoot M, Gwadz M (2003). Four-year behavioral outcomes of an intervention for parents living with HIV and their adolescent children. *AIDS* 17(8):1217–1225.

Rotheram-Borus MJ, Lee M, Lin YY, Lester P (2004). Six-year intervention outcomes for adolescent children of parents with the human immunodeficiency virus. *Arch Pediatr Adolesc Med* 158(8):742–748.

Rotheram-Borus MJ, Lester P, Song J, Lin YY, Leonard NR, Beckwith L, Ward MJ, Sigman M, Lord L (2006). Intergenerational benefits of family-based HIV interventions. *J Consult Clin Psychol* 74(3):622–627.

Rousseau P (2000). Spirituality and the dying patient. *J Clin Oncol* 18:2000–2002.

Schroeder JR, Epstein DH, Umbricht A, Preston KL (2006). Changes in HIV risk behaviors among patients receiving combined pharmacological and behavioral interventions for heroin and cocaine dependence. *Addict Behav* 31(5):868–879.

Sherman AC, Leszcz M, Mosier J, Burlingame GM, Cleary T, Ulman KH, Simonton S, Latif U, Strauss B, Hazelton L (2004). Group interventions for patients with cancer and HIV disease: part II. Effects on immune, endocrine, and disease outcomes at different phases of illness. *Int J Group Psychother* 54(2):203–233.

Shoptaw S, Reback CJ, Peck JA, Yang X, Rotheram-Fuller E, Larkins S, Veniegas RC, Freese TE, Hucks-Ortiz C (2005). Behavioral treatment approaches for methamphetamine dependence and HIV-related sexual risk behaviors among urban gay and bisexual men. *Drug Alcohol Depend* 78:125–134.

Sikkema KJ, Hansen NB, Kochman A, et al. (2004a). Outcomes from a randomized controlled trial of a group intervention for HIV positive men and women coping with AIDS-related loss and bereavement. *Death Stud* 28:187–209.

Sikkema KJ, Hansen NB, Tarakeshwar N, Kochman A, Tate DC, Lee RS (2004b). The clinical significance of change in trauma-related symptoms following a pilot group intervention for coping with HIV-AIDS and childhood sexual trauma. *AIDS Behav* 8(3):277–291.

Temoshok LR, Wald RL, Synowski S, Garzino-Demo A (2008). Coping as a multisystem construct associated with pathways mediating HIV-relevant immune function and disease progression. *Psychosom Med* 70(5):555–561.

Thompson NJ, Potter JS, Sanderson CA, Maibach EW (1997). The relationship of sexual abuse, and HIV risk behaviors among heterosexual adult female STD patients. *Child Abuse Neglect* 21:149–156.

Weiss JJ (1997). Psychotherapy with HIV-positive gay men: a psychodynamic perspective. *Am J Psychother* 51(1):31–44.

Weiss JJ, Mulder CL, Antoni MH, de Vroome EM, Garssen B, Goodkin K (2003). Effects of a supportive-expressive group intervention on long-term psychosocial adjustment in HIV-infected gay men. *Psychother Psychosom* 72(3):132–140.

Wingood GM, DiClemente RJ (1997). Child sexual abuse, HIV sexual risk, and general relations of African-American women. *Am J Prev Med* 13:380–384.

Zisook S, Peterkin J, Goggin KJ, et al. (1998). Treatment of major depression in HIV-seropositive men. HIV Neurobehavioral Research Center Group. *J Clin Psychiatry* 59:217–224.

9

Symptoms Associated with HIV and AIDS

Harold W. Goforth and Mary Ann Cohen

Many persons with HIV and AIDS have symptoms that are unrelated to underlying psychiatric disorders but may masquerade as such. These symptoms may include insomnia, fatigue, nausea, or other troubling symptoms, and often result in suffering for patients, their families, and loved ones. The symptoms are common throughout the course of HIV and AIDS, from onset of infection to late-stage and end-stage AIDS. They need to be addressed whenever they occur and not only as part of end-of-life care. We present protocols to ameliorate or eliminate these symptoms and alleviate suffering.

FATIGUE

Fatigue is one of the most prevalent but underreported and undertreated aspects of HIV disease. The prevalence of fatigue in an HIV population has been estimated to affect at least 50% of seropositive individuals (Breitbart et al., 1998) and may affect up to 80% of the population. Darko and colleagues (1992) found that HIV-seropositive individuals were more fatigued, required more sleep and daytime naps, and showed less alert morning functioning than did persons who are HIV-seronegative. While the symptom of fatigue may fluctuate with increasing viral loads, there is no evidence base for a consistent correlation between fatigue and viral load. Fatigue is a pseudo-specific symptom common to a variety of disabilities found in an HIV population, and it has been linked to a variety of other AIDS-related disabilities including pain, anemia, impaired physical function, psychological distress, and depression. Hormonal alterations, such as those in testosterone and thyroxin, that occur in the context of HIV infection are also common in this group. While these findings are further discussed in Chapter 10, it is worth noting here that they can contribute substantially to tiredness and fatigue in this population. Other sources of fatigue include multimorbid chronic illnesses (opportunistic infections and cancers, chronic renal insufficiency, hepatitis C and other hepatic illnesses, and chronic obstructive pulmonary disease [COPD]) and some of their treatments (notably interferon/ribavirin for hepatitis C and cancer chemotherapy). Substances such as recreational drugs, nicotine, and caffeine are also factors in HIV-related fatigue.

Depression remains high on the differential diagnosis of fatigue-related complaints. The relationship between depression and fatigue is bidirectional, with each worsening the other. Barroso and colleagues (2002) found depression and anxiety to be statistically correlated with fatigue severity, illustrating the link between the two. However, it is erroneous to assume that all fatigue is related to depression or other psychiatric illness; Breitbart and colleagues (1998) found that only approximately half of fatigued subjects concurrently met criteria for depression. Aspects of depression that may help the practitioner to distinguish it from fatigue per se is the presence of anhedonia, or the inability to experience pleasure, instead of the inability to perform activities simply because of tiredness. Anhedonia nearly inevitably accompanies depression and persists even with the possibility of engaging in normally enjoyable activities and the energy level with which to do so. Treatment of depression is covered in more detail in Chapters 7 and 8 of this handbook.

Anemia is often characterized by a sense of persistent physical tiredness, mental exhaustion, impaired strength, and nonspecific symptoms such as dizziness. HIV-related myelosuppression is quite common, and HIV-seropositive individuals who have a low hematocrit or hemoglobin experience more fatigue than noninfected controls (Barroso et al., 2002). Commonly used antiretroviral agents (zidovudine, lamivudine) also can induce myeloid suppression that may add to that induced by viral toxicity. In addition to antiretroviral therapy, other medications that cause HIV-associated anemia include interferon/ribavirin for hepatitis C coinfection, chemotherapeutic agents used for cancers, and medications for multimorbid medical conditions. Other common causes of anemia in this population include erythropoietin deficiency that can occur secondary to HIV-associated nephropathy and renal involvement as well as anemia due to chronic disease (Sullivan et al., 1998). Persons with HIV/AIDS are also at increased risk for anemia due to B_{12} and folate deficiencies as a result of poor nutrition or inadequate intake. These conditions are associated with poverty and concurrent substance abuse patterns involving food neglect (Remacha and Cadafalch, 1999).

Multimorbid illness including opportunistic infections remains high on the list of differential diagnoses of fatigue in HIV. This is especially true of acute-onset fatigue or fatigue that has substantially changed in character from that previously experienced. In addition, endocrine abnormalities identified in patients with HIV are common causes of fatigue in this population (Rabkin et al., 2000; Soffer et al., 2008). Common differential diagnoses of fatigue are presented in Table 9.1. For a more complete discussion of medical multimorbidities, please see Chapter 10 of this handbook.

TABLE 9.1 Differential Diagnosis of Fatigue and Suggested Interventions

Differential Diagnosis	Intervention
Pain	• Diagnostic workup to address cause of pain complaint as well as treat pain according to WHO pain ladder (World Health Organization, 1986) See Chapter 12 of this handbook for details on stepwise treatment of pain
Anemia • HIV-related myelosuppression • Iatrogenic (ART related) • Erythropoetin deficiency due to HIV nephropathy or other renal disease • Anemia due to chronic disease • Nutritional (B_{12}/folate) deficiency • Ongoing blood loss	• Review history, physical exam • CBC with differential • Iron studies (serum Fe, ferritin, TIBC) • Folate, B_{12}, methylmalonic acid serum levels • Folate, B_{12} replacements if needed • Consider hematology–oncology consultation • Consider bone marrow biopsy in refractory cases • Complete evaluation for ongoing losses (e.g., upper and lower GI endoscopy, fecal occult blood loss) • Erythropoietin replacement therapy • Blood transfusions
Debility	• Diagnostic workup to address cause of debility • Physical or occupational therapy for reconditioning
Depression	• Diagnostic workup to establish cause depression. • Thyroid panel (TSH, free T4) • Gonadal panel (free testosterone, LH See Chapters 7 and 8 for treatment of HIV-associated depression

(continued)

Table 9.1 (Continued)

Differential Diagnosis	Intervention
Hypothyroidism	• TSH • Free T4 • Thyroid replacement with levothyroxine, based on laboratory scores and data • Reassess TSH, free T4 every 2–3 months after dosage change See Chapter 10 for further information
Hypogonadism	• Testosterone levels • Free testosterone level • LH level • Androgen replacement therapy
Opportunistic infections	• Diagnostic workup based on history and physical examination • Treatment based on particular diagnosis See Chapter 10 for further information on medical comorbidities
Substances of abuse	• Diagnostic workup based on history and physical examination • Treatment based on particular diagnosis See Chapter 6 for treatment of substance abuse

ART, antiretroviral therapy; CBC, complete blood count; GI, gastrointestinal; LH, luteinizing hormone; TIBC, total iron-binding capacity; TSH, thyroid-stimulating hormone; T4, thyroxine. *Source:* World Health Organization (1986); Henry (1998); Wagner et al. (1998); Breitbart et al. (2001); Afhami et al. (2007); Dickerman et al. (2008).

Sleep Disorders

Insomnia can be defined as persistent difficulty falling asleep or staying asleep, or as non-restorative sleep that is associated with decreased daytime function (Edinger et al., 2004). Insomnia is common in the general population with a prevalence estimated to be about 30%; the prevalence of insomnia in HIV-positive individuals has been reported to be decidedly higher (Rubinstein, 1998). It is tempting to assume that HIV-associated insomnia is due to the stress of a highly stigmatized physical illness, but that assumption is only partially correct and is negated somewhat by the observation that insomnia is a common initial complaint in otherwise asymptomatic HIV infection (Norman et al., 1992). A biopsychosocial approach to insomnia entails a comprehensive approach to both diagnosis and treatment (O'Dowd and Gomez, 2008).

The pathophysiology of insomnia in HIV is equally unclear. It is agreed that insomnia becomes a ubiquitous complaint in the latter stages of HIV infection (Moeller et al., 1991), which strongly supports HIV itself impacting biological sleep centers. However, other potential compounding factors associated with HIV along the life cycle include medication effects (e.g. efavirenz) (Nuñez et al., 2001; Fumaz et al., 2002), opportunistic infections, central nervous system disease, and chronic bereavement in the context of cumulative loss of function. One study of nonadherence in HIV patients showed that 10% of nonadherent subjects reported insomnia as a cause (Ammassari et al., 2001).

Persons with HIV have a high rate of multimorbid HIV and substance abuse disorders, both of which can exacerbate sleep disturbances substantially. Sleep disturbances are one of the strongest predictors of both current and future depressive disorders and manic-depressive syndromes. Substance abuse disorders involving psychostimulants or hallucinogens such as cocaine/methamphetamine and PCP can often present with sleeplessness as a common complaint, and these states of intoxication can often resemble manic or psychotic episodes. Similarly, even though alcohol, opiates, and marijuana are CNS depressants, impaired sleep is a highly common manifestation of abuse or dependence, and impaired sleep has been identified as one of the driving factors for nocturnal use of alcohol and marijuana in efforts to self-medicate a perceived sleep disturbance (Srisurapanont and Jarusuraisin, 1998; Arnedt et al., 2007).

Withdrawal states can also present with significant sleep disruption, and while many withdrawal states are self-limited (e.g. cocaine), many patients will continue to experience sleep disturbances up to many months after their initial detoxification from alcohol, opiates, and marijuana. This places them at higher risk of substance-related relapse and secondary depression unless the sleep disturbance is adequately identified and treated (Arnedt et al., 2007).

For a more comprehensive review of sleep disturbances, we refer the reader to a textbook chapter on the subject (O'Dowd and Gomez, 2008).

Disorders involving excessive daytime sleepiness are also important to consider when evaluating sleep complaints, and these diagnoses differ substantially from typical insomnia. Patients with insomnia frequently are tired yet cannot sleep, whereas those with excessive daytime sleepiness are tired and sleep too much. The most common disorders presenting as excessive daytime sleepiness include nonspecific fatigue, circadian shift disorders, sleep-related breathing disorders (Epstein et al., 1995; Lo Re et al., 2006), movement disorders, and narcolepsy spectrum disorders. Movement disorders can also produce excessive daytime sleepiness due to frequent nocturnal microarousals, with common causes including restless legs syndrome (RLS) or periodic limb movement disorder (PLMD).

It is also important to note important drug–drug interactions with antiviral agents when prescribing medications. In general, sleep agents with a high degree of dependency on the P450 3A4 system should be avoided in patients on protease inhibitors, given the rather marked increases in half-lives and duration noted with triazolam, alprazolam, and, to a lesser extent, zolpidem. These increased durations of action would likely be greater still in those with comorbid hepatic disease (Greenblatt et al., 1999). Safer choices include use of benzodiazepines that are conjugated only, such as lorazepam, oxazepam, or temazepam; however, use of benzodiazepines can also be problematic because of potential cognitive dysfunction, disinhibition, paradoxical agitation and confusion, and dosing in those with comorbid substance abuse. While cautious trials of trazodone may be considered in patients with sleep disorders, it should be kept in mind that trazodone is metabolized to a psychoactive metabolite (m-CPP) by the 3A4 system; m-CPP is further metabolized via the 2D6 isozyme. Any agent that promotes accumulation of m-CPP by either inducing the 3A4 pathway or inhibiting the 2D6 pathway may worsen insomnia complaints in these patients. See Table 9.2 for further details and a summary of differential diagnoses of insomnia.

TABLE 9.2 Differential Diagnosis of Insomnia and Interventions

Differential Diagnosis	Intervention
Disorders of Sleep Onset and Maintenance	
All disorders of sleep onset and maintenance	• Careful psychiatric history and examination
	• Assessment of patterns of eating and drinking
	• Caffeine and other stimulant use
	• Use and amount of substances containing caffeine such as coffee, tea, chocolate, and stimulating vitamin and soda drinks, e.g., colas
	• Assessment of use of prescribed and over-the-counter stimulants such as modafanil, methylphenidate, decongestants such as phenylephrine, and bronchodilators
	• Urine drug testing
	• Thyroid panel
Insomnia	• Relaxation response, meditation, yoga
	• Attention to basic concepts of sleep hygiene

	• Assessment of relative sleep comfort such
	• as sound, light, room temperature, sleeping conditions
	• Adequate daytime activity and exercise
	• Limitation or elimination of daytime napping
	• Cognitive therapy, if available
	• Atypical benzodiazepines, trazodone, and certain benzodiazepines (lorazepam, oxazepam, clonazepam) dosed to effect and with considerations of side effects as noted in text; cognitive therapy if available
Depression	See Chapters 6 and 7
Anxiety	See Chapters 6 and 7
Substance use disorders	See Chapters 6 and 7
Medical conditions	Treat medical condition underlying insomnia complaints occurring during use of hypnotics on short-term basis while underlying disorder is being corrected
Disorders of Excessive Daytime Somnolence	
All disorders of excessive daytime somnolence	• Careful history and physical examination
	• Polysomnography to diagnose obstructive/central sleep apnea, narcolepsy, idiopathic hypersomnia, PLMD
	• Electroencephalography if epilepsy being considered
Obstructive/central sleep apnea	Continuous positive airway pressure (CPAP) device titrated to effect on PSG, dental appliances, weight loss, psychostimulants
Narcolepsy and idiopathic hypersomnia	Psychostimulants. Strongly recommend referral to sleep specialist
Seizure disorders/epilepsy	Refer to epilepsy specialist for appropriate diagnosis and treatment
Circadian shift disorders	Cognitive-behavioral sleep therapy
Movement disorders (restless legs syndrome [RLS], periodic limb movement disorder [PLMD])	Dopamine agonists, clonazepam, and/or gabapentin titrated to effect

DISTURBANCES OF APPETITE AND NUTRITIONAL INTAKE

Disturbances of appetite and adequate nutritional intake also pose severe challenges to persons with HIV/AIDS. Cachexia remains a major cause of weight loss and increased morbidity and mortality, particularly in persons with AIDS who lack access to experienced HIV clinicians and antiretroviral therapy (ART) or who are unable to access care as a result of untreated psychiatric disorders. Cachexia manifests clinically with excessive weight loss in the setting of medical illnesses and is characterized by disproportionate muscle mass wasting. Cachexia is distinguished from starvation in that starvation results from direct caloric insufficiency and often results in fat loss with relatively greater preservation of muscle mass. Sarcopenia is another weight-loss syndrome resulting from muscle atrophy due to a variety of causes. Dehydration constitutes a fourth major category that is characterized by decreasing weight primarily due to fluid loss (Morley et al., 2006).

Cachexia identified within HIV/AIDS remains highly predictive of death. Common causes include depression, medications, opportunistic infections, and hypogonadism. This syndrome is highly debilitating for the sufferer, for with it invariably comes severe fatigue, markedly decreased quality of life, and a high risk of adverse events. The treatment of HIV-associated cachexia includes anabolic steroids, resistance exercise training, megestrol, dronabinol, and corticosteroids. However, even with these treatments, the syndrome is often highly refractory to treatment and is a leading cause of morbidity in persons with AIDS.

Both testosterone and nandrolone have demonstrated efficacy in improving lean-body mass, especially when combined with exercise and resistance training. The emerging risks of adverse events associated with megestrol, including thromboembolism, are significant as they may portend an increased mortality rate among chronic users or in patients who are not already in the terminal stages of their disease. While megestrol continues to have a place among orexigenic agents, its use must be carefully considered in the target population (Bodenner et al., 2007). The disproportionate fat gain associated with megestrol is difficult to accept for most patients, especially in an HIV population that may have many years to live if stabilized on antiviral therapy and who already have significant dyslipidemias.

Loss of appetite without cachexia (starvation) is also an important issue for persons with HIV, and determination of the etiology of the anorexia is paramount to appropriate treatment. Loss of appetite is a common presentation from a variety of factors including anatomic concerns, pain, iatrogenic, depression, and idiopathic causes. Anatomic factors that should be considered include oral infections with thrush and other opportunistic infections as well as side effects from concurrent treatments such as radiation or chemotherapy.

Similarly, nausea and vomiting can produce significant appetite loss; these symptoms are addressed in the following section.

Mirtazapine is an atypical antidepressant with a variety of effects including strong antihistiminergic effects with minimal anticholinergic function. This antidepressant may be a good choice for patients who demonstrate either prominent anorexia secondary to depression or anxiety or idiopathic disease with only a minimal risk of cognitive impairment. Additionally, it also possesses 5-HT$_3$ antagonist properties, making it a potential choice for nausea and vomiting (Theobald et al., 2002). Olanzapine can be useful in treating anorexia and may cause increased appetite as well as weight gain (Cohen and Alfonso, 2004). Other options include cyproheptadine and dronabinol (Pawlowski, 1975; Rahman, 1975; Bruera, 1992; Beal et al., 1995). Corticosteroids can be used as a brief pulse type of therapy designed to stimulate appetite, but they are generally not recommended for chronic therapy.

For a summary of differential diagnoses of appetite loss and interventions, see Table 9.3.

TABLE 9.3 Differential Diagnosis of Appetite Loss and Interventions

Diagnosis	Intervention
Cachexia Highly predictive of poor outcome Address issues of end-of-life care, advance directives	• Careful history and physical exam with attention to current medications, possibility of opportunistic infections, late-stage disease, and hypogonadism • *Anabolic steroids:* testosterone or nandrolone therapy. In females, may combine with estrogens to minimize masculinizing effect • *Resistance exercise training:* best results when combined with anabolic steroids • *Megestrol:* disproportionate adipose tissue increase and fluid retention account for most of weight gain. May still have place as appetite stimulant in terminal disease • *Dronabinol:* increases appetite, but no data available for muscle mass increase as related specifically to cachexia. Caution: may produce psychomimetic side effects • *Corticosteroids:* increases appetite on short-term basis, but not intended for long-term use. Can exacerbate muscle atrophy

(*continued*)

TABLE 9.3 (Continued)

Diagnosis	Intervention
Starvation Inadequate caloric intake, primarily loss of adipose tissue, appetite loss without wasting	If due to depressive disorder, refer to Chapters 6 and 7 for further details on management of severe depression • Aggressive psychopharmacological intervention indicated, including potential role of electroconvulsive therapy (ECT) • *Megestrol:* disproportionate adipose tissue increase and fluid retention account for most of weight gain. May still have place as appetite stimulant in terminal disease • *Olanzapine:* increases appetite, may increase carbohydrate cravings and is associated with weight gain • *Dronabinol:* increases appetite, but no data available for muscle mass increase as related specifically to cachexia. Caution: may produce psychomimetic side effects. • *Corticosteroids:* increases appetite on short-term basis, but not intended for long-term use. Can exacerbate muscle atrophy • *Mirtazapine:* Sedating. Stimulates appetite through antihistaminergic mechanisms. Serotonergic antagonism at 5-HT$_3$ useful for concurrent nausea/vomiting • *Cyproheptadine:* Sedating. Stimulates appetite primarily through antihistaminergic mechanisms • Consider need for percutaneous endoscopic gastrostomy (PEG) tube in accordance with patient's wishes and advanced directives
Dehydration	• Intravenous fluid replacement acutely, then transition to improved po fluid intake • Consider need for percutaneous endoscopic gastrostomy (PEG) tube in accordance with patient's wishes and advanced directives

Nausea and Vomiting

Nausea and vomiting in persons with HIV can arise from a variety of factors, including central nervous system disease (lymphoma, space-occupying lesions), HIV-related chemotherapy, antiretroviral therapy, and other medical conditions such as immune reconstitution syndrome. Symptomatic management of new-onset nausea and vomiting should not be undertaken without an etiological search for the underlying condition producing these problematic symptoms and attempts to address these issues prior to reflexively prescribing an antiemetic agent.

The management of nausea and vomiting, with the exception of that deriving from motion sickness, generally focuses on agents that either provide dopamine antagonism or 5-HT$_3$ antagonism (Karim et al., 1996) at the chemoreceptor trigger zone (CTZ), such as olanzapine (Pirl and Roth, 2000; Passik et al., 2002, 2003; Jackson, 2003; Cohen and Alfonso, 2004; Navari et al., 2005; Cohen, 2006; Dickerman et al., 2008), promethazine, prochlorperazine, droperidol, ondansetron, granisetron, and others (Lohr, 2008). Historically, phenothiazines have been widely used, but they are quite sedating from prominent antihistaminic effects, which can lead to difficulty tolerating the medication when needed for prolonged periods of time. Persons with HIV and AIDS are also exquisitely vulnerable to the extrapyramidal side effects of phenothiazines because the virus has a special affinity for the basal ganglia (Cohen and Alfonso, 2004). These extrapyramidal side effects along with other factors limit the tolerability of droperidol and haloperidol, both of which have been reported as effective antiemetic agents (Mitsunari et al., 2007; Rosow et al., 2008). Serotonergic antagonists such as ondansetron and granistron are typically very well tolerated (Cohen and Alfonso, 2004; Dickerman et al., 2008), but a significant disadvantage includes the high cost for these agents. Olanzapine was found to be the most efficacious medication in combination with ondansetron or megesterol for intractable chemotherapy-induced nausea and vomiting (Pirl and Roth, 2000; Navari et al., 2005; Navari and Brenner, 2009) and has been found to be effective in persons with HIV and AIDS (Cohen and Alfonso, 2004). Metoclopramide is another option that acts both as a prokinetic agent and as a partial dopamine antagonist. Finally, dexamethasone has been used with some success as well to control nausea and vomiting, especially in cases where increased intracranial pressure is the etiology.

Symptom management in reducing nausea and vomiting is an important part of any palliative care practice. Successful reduction of symptoms may allow continuation of antiviral therapies and eventual viral suppression. At the very least, it will improve quality of life and decrease the overall burden of illness experienced by these patients.

See Table 9.4 for a summary of the differential diagnosis of and inter-ventions for nausea and vomiting in persons with HIV.

TABLE 9.4 Differential Diagnosis of Nausea and Vomiting and Interventions

Diagnosis	Intervention
CNS disease (lymphoma, space-occupying lesions) HIV-related chemotherapy, antiretroviral therapy Effect of chronic disease	Potential interventions at site of chemoreceptor trigger zone: *Dopamine Antagonists* (listed in order of preferred treatment) • Olanzapine: advantageous in that it combines both dopaminergic antagonism and 5-HT$_3$ antagonism. Better tolerated than other neuroleptics, but high cost • *Promethazine:* sedating, inexpensive, potential extrapyramidal effects • *Prochlorperazine:* sedating, inexpensive, potential extrapyramidal effects • *Droperidol:* moderately sedating, higher risk for extrapyramidal effects in HIV/AIDS patients • *Haloperidol:* higher risk for extrapyramidal side effects in HIV/AIDS patients • *Metoclopramide:* prolonged use may predispose to tardive syndromes similar to extrapyramidal side effects caused by other dopamine antagonists *Serotonin Antagonists* (listed in order of preferred treatment) • *Ondansetron:* well tolerated, high cost • *Granisetron:* well tolerated, high cost • *Mirtazapine:* sedating, lower cost *Antihistamines* (listed in order of preferred treatment) • *Diphenhydramine:* highly anticholinergic, may induce delirium • *Mirtazapine:* sedating, lower cost, stimulates appetite in many patients *Corticosteroids* These are especially useful in cases of nausea/vomiting due to increased intracranial pressure (in order of preferred treatment): • Dexamethasone • Prednisone

Source: Allen (1992); Aapro et al. (2003); Bruera et al. (2004); Navari et al. (2005); Sarcev et al. (2007).

Conclusion

Symptom management is a central part the comprehensive and compassionate care of persons with HIV and AIDS. AIDS psychiatrists are in a unique position to provide significant relief of distressing symptoms, improve patients' quality of life, and maximize life potential at every stage of illness, from onset of infection to end of life. Attention to symptom management should begin with a medically sound evaluation and proceed rapidly to mitigation of distressing symptoms, followed by facilitation of maximal adherence to medical care and ART.

References

Aapro MS, Thuerlimann B, Sessa C, De Pree C, Bernhard J, Maibach R; Swiss Group for Clinical Cancer Research (2003). A randomized double-blind trial to compare the clinical efficacy of granisetron with metoclopramide, both combined with dexamethasone in the prophylaxis of chemotherapy-induced delayed emesis. *Ann Oncol* 14:291–297.

Afhami S, Haghpanah V, Heshmat R, Rasoulinejad M, Izadi M, Lashkari A, Tavangar SM, Hajiabdolbaghi M, Mohraz M, Larijani B (2007). Assessment of the factors involving in the development of hypothyroidism in HIV-infected patients: a case–control study. *Infection* 35:334–338.

Allan SG (1992). Antiemetics. *Gastroenterol Clin North Am* 21(3):597–611.

Ammassari A, Murri R, Pezzotti P, Trotta MP, Ravasio L, De Longis P, Lo Caputo S, Narciso P, Pauluzzi S, Carosi G, Nappa S, Piano P, Izzo CM, Lichtner M, Rezza G, Monforte A, Ippolito G, Moroni M, Wu AW, Antinori A; AdiCONA Study Group (2001). Self-reported symptoms and medication side effects influence adherence to highly active antiretroviral therapy in persons with HIV infection. *J Acquir Immune Defic Syndr* 28:445–449.

Arnedt JT, Conroy DA, Brower KJ (2007). Treatment options for sleep disturbances during alcohol recovery. *J Addict Dis* 26:41–54.

Barroso J, Preisser JS, Leserman J, Gaynes BN, Golden RN, Evans DN (2002). Predicting fatigue and depression in HIV-positive gay men. *Psychosomatics* 43:317–325.

Beal JE, Olson R, Laubenstein L, Morales JO, Bellman P, Yangco P, Lefkowitz L, Plasse TF, Shepard KV (1995). Dronabinol as a treatment for anorexia associated with weight loss in patients with AIDS. *J Pain Symptom Manage* 10(2):89–97.

Bodenner D, Spencer T, Riggs AT, Redman C, Strunk B, Hughes T (2007). A retrospective study of the association between megestrol acetate administration and mortality among nursing home residents with clinically significant weight loss. *Am J Geriatr Pharmacother* 5(2):137–146.

Breitbart W, McDonald MV, Rosenfeld B, Monkman ND, Passik S (1998). Fatigue in ambulatory AIDS patients. *J Pain Symptom Manage* 15:159–167.

Breitbart W, Rosenfeld B, Kaim M, Funesti-Esch J (2001). A randomized, double-blind, placebo-controlled trial of psychostimulants for the treatment of fatigue in ambulatory patients with human immunodeficiency virus disease. *Arch Intern Med* 161:411–420.

Bruera E (1992). Clinical management of anorexia and cachexia in patients with advanced cancer. *Oncology* 49(Suppl. 2):35–42.

Bruera E, Moyano JR, Sala R, Rico MA, Bosnjak S, Bertolino M, Willey J, Strasser F, Palmer JL (2004). Dexamethasone in addition to metoclopramide for chronic nausea in patients with advanced cancer: a randomized controlled trial. *J Pain Symptom Manage* 28:381–388.

Cohen MA (2006). Suicide and end-of-life care. In F Fernandez and P Ruiz (eds.), *Psychiatric Aspects of HIV/AIDS* (pp. 383–392). Philadelphia: Lippincott Williams & Wilkins.

Cohen MA, Alfonso CA (2004). AIDS psychiatry: psychiatric and palliative care, and pain management. In GP Wormser (ed.), *AIDS and Other Manifestations of HIV Infection*, fourth edition (pp. 537–576). New York: Elsevier.

Darko DF, McCutchan JA, Kripke DF, Gillin JC, Golshan S (1992). Fatigue, sleep disturbance, disability, and indices of progression of HIV infection. *Am J Psychiatry* 149:514–520.

Dickerman AL, Breitbart B, Chochinov HM (2008). Palliative and spiritual care of persons with HIV and AIDS. In MA Cohen and JM Gorman (eds.), *Comprehensive Textbook of AIDS Psychiatry* (pp. 417–439). New York: Oxford University Press.

Edinger JD, Bonnet MH, Bootzin RR, et al. (2004). Derivation of research diagnostic criteria for insomnia: report of an American Academy of Sleep Medicine Work Group. *Sleep* 27:1567–1596.

Epstein LJ, Strollo PJ Jr, Donegan RB, Delmar J, Hendrix C, Westbrook PR (1995). Obstructive sleep apnea in patients with human immunodeficiency virus (HIV) disease. *Sleep* 18:368–376.

Fumaz CR, Tuldra A, Ferrer MJ, Paredes R, Bonjoch A, Jou T, Negredo E, Romeu J, Sirera G, Tural C, Clotet B (2002). Quality of life, emotional status, and adherence of HIV-1-infected patients treated with efavirenz versus protease inhibitor–containing regimens. *J Acquir Immun Defic Syndr Hum Retrovirol* 29:244–253.

Greenblatt DJ, von Moltke LL, Daily JP, Harmatz JS, Shader RI (1999). Extensive impairment of triazolam and alprazolam clearance by short-term low-dose ritonavir: the clinical dilemma of concurrent inhibition and induction. *J Clin Psychopharmacol* 19:293–296.

Henry DH (1998). Experience with epoetin alfa and acquired immunodeficiency syndrome anemia. *Semin Oncol* 25(3 Suppl. 7):64–68.

Jackson WC, Tavernier L (2003). Olanzapine for intractable nausea in palliative care patients. *J Palliat Med* 6:251–255.

Karim F, Roerig S, Saphier D (1996). Role of 5-HT3 antagonists in the prevention of emesis caused by anticancer therapy. *Biochem Pharmacol* 52:685–692.

Lo Re V 3rd, Schutte-Rodin S, Kostman JR (2006). Obstructive sleep apnoea among HIV patients. *Int J STD AIDS* 17:614–620.

Lohr L (2008). Chemotherapy-induced nausea and vomiting. *Cancer J* 14:85–93.

Moeller AA, Oechsner M, Backmund HC, Popescu M, Emminger C, Holsboer F (1991). Self-reported sleep quality in HIV infection: correlation to the stage of infection and zidovudine therapy. *J Acquir Immune Defic Syndr* 4:1000–1003.

Mitsunari H, Ashikari E, Tanaka K (2007). The use of droperidol decreases postoperative nausea and vomiting after gynecological laparoscopy. *J Anesth* 21:507–509.

Morley JE, Thomas DR, Wilson MM (2006). Cachexia: pathophysiology and clinical relevance. *Am J Clin Nutr* 83:735–743.

Navari RM, Brenner MC (2009). Treatment of cancer-related anorexia with olanzapine and megestrol acetate: a randomized trial. *Support Care Cancer* [Epub ahead of print September 11, 2009].

Navari RM, Einhorn LH, Passik SD, Loehrer PJ Sr, Johnson C, Mayer ML, McClean J, Vinson J, Pletcher W (2005). A phase II trial of olanzapine for the prevention of chemotherapy-induced nausea and vomiting: a Hoosier Oncology Group study. *Support Care Cancer* 13:529–534.

Norman SE, Chediak AD, Freeman C, Kiel M, Mendez A, Duncan R, Simoneau J, Nolan B (1992). Sleep disturbances in men with asymptomatic human immunodeficiency (HIV) infection. *Sleep* 15:150–155.

Nuñez M, de Requena DG, Gallego L, Jiménez-Nácher I, González-Lahoz J, Soriano V (2001). Higher efavirenz plasma levels correlate with development of insomnia. *J Acquir Immun Defic Syndr Hum Retrovirol* 28:399.

O'Dowd MA, Gomez MF (2008). Insomnia and HIV: a biopsychosocial approach. In MA Cohen and JM Gorman (eds.), *Comprehensive Textbook of AIDS Psychiatry* (pp. 163–172). New York: Oxford University Press.

Passik SD, Kirsh KL, Theobald DE, et al. (2003). A retrospective chart review of the use of olanzapine for the prevention of delayed emesis in cancer patients. *J Pain Symptom Manage* 25:485–488.

Passik SD, Lundberg J, Kirsh KL, et al. (2002). A pilot exploration of the antiemetic activity of olanzapine for the relief of nausea in patients with advanced cancer and pain. *J Pain Symptom Manage* 23:526–532.

Pawlowski GJ (1975). Cyproheptadine: weight-gain and appetite stimulation in essential anorexic adults. *Curr Ther Res Clin Exp* 18:673–678.

Pirl WF, Roth AJ (2000). Remission of chemotherapy-induced emesis with concurrent olanzapine treatment: a case report. *Psychooncology* 9:84–87.

Rabkin JG, Wagner GJ, Rabkin R (2000). A double-blind, placebo-controlled trial of testosterone therapy for HIV-positive men with hypogonadal symptoms. *Arch Gen Psychiatry* 57:141–147.

Rahman KM (1975). Appetite stimulation and weight gain with cyproheptadine (periactin) in tuberculosis patients (double-blind clinical study). *Med J Malaysia* 29:270–274.

Remacha AF, Cadafalch J (1999). Cobalamin deficiency in patients infected with the human immunodeficiency virus. *Semin Hematol* 36:75–87.

Rosow CE, Haspel KL, Smith SE, Grecu L, Bittner EA (2008). Haloperidol versus ondansetron for prophylaxis of postoperative nausea and vomiting. *Anesth Analg* 106:1407–1409.

Rubinstein S (1998). High prevalence of insomnia in an outpatient population with HIV infection. *J Acquir Immune Defic Syndr Hum Retrovirol* 19:260–265.

Sarcev T, Secen N, Povazan Dj, Sabo A, Popovic J, Bursac D, Kakas M, Zaric B, Milovancev A (2007). The influence of dexamethasone in the decrease of chemotherapy-induced nausea and vomiting. *J BUON* 2:245–252.

Soffer J, Lux JZ, Mullen MP (2008). Endocrine comorbidities in persons with HIV. In MA Cohen and JM Gorman (eds.), *Comprehensive Textbook of AIDS Psychiatry* (pp. 513–528). New York: Oxford University Press.

Srisurapanont M, Jarusuraisin N (1998). Amitriptyline vs. lorazepam in the treatment of opiate-withdrawal insomnia: a randomized double-blind study. *Acta Psychiatr Scand* 97:233–235.

Sullivan PS, Hanson DL, Chu SY, Jones JL, Ward JW (1998). Epidemiology of anemia in human immunodeficiency virus (HIV)-infected persons: results from the multistate adult and adolescent spectrum of HIV disease surveillance project. *Blood* 91:301–308.

Theobald DE, Kirsh KL, Holtsclaw E, Donaghy K, Passik SD (2002). An open-label, crossover trial of mirtazapine (15 and 30 mg) in cancer patients with pain and other distressing symptoms. *J Pain Symptom Manage* 23:442–447.

Wagner GJ, Rabkin JG, Rabkin R (1998). Testosterone as a treatment for fatigue in HIV+ men. *Gen Hosp Psychiatry* 20:209–213.

World Health Organization (1986). *Cancer Pain Relief*. Geneva: World Health Organization.

10

HIV, AIDS, and Medical Multimorbid Illnesses

Joseph Z. Lux and Harold W. Goforth

Since the introduction of combination antiretroviral therapy, clinicians have seen a sharp decrease in the incidence of many HIV-associated comorbidities, and patients with access and adherence to combination antiretroviral therapy are living longer and healthier lives. However, the frequency of endocrine, metabolic, cardiovascular, renal, dermatological, neoplastic, hepatic, renal, pulmonary, and gastrointestinal multimorbid medical conditions remains very significant and in some cases is increasing. Although the incidence of particular HIV-associated comorbidities such as cytomegalovirus (CMV) retinitis has declined considerably, it remains a significant source of distress and suffering for persons with AIDS. This chapter is not intended to provide a lengthy discourse on each topic addressed, but rather be a general overview that will give the reader a basic working knowledge of multimorbid medical conditions and enhance the understanding of associated psychiatric complications and psychological distress. For a summary of these conditions and their respective features and treatment, see Table 10.1.

ENDOCRINE ABNORMALITIES IN HIV INFECTION

HIV and AIDS have been associated with a wide spectrum of endocrine abnormalities that underscore the complex relationships between immunological, endocrinological, and psychological systems. Endocrinopathies are great mimickers of psychiatric disorders, manifesting in some cases as disturbances of mood, sleep, appetite, thought process, energy level, or general sense of well-being. Endocrinopathies may present insidiously or abruptly, in

Table 10.1 HIV-Associated Multimorbidities and Their Treatments

Multimorbidity	Clinical Features	Psychiatric Symptoms	Suggested Treatment
Adrenal insufficiency	Nausea, vomiting, orthostatic hypotension	Fatigue, anorexia, lethargy, apathy, irritability, crying, and impaired sleep, decreased concentration, decreased memory, episodic confusion	Adrenal replacement with glucocorticoids and/or mineralocorticoids
Hypothyroidism	Intolerance to cold, bradycardia, skin thickening, edema, hair loss	Inattentiveness, slowed thought process, impaired memory, depression	Thyroid hormone replacement
Hyperthyroidism	Tachycardia, intolerance to heat, anxiety	Anxiety, irritability, nervousness	Antithyroid medication versus ablation
Hypogonadism	Decreased male-pattern hair, testicular atrophy, decreased libido, gynecomastia	Fatigue, decreased energy, depressed affect, poor self-image	Testosterone replacement therapy
Osteoporosis	Decreased bone mineral density, fractures	Increased rates of anxiety, depression, alexithymia	Bisphosphonates, calcium, vitamin D_3
Lipodystrophy	Central and dorsocervical fat accumulation, limb and facial subcutaneous fat atrophy, and associated metabolic complications such as insulin resistance and diabetes, lactic acidosis, osteopenia, dyslipidemia	Decreases in sexual activity, enjoyment of sex, and confidence in relationships; poor body image and social isolation; feelings of shame	Plastic/cosmetic surgery; consider switching antiretrovirals
Hyperglycemia/ diabetes mellitus	Impaired regulation of blood glucose, polydipsia, polyuria	Depression; alterations in mental status (delirium) if glucose is highly elevated	Lifestyle changes, change in antiretroviral treatment, and treatment with insulin-sensitizing medications

Cardiovascular disease	Dyslipidemia and insulin resistance, myocardial infarction risk	Severe physical limitations that isolate and limit ability to perform previously enjoyable coping activities	Consider switching to another antiretroviral, statins, aspirin, ACE inhibitors
Dermatological disease	Itching, dermatological changes, increased risk of adverse drug reactions	Marked reductions in quality of life in terms of social functioning, emotional capacity, impaired confidence, social withdrawal, anxiety, depression	Attention to symptom management
Oncological disease	Cutaneous and visceral manifestations, pain, cachexia, side effects of radiation and chemotherapy	Fatigue, anxiety, depression, cognitive slowing, mania, delirium	Oncological consultation
Ophthalmological disease	Visual loss, pain, blindness	Marked reductions in quality of life in terms of social functioning and emotional capacity; impaired confidence, social withdrawal, anxiety, depression	Emergent ophthalmological consultation; antivirals for CMV
Hepatitis C infection	Elevated transaminases, hyperbilirubinemia	Inattentiveness, slowed thought process, impaired memory, depression Encephalopathy if later stages of disease	IFN and ribavirin dosed concurrently with SSRI Lactulose, neomycin, or rifaximin for hepatic encephalopathy Liver transplantation
IFN/ribavirin treatment	Potential bone marrow suppression	Mood disturbance, irritability, tearfulness, rage, and anhedonia are predominant symptoms Insomnia, increased anxiety, decreased frustration tolerance, mania/hypomania	Stop IFN/ribavirin therapy; atypical antipsychotics, mood stabilizers, antidepressants if indicated

(continued)

TABLE 10.1 (Continued)

Multimorbidity	Clinical Features	Psychiatric Symptoms	Suggested Treatment
Nephropathy	Proteinuria, progressive renal failure	Severe physical limitations that isolate and limit ability to perform previously enjoyable coping activities	Initiation of ART therapy Dialysis if indicated Renal transplantation
Pulmonary disease	Dyspnea, cough, weight loss, fever, hypoxia	Severe physical limitations that isolate and limit ability to perform previously enjoyable coping activities	Antibiotics, oxygen, supportive therapy, curative therapies depending on etiologies
Esophagitis	Pain on swallowing	Anorexia, pain, discomfort, reactive depression	Empiric therapy with fluconazole; endoscopy if atypical presentation or treatment failure
Diarrhea	Multiple loose stools daily	Severe physical limitations that isolate and limit ability to perform previously enjoyable coping activities	Antibiotics if clinically indicated; antidiarrheal agents to prevent dehydration

ART, antiretroviral therapy; CMV, cytomegalovirus; IFN, interferon; SSRI, selective serotonin reuptake inhibitor.

either case with potentially tragic consequences when misdiagnosed as psychopathology. Prompt recognition of reversible alterations in endocrine function is essential to prevent unnecessary morbidity and mortality. An understanding of the complex interactions between endocrine and psychological systems may improve recognition and treatment of endocrinopathies, diminish suffering, and enhance quality of life and longevity in persons with HIV and AIDS.

Adrenal gland in HIV infection

Many studies have demonstrated alterations in adrenal function in patients with HIV and AIDS. Associated infections and tumors, as well as direct invasion of the adrenal glands by the virus, partly explain these changes. Patients are also commonly prescribed drugs that alter steroid synthesis or metabolism; for example, ketoconazole decreases steroid synthesis, megesterol acetate suppresses pituitary secretion of corticotropin, and rifampin increases p450 activity, leading to increased metabolism of cortisol. Ritonavir administration with inhaled corticosteroids can cause iatrogenic Cushing's syndrome (Samaras et al., 2005; Pessanha et al., 2007). The altered cytokine milieu in immune deficiency states may also affect the hypothalamic–pituitary–adrenal (HPA) axis.

In the 1980s, many postmortem studies demonstrated high rates of adrenal involvement in patients dying from AIDS (Welch et al., 1984; Laulund et al., 1986). Cytomegalovirus has been the most common associated infectious agent, found in the adrenal glands in 33%–88% of cases (Glasgow et al., 1985, Pulakhandam and Dincsoy, 1990; Marik et al., 2002). Less common agents observed in autopsy studies include *Cryptococcus*, *Toxoplasma*, *Histoplasma*, *Mycobacteria*, and neoplasms such as lymphoma and Kaposi's sarcoma.

Clinical symptoms of adrenal insufficiency in patients with HIV, in contrast, are much less commonly observed, probably because more than 80% to 90% of the adrenal glands must be destroyed before the appearance of symptoms. In fact, despite the association of HIV with adrenal dysfunction and blunted stress responses, most studies have found normal or more commonly elevated basal cortisol levels in patients with HIV infection (Villette et al., 1990; Biglino et al., 1995; Sellmeyer and Grunfeld, 1996; Christeff et al., 1997). Multiple factors could explain the hypercortisolism commonly observed in patients with HIV infection, including comorbid depression and severe psychosocial stress, both of which are associated with increased levels of cortisol. Increased levels of cytokines present during HIV infection may also stimulate cortisol production by the adrenal glands.

Most clinicians would agree that adrenal insufficiency is relatively common in patients with advanced-stage AIDS, especially those positive for CMV. Normal findings on adrenal stimulation in the presence of clinical signs and symptoms of insufficiency should be interpreted with caution. Finally, glucocorticoid replacement is crucial for all patients with a diagnosis of adrenal insufficiency and should be considered and increased in AIDS patients during times of febrile illness or worsening infection.

There can be considerable overlap between symptoms of HIV itself, adrenal insufficiency, and psychiatric illness, including fatigue, anorexia, nausea, vomiting, and orthostatic hypotension. Some patients report a sensation of heavy and weak muscles, dizziness, and tachycardia, which may be confused with a depressive or anxiety disorder. Patients with adrenal insufficiency have been misdiagnosed with hypochondriasis, conversion disorder, and anorexia nervosa. Associated behavioral changes in patients with adrenal insufficiency may include lethargy, apathy, irritability, crying, and impaired sleep. Cognitive difficulties have also been reported, including decreased concentration, decreased memory, and episodic confusion. Impaired thought process can worsen to frank psychosis during an adrenal crisis (Starkman, 2003).

Thyroid gland in HIV infection

Patients with HIV and AIDS often manifest abnormalities in thyroid function tests. Recent studies have demonstrated approximately 7% rates of subclinical hypothyroidism in patients with HIV (Beltran et al., 2003), with rates of overt hypothyroidism ranging between 2% and 9%. Isolated low free T4 levels with normal thyroid-stimulating hormone (TSH) levels has been found among HIV-infected individuals (Collazos et al., 2003; Hoffman and Brown, 2007) and associated with the use of stavudine, didanosine, and ritonavir (Beltran et al., 2006). There have been other reports of thyroid dysfunction with antiretroviral therapy, including one study in which receipt of stavudine was associated with hypothyroidism (Beltran et al., 2003). Thyroid function patterns consistent with nonthyroidal illness or "sick euthyroid syndrome" may develop in patients with severe medical illness (Hoffman and Brown, 2007). There have been recent reports of autoimmune thyroid disease, particularly Graves' disease, developing in association with immune reconstitution (Vos et al., 2006).

Alterations in thyroid function have also been associated with infections and tumors, particularly in the early literature. There have been isolated case reports of *Pneumocystis* infection of the thyroid gland (Ragni et al., 1991; Guttler et al., 1993). Clinically, many of these cases presented with symptoms or signs of hypothyroidism (Ragni et al., 1991; Spitzer et al., 1991; McCarty et al., 1992) and/or as a neck mass or thyroid goiter (Battan et al., 1991; Ragni et al., 1991). Other cases of Kaposi's sarcoma invading the thyroid gland and causing clinical hypothyroidism (Mollison et al., 1991) or a palpable thyroid mass (Krauth and Katz, 1987) have been reported. Autopsy studies have also found CMV inclusions in the thyroid follicles of patients dying of AIDS (Frank et al., 1987), in addition to other infections.

Medications prescribed for patients with HIV may have an impact on thyroid function. Interferon-alpha has been associated with thyroid dysfunction, possibly through an autoimmune mechanism. Medications that induce hepatic p450 enzyme systems, such as rifampin and ketoconazole, increase excretion of thyroid hormones, and patients treated with these medications who are receiving thyroid replacement may need higher doses.

True clinical hypothyroidism can cause multiple neuropsychiatric symptoms and signs that the psychiatrist should be aware of, most commonly cognitive dysfunction and depression. Severe forms can be manifested by psychotic and delusional symptoms, including visual and auditory hallucinations. Cognitive changes can include inattentiveness, slowed thought process, and impaired memory; mood changes can include anxiety, irritability, and emotional lability in addition to other depressive symptoms (Bauer et al., 2003). While these changes are not specific to patients with HIV, the presence of other HIV-associated medical and psychiatric comorbidities increases the challenge and complexity of identifying and treating such symptoms.

Graves' disease is associated with a myriad of psychiatric symptoms such as depression, anxiety, cognitive slowing, hypomania, and psychosis (Bunevicius and Prange, 2006). Patients often require psychotropic medications in conjunction with antithyroid therapy.

Gonadal function in HIV infection

Hypotestosteronemia has been one of the most prevalent endocrine abnormalities observed in patients with HIV. Testosterone is important for the maintenance of normal bone health, muscle mass, strength, energy level, and general sense of well-being. As the population infected with HIV ages, given the success of antiretroviral therapy (ART) in decreasing mortality, normal declining testosterone levels will be compounded by HIV-associated decreases in testosterone.

Early studies documented approximately 50% of men with AIDS to have hypogonadism (Dobs et al., 1988). The prevalence of hypogonadism is felt to be lower but still significant in the era of ART (Crum et al., 2005) and may not resolve with ART (Wunder et al., 2007). Limited studies have indicated that hypoandrogenic states are present in women with HIV at similar rates to those observed in men.

There have been inconsistent reports linking hypogonadism with ART. Besides antiretrovirals, other medications commonly used by patients with HIV might have an impact on the HPG axis. Ketoconazole inhibits gonadal production of steroids. Megestrol acetate (a progestational agent), glucocorticoids, and anabolic steroids can all reduce secretion of gonado-tropins (Mylonakis et al., 2001). Patients on methadone replacement (and those using heroin) have been found to have lower gonadotropin and testos-terone levels (Celani et al., 1984).

There are currently many available forms of testosterone replacement, including intramuscular injection, transdermal patch, and gel. In general, testosterone supplementation is fairly safe but should be avoided in patients with polycythemia or prostate cancer and used cautiously in patients with prostrate enlargement. Treatment options for hypogonadism in women are still limited. Oral contraceptives or isolated estrogen or progesterone pre-parations have traditionally been used for replacement. A pilot study for a transdermal test of testosterone replacement in women showed promising results, but more research is needed (Miller et al., 1998).

The diagnosis of hypogonadism can present a challenge, as many symp-toms are nonspecific and overlap with those of depression or chronic illness. These include fatigue, decreased energy, depressed affect, and poor self-image (Mylonakis et al., 2001). More specific symptoms can include decreased male-pattern hair, testicular atrophy, decreased libido, and gynecomastia (Crum et al., 2005). In some early studies of antidepressants for the treatment of depression in men with HIV, patients reported improved mood but residual diminished libido and low energy. Since then, considerable evidence has amassed supporting the beneficial effect of testosterone supplementation on mood and energy level in patients with HIV and depression.

Bone and mineral metabolism in HIV infection

In recent years, an extensive body of literature has emerged demonstrating the high prevalence of changes in bone and mineral metabolism in patients with HIV (Brown and Qaqish, 2006). These are likely due to multiple etiologies, including direct interactions of the virus with bone and marrow cells, as well as indirect effects through immune system activation and altered cytokine pro-duction. Associated illness and adverse effects of drugs used to treat HIV may also contribute to altered bone metabolism. Decreased physical activity, hypogonadism, and malabsorption of calcium and vitamin D, all common in patients with HIV infection, might additionally lead to decreases in bone mineral density (BMD). In the subpopulation of HIV patients who are on methadone or using heroin, effects may be more pronounced, as opiates can contribute to lowered BMD (Pedrazzoni et al., 1993).

Several studies have indicated the efficacy of bisphosphonates for the treatment of osteopenia and osteoporosis in the HIV population (Guaraldi et al., 2004; Negredo et al., 2005; McComsey et al., 2007). Appropriate calcium and vitamin D3 supplementation should be provided as well. Recent studies, however, have raised the specter of a rare risk of osteonecrosis of the jaw in association with bisphosphonate use (Woo et al., 2006; Pazianas et al., 2007).

Mood disorders such as major depression, in some cases associated with high levels of cortisol, have been reported to increase the risk of developing osteoporosis. One study examined psychoaffective and psychodynamic aspects in patients with osteoporosis, finding increased rates of anxiety, depression, and alexithymia (Zonis De Zukerfeld et al., 2003–2004). There was also association of osteoporosis with early childhood trauma, decreased support networks, and lower reported quality of life. Both psychosocial support and specific intervention programs can improve independence and the quality of life in patients with osteoporosis (Bayles et al., 2000). There is a paucity of literature specifically addressing the psychosocial implications of osteoporosis in patients with HIV.

Growth hormone abnormalities in HIV infection

AIDS-associated wasting is linked with growth hormone (GH) resistance, with increased GH and reduced insulin-like growth factor 1 levels (IGF-1) (Stanley and Grinspoon, 2008). Recombinant human GH has been used to treat patients with AIDS-associated wasting (Schambelan et al., 1996), but its use is controversial, it is expensive, and it may cause adverse reactions such as edema, insulin resistance, and diabetes. There is evidence that patients with HIV lipodystrophy and central adiposity have reduced GH secretion (Stanley and Grinspoon, 2008). Recent clinical trials in lipodystrophic patients with low-dose physiological GH (Lo et al., 2008) or tesamorelin, a GH-releasing factor analogue (Falutz et al., 2007), have reduced visceral fat and improved dyslipidemia with fewer side effects. The future role of these agents for the treatment of HIV lipodystrophy and visceral adiposity remains to be determined.

Lipodystrophy, Metabolic Disorders, and Cardiovascular Disorders in HIV Infection

Lipodystrohy

HIV-associated lipodystrophy is a syndrome of fat redistribution associated with antiretroviral therapy. Although many of the complications occur most commonly with protease inhibitors, lipodystrophy is associated with all antiretroviral classes. Lipodystrophy is associated with a number of changes in fat redistribution including central and dorsocervical fat accumulation, limb and facial subcutaneous fat atrophy, and associated metabolic complications such as insulin resistance and diabetes, lactic acidosis, osteopenia, and dyslipidemia. The presentation is heterogeneous; patients may develop one or a number of these complications. Potential effects on cardiovascular risk and events have also gained increasing attention.

The optimal management of lipodystrophy is still unclear. Expert guidelines have been published to assist clinicians in managing antiretroviral-associated metabolic complications (Schambelan et al., 2002). The three main approaches are initiation of antiretroviral therapy later to postpone the metabolic side effects, switching to a less metabolically toxic agent, and continuation of the current treatment but treating the metabolic effect.

The impact of switching antiretroviral medications, particularly protease inhibitors and thymidine analogues such as stavudine, has been studied. Although switching from a protease inhibitor may improve lipodystrophy (Barreiro et al., 2000), switching from a thymidine analogue appears to be the intervention that most consistently improves peripheral fat loss (Carr et al., 2002; McComsey et al., 2004; Moyle, et al., 2006). There is some evidence that the use of a GH-releasing factor analogue may be effective in reducing visceral adipose tissue (Falutz et al., 2007).

Plastic surgery is a tested option for patients with lipodystrophy. Liposuction for central accumulation and treatment of buffalo hump can be helpful (Gervasoni et al., 2004), although reaccumulation may occur. Facial lipoatrophy can be particularly psychologically disabling, and filler injections have been used in this situation. Polylactic acid injections, which have been approved by the U.S. Food and Drug Association (FDA) for this indication, have been satisfying for patients with minimal adverse effects (Burgess and Quiroga, 2005; Barton et al., 2006). Unfortunately, plastic surgery is generally considered cosmetic by private health insurance companies as well as by Medicaid and Medicare and is therefore not reimbursed. As a result, for those without significant financial means, surgical correction is not a feasible option for patients who suffer the consequences of disfigurement from lipodystrophy.

The visible effects of lipodystrophy and its association with HIV infection lead to a range of psychological issues. Studies investigating the psychological effects of HIV-associated lipodystrophy have revealed that those experiencing this disorder may experience decreased quality of life (Rajagopalan et al., 2008) with less sexual activity, less enjoyment of sex, decreased confidence in relationships (Dukers et al., 2001), poor body image and social isolation (Power et al., 2003), and feelings of shame (Blanch et al., 2004). Another commonly expressed concern among patients is that as the signs of lipodystrophy become more recognizable they may serve to "out" people as being HIV positive. Clinicians who treat persons with HIV infection should focus not only on the physical issues related to lipodystrophy, but also on any associated issues of anxiety, depression, social isolation, altered body image, or medication nonadherence.

Lactic acidosis

Lactic acidosis is a potentially life-threatening metabolic complication associated with lipodystrophy. Antiretroviral nucleoside therapy is associated with mitochondrial dysfunction. Mitochondrial pathology is associated with hyperlactatemia, lactic acidosis, lipoatrophy, hepatic steatosis, peripheral neuropathy, neuromuscular weakness, pancreatitis, and myopathies (McComsey and Lonergan, 2004). Asymptomatic hyperlactatemia is common in patients taking antiretrovirals, but lactic acidosis is infrequent (Boubaker et al., 2001; John et al., 2001; Imhof et al., 2005). Clinical symptoms with severe lactatemia include fatigue, dyspnea, tachycardia, abdominal pain, weight loss, and peripheral neuropathy (Carr et al., 2000; Gerard et al., 2000; Falco et al., 2002; Imhof et al., 2005).

The mechanism of nucleoside reverse transcriptase inhibitor (NRTI)-associated lactic acidosis is likely related to mitochondrial toxicity. The more potent NRTI inhibitors of mitochondrial synthesis, in decreasing order, are zalcitabine, didanosine, stavudine, and zidovudine (Birkus et al., 2002). Other nucleoside/nucleotide reverse transcriptase inhibitors such as lamivudine, abacavir, and tenofovir are less potent inhibitors of mitochondrial synthesis (Birkus et al., 2002). Administration with essential cofactors, including thiamine, riboflavin, L-carnitine, prostaglandin E, uridine, and coenzyme Q, that are thought to improve mitochondrial function for mitochondrial illnesses have been used to treat nucleoside-associated lactic acidosis with promising but still unproven benefit (Falco et al., 2002).

Diabetes

Hyperglycemia is increasingly seen in HIV-infected patients, particularly those on protease inhibitor therapies (Dube et al., 1997). Lipodystrophy is associated with insulin resistance and the development of diabetes. Advanced HIV illness may itself predispose patients to insulin resistance. In HIV antiretroviral-naive patients, a lower CD4 count is associated with increased insulin resistance (El-Sadr et al., 2005). The incidence of diabetes among HIV-infected individuals receiving antiretrovirals ranges between 1% and 7% (Carr et al., 1999; Palacios et al., 2003), with a higher percentage, in one study 16%, developing impaired glucose tolerance (Carr et al., 1999). Risk factors for development of diabetes include obesity, duration of treatment on protease inhibitors, and lipodystrophy (Palacios et al., 2003).

Different protease inhibitors appear to pose different risks. While atazanavir appears to have minimal or no effect on insulin sensitivity, indinavir causes a substantial decline in glucose disposal with just one dose (Hruz et al., 2002; Noor et al., 2002), and lopinavir/ritonavir worsened glucose tolerance after a 4-week trial (Lee et al., 2004). Amprenavir-treated patients exhibited a trend toward insulin resistance after 48 weeks (Dube et al., 2002). Other antiretroviral classes may also be a factor in developing insulin resistance and glucose tolerance. Cumulative NRTI therapy, particularly stavudine, is associated with increased insulin levels (Brown et al., 2005).

Strategies to address glucose intolerance, insulin resistance, and diabetes include lifestyle changes, change in antiretroviral treatment, and treatment with insulin-sensitizing medications. Exercise may improve hyperinsulinemia (Driscoll et al., 2004). Metformin therapy reduces insulin resistance in HIV-infected patients with lipodystrophy and impaired glucose metabolism (Hadigan et al., 2000). The strategy of switching from a protease inhibitor–based regimen to nevirapine is useful in lowering glucose and insulin resistance (Martinez et al., 1999). However, the use of switch strategies must be approached cautiously to avoid virological failure. Finally, numerous studies have reported an association between depression and diabetes, and clinicians should inquire about symptoms of depression in patients who develop diabetes or poor glycemic control (Lustman et al., 2000).

Hyperlipidemia

Changes in lipid metabolism also occur in HIV-infected individuals. One study showed that HIV seroconversion resulted in marked decreases in high-density lipoprotein (HDL) cholesterol, low-density lipoprotein (LDL) cholesterol, and total cholesterol levels, with a pattern of increases in total and LDL cholesterol after initiation of antiretroviral therapy (Riddler et al., 2003). In a study of 419 antiretroviral-naive patients, an AIDS diagnosis was associated with higher levels of total cholesterol, very-low-density lipoprotein (VLDL) cholesterol, and triglycerides (El-Sadr et al., 2005). Elevated HIV RNA levels were associated with lower concentrations of HDL cholesterol and LDL cholesterol, and higher levels of VLDL cholesterol and triglycerides.

The protease inhibitor class is particularly associated with dyslipidemia, although all antiretroviral classes may induce atherogenic lipid profiles. In one population-based cohort, increased cholesterol or triglyceride concentrations were associated with protease inhibitor use by an adjusted odds ratio of 7.17 (Heath et al., 2002). The effects, however, can vary widely between protease inhibitors. Changes in lipid levels are significantly less in patients treated with atazanvir than those in patients receiving nelfinavir or lopinavir (Wood et al., 2004; Soriano et al., 2008).

A number of studies have been conducted to assess other strategies for minimizing antiretroviral-associated lipid abnormalities. The NRTI tenofovir SR had a more favorable lipid panel than that of stavudine when used in combination with lamivudine and efavirenz (Gallant et al., 2004). The substitution of nevirapine for a protease inhibitor increased HDL cholesterol and decreased total, LDL, and VLDL cholesterol (Negredo et al., 2002). There is a role for dietary interventions as well; increased total protein, animal protein, and trans fat intake, as well as reduced soluble fiber intake worsen the lipid profile in patients with lipodystrophy on protease inhibitor therapy (Shah et al., 2005).

Treatment recommendations have been published for the evaluation and management of dyslipidemia in HIV-infected adults that build on the treatment recommendations for dyslipidemia in the general adult population (Expert Panel, 2001; Dube et al., 2003). Consideration should be given to obtaining baseline and follow-up lipid profiles, assessing for coronary heart disease risk factors, counseling for modifiable risk factors, and changing antiretroviral therapy or beginning lipid-lowering agents as necessary.

Cardiovascular risk

Many of the metabolic abnormalities associated with lipodystrophy are coronary risk factors in non-HIV-infected individuals. The aging of the HIV population and evidence that HIV-infected individuals are more likely to smoke (Shah et al., 2005) are additional factors increasing patients' cardiovascular risk. Overall mortality has decreased since the advent of protease inhibitors, but there have been concerns that cardiovascular risk and events may have risen at the same time. Treatment with antiretrovirals overall appears to lower the total death rate (Bozzette et al., 2003) but predisposes patients, especially those being treated with protease inhibitors, to cardiovascular risk factors such as dyslipidemia and insulin resistance.

There is a significant amount of data suggesting an increased risk of coronary risk and events in HIV-infected patients, both from HIV infection itself and from antiretroviral use, notably those treated with protease inhibitors and certain NRTIs. A series of large, well-designed epidemiological studies have produced conflicting results on the relationship between the rate of coronary events in the HIV-infected population and use of antiretroviral therapy. Some of these studies have noted an association with protease inhibitor use and coronary events (Mary-Krause et al., 2003; D:A:D Study Group, 2007), while others have not observed an increased risk with protease inhibitor use (Klein et al., 2002; Bozzette et al., 2003). One recent study noted a possible association between the use of abacavir and didanosine and myocardial infarctions (D:A:D Study Group, 2008).

Complicating the field further, recent evidence suggests that uncontrolled HIV viremia can increase cardiac risk and that antiretroviral use mitigates this risk (El-Sadr et al., 2006), possibly by reducing endothethial inflammation (Melendez et al., 2008). In weighing the recent literature, a recent antiretroviral treatment guideline (Hammer et al., 2008) has suggested that earlier antiretroviral treatment may be warranted in patients at high risk for cardiovascular disease.

Cardiovascular disease may further isolate HIV-infected individuals and limit individuals' ability to perform previously enjoyable coping activities such as exercise. In advanced cases, it impinges directly on patients' ability to maintain independence and perform activities of daily living, serving as a constant reminder of impending mortality. Studies in populations with coronary artery disease and no HIV infection have found increased mortality in patients with depression, but it remains uncertain whether treatment of depression will improve mortality (Blumenthal et al., 2003; Carney et al., 2008).

DERMATOLOGICAL DISORDERS ASSOCIATED WITH HIV INFECTION

Greater than 90% of HIV-infected individuals will have a dermatological complaint at some time in the course of their illness (Coldiron and Bergstresser, 1989). Acute HIV seroconversion itself is associated with a rash in greater than 70% of patients. Dermatological signs and symptoms can be secondary to bacterial, viral, or fungal infections, in addition to cutaneous drug eruptions and malignancies.

Bacterial agents that have been associated with cutaneous infections in the HIV population are *Bartonella* (bacillary angiomatosis), tuberculosis, and *Mycobacterium avium* complex (MAC) (Tappero et al., 1995; Rigopoulos et al., 2004). Primary syphilis may present atypically with multiple chancres (Rolfs et al., 1997). Secondary syphilis, which is known to occur with increased frequency in HIV infected individuals, can present with a diffuse maculopapular rash involving the palms and soles (Hutchinson et al., 1994).

Viral infections with cutaneous manifestation include *Molluscum contagiosum*, human papillomavirus (HPV), common warts, herpes simplex virus 1 (HSV-1) and HSV-2, *Varicella zoster* (shingles), CMV, Epstein–Barr virus, and human herpesvirus 8 (HHV-8) (Kaposi's sarcoma) (Tappero et al., 1995). Dermatophytes and, to a lesser degree, *Candida*, infect the skin, hair, and nails (Elewski and Sullivan, 1994). Because these infections tend to be chronic and recurrent, they are a frequent source of distress. Deep fungal infections such as *Cryptococcus neoformans*, *Histoplasma capsulatum*, *Coccidioides immitis*, and *Blastomyces dermatitidis* may also present with cutaneous manifestations (Pappas et al., 1992, Tappero et al., 1995).

Other dermatological manifestations include seborrheic dermatitis, a common cutaneous manifestation associated with HIV infection. A hyperkeratotic, highly contagious form of scabies (Norwegian) is also seen more frequently in severely immunocompromised HIV individuals (Portu et al., 1996). A chronic dermatosis associated with severe pruritus, eosinophilic folliculitis, is usually seen with advanced illness (Milazzo et al., 1999), although it can also occur with the initiation of effective antiretroviral therapy as a result of immune reconstitution syndrome. Pruritus is a common complaint in HIV infection and is generally a more significant issue in advanced disease. Studies of distress in relation to HIV disease and itching have not been performed, but quality-of-life studies of chronic urticarial illness have demonstrated marked reductions in quality of life in terms of both social functioning and emotional capacity (Staubach et al., 2006).

HIV-infected individuals also seem to be at increased risk for adverse drug reactions, and this risk increases with advancing immunosuppression (Coopman et al., 1993). Abacavir, a nucleoside analogue reverse transcriptase inhibitor, is associated with a severe hypersensitivity reaction in which a maculopapular or urticarial skin rash can be part of the constellation of symptoms. These reactions are rare in African-American patients and are associated with the presence of the HLA-B*5701 allele. Patients who are screened for this allele and test positive should not receive abacavir, and their allergy to abacavir should be documented in the medical record (Mallal et al., 2008). If the drug is started and discontinued secondary to concern of a hypersensitivity reaction, the patient should never be rechallenged with this agent, since fatalities are known to occur (Hewitt, 2002).

In conclusion, the dermatological manifestations of HIV may range from cosmetic concerns to life-threatening systemic conditions. As a number of HIV-associated dermatological conditions may relapse and remit, it is important that clinicians understand that living with a chronic dermatological condition is associated with impaired confidence, social withdrawal, anxiety, depression, and suicidality (Ginsburg and Link, 1993; Gupta and Gupta, 1998; Hong et al., 2008).

HIV-Associated Ophthalmological Disease

Prior to the development of effective antiretroviral therapy, HIV-associated ocular complications were very common. In fact, CMV retinitis was the most common ocular infection in patients with AIDS, affecting an estimated 20%–45% of patients (Holland et al., 1983). Patients required lifelong therapy and had a mean survival of 6–10 months after diagnosis (Hoover et al., 1993). Currently, largely because of effective antiretroviral therapy, new cases of CMV retinitis are rare, with a decline in incidence of 80%

(Goldberg et al., 2005). Patients with a history of CMV retinitis who have had a successful response to antiretroviral therapy with increasing CD4 lymphocyte count can safely discontinue maintenance therapy with close observation for recurrence (MacDonald et al., 2000). An ocular inflammatory syndrome associated with immune recovery in patients with CMV retinitis is immune recovery uveitis (Jacobson et al., 1997). This syndrome needs to be anticipated and recognized early, since it can result in a substantial loss of vision.

Other ocular diseases that were seen prior to effective antiretroviral therapy were progressive outer retinal necrosis (PORN), acute retinal necrosis (ARN) secondary to herpes zoster virus (HZV) and HSV, toxoplasmosis retinochoroiditis, *Pneumocystis jiroveci (carinii)* choroiditis, syphilitic retinitis, tuberculosis choroiditis, cryptococcal choroiditis, and ocular lymphomas (Moraes, 2002).

Despite the overall decline in prevalence of CMV retinitis in HIV-infected patients, visual loss and blindness from multiple etiologies are still significant causes for concern and sources of distress for persons with HIV (Ng et al., 2000; Kestelyn and Cunningham 2001; Hill and Dubey 2002; Oette et al., 2005). Specific studies examining the quality of life and distress experienced by persons with visual loss have not been performed among persons with HIV disease. However, data on distress among patients with macular degeneration and other acquired forms of visual loss may be used to better understand the sense of isolation, psychological distress, and limitations these patients experience on a routine basis. Data from patients with acquired macular degeneration indicated a strong association between decline in vision and functional impairment, along with high rates of depression, anxiety, and emotional distress (Berman and Brodaty, 2006). In a study focusing on patients' attitudes toward visual loss from subfoveal choroidal neovascularization, patients reported that they would rather suffer medical illnesses such as dialysis-dependent renal failure and AIDS than visual impairment (Bass et al., 2004). Similar findings have been noted in studies of diabetes mellitus–associated visual loss (Cox et al., 1998). Clearly, across multiple medical conditions, acquired visual loss has a profound impact on self-perception of overall health-related quality of life, distress, and suffering.

HIV AND MALIGNANCIES

It is a well-known fact that defects in cell-mediated immunity have been associated with the development of certain tumors. This association has been reported in congenital immunodeficiency disorders, transplant recipients on chronic immunosuppressive medication, and patients with autoimmune disorders (Penn, 1975; Frizzera et al., 1980). Hence, it was no surprise that there would be such an association with HIV infection. The initial reports of Kaposi's sarcoma (KS), a rare vascular tumor, and *Pneumocystis carinii* pneumonia in gay men in San Francisco and New York City in 1981 initiated the beginning of what is now known as the AIDS epidemic (Friedman-Kien et al., 1982). Subsequently, it was noted that there were increasing reports of non-Hodgkin's lymphoma (NHL) and, later, invasive cervical carcinoma in this population, placing these diagnoses in the category of AIDS-defining illnesses (CDC, 1985).

With the development of antiretroviral therapy, the incidence of KS has had such a significant decline that in developed countries it is a rare diagnosis (Hengge et al., 2002), although KS still causes a significant amount of morbidity and even mortality in the developing world. The consensus is that this decline in incidence is most likely due to improved immunity, which in turn influences the host response to the causative agent, HHV-8. Although less dramatic, the incidence of NHL has also shown a decrease since the development of effective antiretroviral therapy (Grulich and Vajdic, 2005; Wood and Harrington, 2005; Polesel et al., 2008). The incidence of invasive cervical cancer has remained unchanged (Clifford et al., 2005)

The diagnosis of KS with cutaneous lesions can be particularly distressing for HIV-infected persons. It can serve as an unwanted exposure of their seropositive status and worsen fears of experiencing HIV and sexual stigma (de Moore et al., 2000). It is important that HIV clinicians not only focus on the diagnosis and treatment of Kaposi's sarcoma but also ask about related psychological distress.

Over the years of the epidemic, there have been other associated malignancies that are not considered AIDS defining but have been reported with some increased frequency, such as Hodgkin's disease, lung cancers, anogenital carcinomas, testicular cancers, gastric cancers, hepatomas, and multiple myeloma (Remick, 1996). These are often complex associations in which other risk factors may play a more significant role than HIV infection itself and may influence the development of these malignancies.. Such factors include the use of tobacco, alcohol, and coinfection with hepatitis B, hepatitis C, and HPV.

Investigators have sought to understand whether the frequency of these non-AIDS cancers has changed in the ART era. Although the literature is sometimes contradictory, recent studies suggest that non-AIDS-defining malignancies are increasing in frequency and causing a larger proportion of overall mortality in HIV-infected persons (D'Souza et al., 2008; Lewden et al., 2008; Long et al., 2008).

When a malignancy is diagnosed, it is important that HIV clinicians be aware that a cancer diagnosis may heighten psychological distress, exacerbate anxiety and depression, and expose the patient to radiation therapy and/or chemotherapeutic agents such as corticosteroids, interferon, and interleukins. These agents are associated with a myriad of neuropsychiatric side effects including fatigue, depression, mania, psychosis, cognitive slowing, and delirium. Psychiatric consultation is warranted when a patient with cancer develops any of these symptoms. Further discussion on the psychopharmacologic and psychotherapeutic treatment of these psychiatric syndromes may be found in Chapters 6, 7, 8, 9, 11, and 12 of this handbook.

HEPATITIS C AND HIV COINFECTION

Hepatitis C virus (HCV) coinfection has also become a major problem among those with HIV and is a significant cause of morbidity and mortality. Of persons injecting drugs for at least 5 years, 60% to 80% are infected with HCV (CDC, 2002). Approximately 50%–60% of HIV injecting drug abusers are also HCV seropositive, with approximately 25%–35% of the overall HIV population coinfected (Everson, 2005; Alter, 2006).

Hepatitis C is a blood-borne virus with predominant parenteral transmission (Koziel and Peters, 2007). Intravenous drug use accounts for the majority of infections; although they can also occur from nosocomial exposure such as sharing of toothbrushes, razors, body piercing, and tattoos. Other risk factors include blood transfusions prior to 1991 and hemodialysis.

Hepatitis C is a single-stranded RNA virus belonging to the *Flaviridiae* family. Genotype 1 is most common in the United States and the most treatment resistant, whereas genotypes 2 and 3 are more responsive to interferon (IFN) treatment. No vaccine is available. Enzyme immune assay testing for the antibody to core protein is usually reactive 4–10 weeks after exposure. Liver function tests are not reliable, as 30% of patients are asymptomatic and have normal liver function results. Treatment is indicated if there is evidence of fibrosis, high inflammatory activity, or high viral load (Jacobson, 2001; Koziel and Peters, 2007).

Treatment with combined pegylated IFN and ribavirin has shown the best results for treatment of hepatitis C. All coinfected patients should be considered candidates for treatment with IFN/ribavirin because of the rapid progression to cirrhosis and higher risk of liver toxicity. Hepatic decompensation, history of active alcohol or drug use, current psychiatric illness, and history of neuropsychiatric complications are relative contraindications, but not absolute contraindications to IFN use (Soriano et al., 2004; Wagner and Ryan, 2005). Side effects include flu-like symptoms including myalgia, chills, fever, headache, loss of appetite, nausea, and diarrhea. As treatment progresses, bone marrow suppression with anemia, neutropenia, and thrombocytopenia can occur. Thyroid dysfunction has also been noted.

At least 20%–40% of patients without any psychiatric history develop neuropsychiatric side effects after 4–6 weeks of treatment, especially fatigue. Mood disturbance, cognitive dysfunction, irritability, tearfulness, rage, and anhedonia are common, and insomnia, increased anxiety, decreased frustration tolerance, and mania/hypomania have also been associated with IFN treatment. Suicidal ideation, suicide attempts, and psychosis have been reported but are rare (Dieperink et al., 2000; Hoffman et al., 2003; Onyike et al., 2004).

Patients who are currently symptomatic with a mood or anxiety disorder need to be stabilized prior to treatment initiation, and prophylactic treatment with a selective serotonin reuptake inhibitor (SSRI) has been effective in reducing mood disturbances during treatment (Musselman et al., 2001). Diagnosis and treatment of IFN-induced mood disorder is critical during HCV treatment, as fatigue and depression are common and serve as major risk factors for discontinuation of IFN (Gleason and Yates, 1999; Trask et al., 2000; Loftis and Hauser, 2003; Raison et al., 2005).

Hepatic Encephalopathy and Liver Transplantation

Hepatic encephalopathy is a common neuropsychiatric condition seen in patients with liver disease or portosystemic shunting. Early hepatic encephalopathy generally presents with personality changes, irritability, and mental rigidity. Alteration in sleep/wake cycles, with fatigue and sleepiness during the day and inability to sleep at night, are also early symptoms. Hepatic encephalopathy eventually progresses to worsening of lethargy, disorientation, inappropriate behavior, asterixis, and abnormal reflexes. Severe cases are characterized by lethargy and obtundation along with a positive Babinski reflex and decerebrate posture.

The definitive treatment for severe hepatic encephalopathy is liver transplantation.

The United Network for Organ Sharing (UNOS), a private, nonprofit organization, is responsible for allocation of organs within the United States. Each year there are at least 20,000 potential deceased donors, but of these only 10%–20% are able to donate organs. Living donation is a possibility for liver (60% of liver is donated in adult-to-adult donation), kidney, and lung transplantation. Currently, there are over 18,000 people waiting for a new liver. In order to provide fair access to organs, patients are stratified according to their health status and probability of death. Introduced in 2002, the MELD system (Model of End Stage Liver Disease) uses a mathematical formula to predict death within 3 months. This system has replaced the Child-Turcotte-Pugh score and eliminated time on the wait list as a factor in obtaining an organ. Total bilirubin, creatinine, and INR (coagulation time) are used to calculate the MELD score, with a higher MELD indicating more severe disease.

Patients are screened for cardiac and pulmonary disease, cancer, and end-organ manifestation of diabetes. They must demonstrate an understanding of their illness, understand the risk and benefits, show good adherence to current medical treatment, and have adequate social support and means of paying for food, rent, medications, and medical care. Patients must have comorbid illnesses under control, and the HIV viral load should be unde-tectable with a CD4 count above 200. There should also be minimal drug resistance to ART. A transplant does not necessarily immediately and mark-edly improve life (Levenson and Olbrisch, 2000).

Assessment of psychiatric disorders prior to transplantation

Alcohol dependence has a lifetime prevalence of 7% to 10% with approxi-mately 10% to 15% of these individuals developing liver cirrhosis. Of all liver transplants, 20% to 40% are for alcoholic cirrhosis, which is the second most common indication after hepatitis C. Alcohol relapse occurs in up to 20% to 30% of patients post-transplant (DiMartini and Trzepacz, 2000; DiMartini et al., 2001), thus post-transplant screening needs to be continued. Similarly, a cocaine abuse history should be of great concern to the treating physician, given that a history of cocaine abuse places patients at higher risk for relapse than any other drug of abuse before or after transplant.

Patients in a methadone program who have demonstrated abstinence from heroin are accepted at most transplant centers, as it is unethical to discontinue methadone treatment because of increased relapse rates. Methadone dosage may need to be lowered to diminish worsening of hepatic encephalopathy as liver disease progresses (Koch and Banys, 2001). Abstinence from nicotine is strongly encouraged, and marijuana use is not acceptable because of the high risk of pulmonary infection with *Aspergillus* post-transplant and the risk of worsening of hepatic encephalopathy.

If patients are diagnosed with a psychiatric illness, they are encouraged to obtain treatment and achieve stability prior to transplantation. Patients with borderline personality disorder have greater difficulty coping with the med-ical demands in the post-transplant period and have higher rates of nonad-herence and graft failure (Shapiro et al., 1995). However, there are no absolute psychiatric contraindications for transplantation other than active substance abuse and untreated psychosis.

Living with immunosuppression

Individuals who have undergone transplantation will be required to take immunosuppressants following transplantation for the rest of their lives. HIV-coinfected patients are particularly sensitive to toxicity of immunosuppression drugs. Drug levels of immunosuppression medication need to be carefully monitored to avoid over-immunosuppression, and inhibition of P450 3A4 enzymes by ART, especially protease inhibitors, will dramatically increase levels of tacrolimus and cyclosporine. Neuropsychiatric effects of immunosuppressants are many, with symptoms in the spectrum of mood disorders, including depression and mania; anxiety symptoms such as irritability or restlessness, and insomnia; and delirium (Beresford, 2001; Wijdicks, 2001).

Persons with HIV and hepatitis C have the burdens of two complex and severe medical illnesses, both with multiorgan and multisystem involvement, including profound psychiatric complications. An integrated team approach and the skills of a psychosomatic medicine psychiatrist can help alleviate suffering and promote adherence to care.

HIV-Associated Nephropathy, End-Stage Renal Disease, Dialysis, and Kidney Transplant

The causes of end-stage renal disease (ESRD) may be multifactorial but are frequently related to HIV-associated nephropathy in addition to concomitant illnesses such as diabetes, hypertension, substance abuse–related (heroin) nephropathy, and primary renal diseases. Similar to AIDS itself, ESRD is also associated with a high prevalence of psychiatric comorbidity and a high rate of suicide.

Approximately 325,000 people in the United States currently require hemodialysis as part of the End-Stage Renal Disease (ESRD) Program, and 100,000 new patients begin treatment each year (U.S. Renal Data System, 2005). Kidney disease in the United States also falls disproportionately on the minority community, with African Americans accounting for greater than 30% of ESRD (Statistics, N.C.f. H., 2005). Ten to fifteen percent of patients with HIV infection have chronically impaired kidney function or disease (CKD); risk factors are older age, black race, hypertension, diabetes, AIDS, injection drug use, and HCV coinfection (Gardner et al., 2003; Gupta et al., 2004; Szczech et al., 2004).

HIV-associated nephropathy (HIVAN) remains the single most common cause of chronic kidney disease in HIV patients (Ross and Klotman, 2004). It is strongly associated with black race as a risk factor with over 90% of affected patients in the United States being of African-American descent. HIVAN is characterized by heavy proteinuria, often in the nephritic range, with varying degrees of renal insufficiency. The clinical course of untreated

HIVAN is marked by progression to renal failure requiring dialysis within weeks to months, but patients receiving antiviral therapy have a more indolent course with some reversal of structural and functional abnormalities if started early. Several studies have demonstrated a slower progression to ESRD with ART (Wali et al., 1998; Winston et al., 2001; Cosgrove et al., 2002; Szczech et al., 2002).

Patients with more advanced kidney disease often present with constitutional symptoms including fatigue and anorexia, which may be confused with HIV-associated symptoms. Treatment must be initiated to control lipid abnormalities, Ca/PO$_4$ metabolism, and anemia. Hypertension must also be treated as kidney function deteriorates, and the therapeutic focus should shift to preparation for renal replacement therapy, as kidney transplantation is a viable option in selected patients with undetectable viral RNA for at least 3 months, CD4 cells >200/μL, and no history of an opportunistic infection or neoplasm. One- and two-year survival for incident ESRD patients has improved dramatically in the ART era; 1-year survival now approaches 80% (Ahuja et al., 2002) and is not substantially different from that for non-HIV-infected controls on peritoneal dialysis (Khanna et al., 2005). Although there are no long-term studies on the survivability of persons with HIV who are on hemodialysis, hemodialysis is widely used in this population even though it is associated with higher arteriovenous fistula failure rates (Schild et al., 2004).

Palliative care

An increasing number of persons with ESRD are choosing to withdraw from dialysis; the percentage of patients choosing this rose from 8.4% in 1988–1990 to 17.8% in 1990–1995 (Leggat et al., 1997). For persons making this decision, it is important that the nephrology, psychiatry, and palliative care teams work together to ensure maximal quality of life. Withdrawal of care is a complex decision even when medically, legally, and ethically justifiable. It often is experienced through a combination of ambivalence, changes in decisions, and needed time to process the decision on an emotional level (Cohen et al., 1997). More comprehensive approaches to palliative and end-of-life care are presented in Chapter 12 of this handbook.

Psychiatric disorders and distress associated with renal disease

When an individual faces both dependency and loss of function as a result of being on dialysis along with the severe distress associated with HIV, the situation can become overwhelming to even the most resilient individuals. People who are very independent do not do well on dialysis, although some tailoring of the procedure is possible for patients with emphasis on self-care such as home dialysis, peritoneal dialysis, or early renal transplantation (Reichsman and Levy, 1972). Work-related difficulties are common to persons with HIV and those on dialysis, with rates of underemployment or unemployment approaching two-thirds in dialysis patients (Cohen et al., 1997). Other sources of distress include restricted diets, discomfort during hemodialysis, dermatological changes, loss of menstrual cycle, infertility, diminished sexual function, and loss of work, school, and housework-related responsibilities. These stressors and losses affect not only the self-esteem of the patient but also their very concept of role identity (Levy, 2000).

The most common psychological problem seen in people with medical or surgical illness is depression, or the combination of anxiety and depression (O'Donnell and Chung, 1997). Persons on dialysis have a higher incidence of suicide than that in the general healthy population or in other persons with chronic medical illnesses (Abram et al., 1975; Haenel et al., 1980). Patients who are HIV positive and suffer end-stage renal failure also have a predisposition to becoming delirious during treatment as a result of electrolyte abnormalities, azotemia, and dysequilibrium syndrome. The accepted and ideal treatment of depression and anxiety is with antidepressants and psychotherapy. Such treatment is covered more extensively in Chapters 6, 7, 8, 9, 11, and 12.

Pharmacokinetics are significantly affected with renal failure. The aspects requiring greatest attention are the effect of renal failure on protein binding (Brater, 1999) and the effect of dialysis on drug levels. In renal failure, there is a decrease in available circulating protein and thus a decrease in binding capacity for most psychiatric medications. Therefore, a rule of thumb is that the maximum dose of a medication used for a patient in renal failure should be no more than two-thirds of the maximum dose used for a patient with normal kidney function.

Renal transplantation

Solid organ transplantation has been noted to be among the triumphs of modern medicine, and current guidelines suggest that it is not justifiable to withhold solid organ transplantation from HIV-seropositive recipients on the basis of their serostatus alone (Roland and Stock, 2006). The increase in organ transplantation, however, is limited to the number of available organs, which has not increased proportionately to the demand for new organs (Belle et al., 1996). The needs of HIV-seropositive patients with concurrent transplantation needs are highly complex. Frequently these patients are subject to not only the psychosocial strain of transplantation but also the significant stressors associated with HIV seropositivity.

Selection of transplant recipients with concurrent HIV is complex given the perceived terminal quality of this illness among many medical practitioners. Current evidence supports ART-treated HIV-seropositive patients undergoing successful transplantation with a low incidence of both acute rejection and infectious complications (Bhagani et al., 2006; Gruber et al., 2008). In addition, long-term survival of HIV patients with kidney transplants is favorable with equal or greater graft rate and patient survival at 1, 3, and 5 years compared to HIV-seronegative counterparts (Qiu et al., 2006). Thus, the AIDS psychiatrist can serve as a potent advocate for those individuals who are otherwise good candidates medically and psychosocially and who have demonstrated good adherence to antiretroviral therapy.

Psychopharmacological considerations are complex in this group. Neurotoxicity associated with cyclosporine-derived compounds is not infrequent and may present as syndromes mimicking neuropsychiatric illness such as toxicity, delirium, and seizures (Estol et al., 1989 Kershner and Wang-Cheng, 1989; Coleman and Norman, 1990; Burkhalter et al., 1994). The practitioner's differential diagnosis is confounded as these patients suffer from both an immunosuppressive disease and pharmacological immunosuppression, so a full assessment of any presenting symptom is required prior to preemptive therapy.

In summary, renal effects of HIV are myriad and complex, requiring close consultation between infectious disease, nephrology, and psychiatric liaison teams. Transplantation guidelines no longer prohibit solid organ transplant in selected HIV patients (Bhagani et al., 2006). In cases of advanced disease, palliative medicine teams should be involved early to provide increased symptom management and end-of-life care for patients with HIV and renal disease. AIDS psychiatrists can provide support to persons with HIV and AIDS by encouraging adherence and treating comorbid psychiatric illness to improve adherence to ART. In addition, psychiatry can assist with behavior change and family support to encourage a comprehensive approach to care.

PULMONARY MANIFESTATIONS OF HIV INFECTION

The spectrum and incidence of AIDS-related pulmonary opportunistic infections have changed significantly over the past 29 years since the first description in 1981 of gay men with *Pneumocystis jiroveci (P. carinii)* pneumonia (PCP) in New York City and San Francisco (Gottlieb et al., 1981; Masur et al., 1981). Development and use of effective combination antiretroviral therapy and prophylaxis with agents targeted against these infections have largely been responsible for the decrease in their incidence (Palella et al., 1998).

Pneumocystis jiroveci (carinii)

Pneumocystis still remains the most common AIDS-associated opportunistic infection in the United States (Jones et al., 1999). The CD4 lymphocyte count has been found to be a good predictor for risk of infection, since 80%–90% of infections are associated with a CD4 count of less than 200 cells/mm^3 (Masur and Kovacs, 1998). Patients can present with a wide array of pulmonary symptomatology, from mild dyspnea on exertion to rapidly progressive respiratory failure. In general, patients have fever, nonproductive cough, hypoxemia, elevated serum lactate dehydrogenase (LDH), and bilateral interstitial infiltrates on chest X-ray (Hoover et al., 1993).

A diagnosis of PCP requires the detection of organisms in sputum or bronchoalveolar lavage fluid. Bronchoalveolar lavage has a sensitivity of 95%–99%, making transbronchial or open lung biopsy rarely necessary (Ognibene et al., 1984). Early diagnosis may prevent hospitalization and progression to respiratory failure (Brenner et al., 1987; Benfield et al., 2001). Trimethoprim-sulfamethoxazole remains the treatment of choice unless the patient has demonstrated a severe hypersensitivity to sulfa in the past (Gluckstein and Ruskin, 1995). Alternative agents include pentamidine, clindamycin-primaquine, atovaquone, trimethoprim-dapsone, and trimetrexate (D'Avignon et al., 2008).

Mycobacterium tuberculosis

Although the incidence of acute tuberculosis is decreasing in the United States, worldwide, *Mycobacterium* tuberculosis (TB) infection is the leading cause of mortality in persons infected with HIV. Tuberculosis has been noted to kill more people with HIV than any other condition (Williams et al., 2008). Of the estimated 40 million persons living with HIV, approximately one-third of them are coinfected (Raviglione et al., 1995). The extensive spread of HIV has had a direct effect on increasing outbreaks of tuberculosis. Similarly, tuberculosis has an adverse effect on HIV progression, accounting for increased rates of AIDS deaths, viral replication, and opportunistic infections (Corbett et al., 2003). The number of combined HIV-TB cases continues to grow; among 20 countries reporting data in 2005, HIV-positive tuberculosis cases increased to 3.3% of the total from 2.1% in 2004 with a nearly 3:1 preponderance of males and young people aged 25–34 years (Lazarus et al., 2008). Alternately, the incidence of tuberculosis in HIV-infected patients has declined steadily with prolonged use of antiretroviral therapy, and patients on effective antiretroviral therapy with acute tuberculosis have been shown to have prolonged survival (Miranda et al., 2007).

The mean CD4 count at tuberculosis presentation is approximately 200–400 cells/mm^3. The course of acute tuberculosis appears to behave similarly in HIV-infected and non-infected individuals when the CD4 count is above 300 cells/mm^3. The typical presentation is pulmonary with fever, weight loss, night sweats, and apical infiltrates that can cavitate. As the CD4 count declines below 200 cells/mm^3, the presentation can be more atypical, making the diagnosis more difficult and increasing the risk of an extrapulmonary manifestation (Jones et al., 1993).

Tuberculosis skin testing (PPD) should be performed on all individuals with HIV infection, regardless of whether a diagnosis of active tuberculosis is suspected. A 5 mm or greater area of induration is considered to be positive; however, in acute tuberculosis the PPD skin test is often falsely negative. A high index of suspicion must be maintained and empiric treatment started in all truly suspected cases followed by sensitivity testing to ensure appropriate therapy (CDC, 2007). Consultation with an experienced infectious disease specialist should be sought to ensure the proper regimen selection.

Drug-resistant tuberculosis in HIV infection is an ongoing issue and therapy should be based on sensitivity testing and infectious disease consultation. Recent CDC data show that institutional outbreaks of MDR-TB have primarily affected HIV-seropositive patients. Factors such as delayed diagnosis, inadequate treatment, and prolonged infectivity contributed greatly to fatality rates in these instances (Wells et al., 2007).

Other HIV-related respiratory illnesses

Retrospective and prospective multicentered trials have shown that HIV-infected individuals have an increased rate of both upper and lower respiratory infections compared to that in uninfected controls (Wolff and O'Donnell, 2001). Infections and other related respiratory illnesses that can occur at any CD4 lymphocyte count include sinusitis, bacterial pneumonia and bronchitis, *Mycobacterium* tuberculosis pneumonia, bronchogenic carcinoma, non-Hodgkins lymphoma, and nonspecific interstitial pneumonitis. When CD4 counts approach 200 cells/mm^3 and below, PCP, *Cryptococcus neoformans* pneumonia, bacterial pneumonia with bacteremia or sepsis, and extrapulmonary or disseminated *Mycobacterium* tuberculosis need to be considered. At CD4 counts fewer than 100 cells/mm^3, bacterial pneumonia due to *Pseudomonas aeruginosa*, *Toxoplasma gondii* pneumonia, and pulmonary Kaposi's sarcoma are more frequently seen. In advanced AIDS, with CD4 counts less than 50 cells/mm^3, disseminated endemic fungal diseases with pneumonia, such as histoplasmosis and coccidioidomycosis, disseminated viral infections, i.e., cytomegalovirus, and disseminated atypical *Mycobacterium* infection with pneumonia should be included in the differential diagnosis (Boyton, 2005). Nosocomial infections in HIV patients are underestimated and continue to constitute a significant source of disability and distress among HIV patients because of their increase in associated comorbidity and mortality (Petrosillo et al., 2005).

Gastrointestinal Manifestations of HIV Infection

Gastrointestinal complaints associated with HIV infection are common and include diarrhea, nausea, vomiting, dysphagia, odonyphagia, wasting, abdominal pain, gastrointestinal bleeding, jaundice, and anorectal ulceration. Disorders can be secondary to opportunistic infection, chronic coinfection with hepatitis B or C, malignancies, drug toxicities, and HIV itself (Wilcox, 1993; Wallace and Brann, 2000).

Esophagitis

Candida albicans is the most common cause of esophagitis in patients with AIDS (Wilcox 1993). Empiric therapy with fluconazole is indicated in patients with esophageal complaints and thrush, reserving endoscopy for treatment failures (Bashir and Wilcox, 1996). Other infectious causes of esophagitis in AIDS are CMV, herpes simplex virus (HSV), and idiopathic esophageal ulceration (IEU) (Monkmuller and Wilcox, 2000a). Although HIV-associated IEU can be seen at the time of acute seroconversion, it is more commonly seen with a CD4 lymphocyte count of fewer than 100 cells/ mm^3 (Kotler et al., 1992). Less common causes of esophagitis in AIDS patients are *Mycobacterium avium* intracellulare (MAI), *Bartonella henselae*, *Cryptosporidium*, *Histoplasma capsulatum*, Epstein–Barr virus, and HPV (Monkemuller and Wilcox, 2000a). HIV-related malignancies, such as non-Hodgkin's lymphoma and Kaposi's sarcoma, and gastroesophageal reflux disease also need to be considered when a patients presents with esophageal symptoms.

Diarrhea

Diarrhea remains the most common gastrointestinal complaint among patients with HIV disease. In its severe form, it is one of the most debilitating symptoms associated with HIV. The etiology of diarrhea is often multi-factorial. A wide array of viruses, bacteria, fungi, and parasites has been implicated in the etiology of diarrhea (Smith et al., 1992). The degree of immunodeficiency makes certain pathogens and refractory disease such as CMV, *Cryptosporidium*, *Microsporidia*, and disseminated MAI more common. Other potential pathogens include *Clostridium difficile*,

Salmonella, *Campylobacter*, and *Shigella* (Navin et al., 1999; Call et al., 2000; Monkemuller and Wilcox 2000b). Antiretroviral agents associated with diarrhea include nelfinavir, lopinavir/ritonavir, saquinavir, and didanosine (buffered formulation). Empiric therapy with antimicrobial and antiparasitic agents is indicated when clinical suspicion is high. Antidiarrheal agents should be considered to prevent dehydration.

HEPATOBILIARY DISEASE

Hepatic disease in HIV infection is a significant cause of morbidity and mortality. Most patients with AIDS will have some evidence of liver dysfunction. Like gastrointestinal disorders, they tend to occur later in the course of HIV infection, reflecting increasing immunosuppression (Cappell, 1991). A wide array of opportunistic infections, including MAI, CMV, HSV, *Mycobacterium* tuberculosis, *Bartonella hensalae*, *Pneumocystis*, and disseminated fungal disease, and HIV-associated malignancies, such as Kaposi's sarcoma and non-Hodgkin's lymphoma, have all been shown to involve the liver (Perkocha et al., 1990; Bonacini, 1992). Hepatotoxicity can also be due to antiretroviral therapy, idiosyncratic or immunoallergic mechanisms, or direct cytotoxicity due to underlying liver disease. There is an increased risk of chronic active hepatitis progressing to cirrhosis and the development of hepatocellular carcinoma in the presence of comorbid HIV infection. Therefore, all coinfected patients should limit alcohol and hepatotoxic agents. The HAV and HBV vaccine should be offered to all seronegative patients.

AIDS cholangiopathy has been seen largely in patients with advanced disease and presents with right upper quadrant pain, jaundice, and hepatomegaly with elevated serum alkaline phosphatase levels. All clinical syndromes can be diagnosed by endoscopic retrograde cholangiopancreatography (ERCP). *Cryptosporidium*, *Microsporidia*, CMV, and *Cyclospora* have all been associated but without a clear link. If possible, the offending pathogens should be treated, although often the treatment requires biliary stenting. In general, the prognosis is poor (Yusuf and Barron, 2004).

CONCLUSION

This chapter has provided the reader with a basic working knowledge of medical multimorbidities associated with HIV infection. While patients effectively treated with antiretroviral therapy are living longer lives, in order to optimize health and minimize multimorbid medical complications, it is important that clinicians encourage HIV-infected individuals to maintain a healthy lifestyle that includes a well-balanced diet, exercise, and avoidance of alcohol and tobacco. Clinicians must focus on not only the physical issues related to multimorbid illnesses but also the associated psychiatric disorders and psychological distress. When unrecognized, such disorders and stress can cause additional suffering and may worsen medical outcomes. Recognition and treatment of multimorbid medical psychiatric disorders can contribute to maximizing life potentials in persons with HIV and AIDS.

REFERENCES

Abram HS, Moore GL, Westervelt BS Jr (1975). Suicidal behavior in chronic dialysis patients. *Am J Psychiat* 127(9):1199–1204.

Ahuja TS, Grady J, Khan S (2002). Changing trends in the survival of dialysis patients with human immunodeficiency virus in the United States. *J Am Soc Nephrol* 13(7):1889–1893.

Alter MJ (2006). Epidemiology of viral hepatitis and HIV co-infection. *J Hepatol* 44(Suppl.1):S6–S9.

Barreiro P, Soriano V, Blanco F, Casimiro C, de la Cruz JJ, Gonzalez-Lahoz J (2000). Risks and benefits of replacing protease inhibitors by nevirapine in HIV-infected subjects under long-term successful triple combination therapy. *AIDS* 14(7):807–812.

Barton SE, Engelhard P, Conant M (2006). Poly-L-lactic acid for treating HIV-associated facial lipodystrophy: a review of the clinical studies. *Int J STD AIDS* 17(7):429–435.

Bashir RM, Wilcox CM (1996). Symptom-specific use of upper gastrointestinal endoscopy in human immunodeficiency virus–infected patients yields high dividends. *J Clin Gastroenterol* 23(4):292–298.

Bass EB, Marsh MJ, Mangione CM, Bressler NM, Childs AL, Dong LM, Hawkins BS, Jaffee HA, Miskala P (2004). Submacular Surgery Trials Research Group. Patients' perceptions of the value of current vision: assessment of preference values among patients with subfoveal choroidal neovascularization. The Submacular Surgery Trials Vision Preference Value Scale: SST Report No. 6. *Arch Ophthalmol* 122(12):1856–1867.

Battan R, Mariuz P, Raviglione MC, Sabatini MT, Mullen MP, Poretsky L (1991). *Pneumocystis carinii* infection of the thyroid in a hypothyroid patient with AIDS: diagnosis by fine needle aspiration biopsy. *J Clin Endocrinol Metab* 72(3):724–726.

Bauer M, Szuba MP, Whybrow PC (2003). Psychiatric and behavioral manifestations of hyperthyroidism and hypothyroidism. In OM Wolkowitz and AJ Rothschild (eds.), *Psychoneuroendocrinology: The Scientific Basis of Clinical Practice* (pp. 419–444). Arlington VA: American Psychiatric Publishing.

Bayles CM, Cochran K, Anderson C (2000). The psychosocial aspects of osteoporosis in women. *Nurs Clin North Am* 35(1):279–286.

Belle SH, Beringer KC, Detre DM (1996). Recent findings concerning liver transplantation in the United States. *Clin Transplant* 10:15–29.

Beltran S, Lescure FX, Desailloud R, Douadi Y, Smail A, El Esper I, Arlot S, Schmit JL; Thyroid and VIH Group (2003). Increased prevalence of hypothyroidism among human immunodeficiency virus–infected patients: a need for screening. *Clin Infect Dis* 37(4):579–583.

Beltran S, Lescure FX, El Esper I, Schmit JL, Desailloud R (2006). Subclinical hypothyroidism is not an autoimmune disease. *Horm Res* 66(1):21–26.

Benfield TL, Helweg-Larsen J, Bang D, Junge J, Lundgren JD (2001). Prognostic markers of short-term mortality in AIDS-associated. *Pneumocystis carinii* pneumonia. *Chest* 119(3):844–851.

Beresford T (2001). Neuropsychiatric complications of liver and other solid organ transplantation. *Liver Transplant* 7(11 Suppl.1):S36–S45.

Berman K, Brodaty H (2006). Psychosocial effects of age-related macular degeneration. *Int Psychogeriatr* 18(3):415–428.

Bhagani S, Sweny P, Brook G; British HIV Association (2006). Guidelines for kidney transplantation in patients with HIV disease. *HIV Med* 7(3):133–139.

Biglino A, Limone P, Forno B, Pollona A, Cariti G, Molinatti GM, Gioannini P (1995). Altered adrenocorticotropin and cortisol response to corticotropin-releasing hormone in HIV-1 infection. *Eur J Endocrinol* 133(2):173–179.

Birkus G, Hitchcock MJM, Cihlar T (2002). Assessment of mitochondrial toxicity in human cells treated with tenofovir: comparison with other nucleoside reverse transcriptase inhibitors. *Antimicrob Agents Chemother* 46(3):716–723.

Blanch J, Rousaud A, Martinez E, De Lazzari E, Milinkovic A, Peri JM, Blanco JL, Jaen J, Navarro V, Massana G, Gatell JM (2004). Factors associated with severe impact of lipodystrophy on the quality of life of patients infected with HIV-1. *Clin Infect Dis* 38(10):1464–1470.

Blumenthal JA, Lett HS, Babyak MA, White W, Smith PK, Mark DB, Jones R, Mathew JP, Newman MF; NORG Investigators (2003). Depression as a risk factor for mortality after coronary artery bypass surgery. *Lancet* 362 (9384):604–609.

Bonacini M (1992). Hepatobiliary complications in patients with human immunodeficiency virus infection. *Am J Med* 92(4):404–411.

Boubaker K, Flepp M, Sudre P, Furrer H, Haensel A, Hirschel B, Boggian K, Chave JP, Bernasconi E, Egger M, Opravil M, Rickenbach M, Francioli P, Telenti A; Swiss HIV Cohort Study (2001). Hyperlactatemia and antiretroviral therapy: the Swiss HIV cohort study. *Clin Infect Dis* 33(11):1931–1937.

Boyton RJ (2005). Infectious lung complications in patients with HIV/AIDS. *Curr Opin Pulm Med* 11(3):203–207.

Bozzette SA, Ake CF, Tam HK, Chang SW, Louis TA (2003). Cardiovascular and cerebrovascular events in patients treated for human immunodeficiency virus infection. *N Engl J Med* 348(8):702–710.

Brater DC (1999). Drug dosing in renal failure. In Brady HR and Wilcox CS (eds.), *Therapy in Nephrology and Hypertension: A Companion to Brenner and Rector's the Kidney*, fifth edition (pp. 641–653). Philadelphia: WB Saunders.

Brenner M, Ognibene FP, Lack EE, Simmons JT, Suffredini AF, Lane HC, Fauci AS, Parrillo JE, Shelhamer JH, Masur H (1987). Prognostic factors and life expectancy of patients with acquired immunodeficiency syndrome and *Pneumocystis carinii* pneumonia. *Am Rev Respir Dis* 136(5):1199–1206.

Brown TT, Li X, Cole SR, Kingsley LA, Palella FJ, Riddler SA, Chmiel JS, Visscher BR, Margolick JB, Dobs AS (2005). Cumulative exposure to nucleoside analogue reverse transcriptase inhibitors is associated with insulin resistance markers in the Multicenter AIDS Cohort Study. *AIDS* 19(13):1375–1383.

Brown TT, Qaquish RB (2006). Antiretroviral therapy and the prevalence of osteopenia and osteoporosis. *AIDS* 20(17):2165–2174.

Bunevicius R, Prange AJ (2006). Psychiatric manifestations of Graves' hyperthyroidism: pathophysiology and treatment options. *CNS Drugs* 20(11):897–909.

Burgess CM, Quiroga RM (2005). Assessment of the safety and efficacy of poly-L-lactic acid for the treatment of HIV-associated facial lipoatrophy. *J Am Acad Dermatol* 52(2):233–239.

Burkhalter EL, Starzl TE, Van Thiel DH (1994). Severe neurological complications following orthotopic liver transplant in patients receiving FK-506 and prednisone. *J Hepatol* 21(4):572–577.

Call SA, Heudebert G, Saag M, Wilcox CM (2000). The changing etiology of chronic diarrhea in HIV-infected patients with CD4 cell counts less than 200 cells/mm^3. *Am J Gastroenterol* 95(11):3142–3146.

Cappell MS (1991). Hepatobiliary manifestations of the acquired immune deficiency syndrome. *Am J Gastroenterol* 86(1):1–15.

Carney RM, Freedland KE, Steinmeyer B, Blumenthal JA, Berkman LF, Watkins LL, Czajkowski SM, Burg MM, Jaffe AS (2008). Depression and five-year survival following acute myocardial infarction: a prospective study. *J Affect Disord* 109(1-2):133–138.

Carr A, Miller J, Law M, Cooper DA (2000). A syndrome of lipoatrophy, lactic acidaemia, and liver dysfunction associated with HIV nucleoside analogue therapy: contribution to protease inhibitor–related lipodystrophy syndrome. *AIDS* 14(3):F25–F32.

Carr A, Samaras K, Thorisdottir A, Kaufman GR, Chisholm DJ, Cooper DA (1999). Diagnosis, prediction, and natural course of HIV-1 protease-inhibitor-associated lipodystrophy, hyperlipidaemia, and diabetes mellitus: a cohort study. *Lancet* 353(9170):2093–2099.

Carr A, Workman C, Smith DE, Hoy J, Hudson J, Doong N, Martin A, Amin J, Freund J, Law M, Cooper DA (2002). Mitochondrial Toxicity (MITOX) study group: abacavir substitution for nucleoside analogs in patients treated with HIV lipoatrophy: a randomized trial. *JAMA* 288(2):207–215.

Celani MF, Carani C, Montanini V, Baraghini GF, Zini D, Simoni M, Ferretti C, Marrama P (1984). Further studies on the effects of heroin addiction on the hypothalamic–pituitary–gonadal function in man. *Pharmacol Res Commun* 16(12):1193–1203.

[CDC] Centers for Disease Control and Prevention (1985). Revision of the case definition of acquired immunodeficiency syndrome for national reporting–United States. *MMWR Morb Mortal Wkly Rep* 34(25):373–375.

[CDC] Centers for Disease Control and Prevention (2002). Viral hepatitis and injection drug users. IDU HIV Prevention Fact Sheet Series. Retrieved September 24, 2009, from http://www.cdc.gov/idu/hepatitis/viral_hep_drug_use.htm

[CDC] Centers for Disease Control and Prevention (2007). Extensively drug-resistant tuberculosis—United States, 1993–2006. *MMWR Morb Mortal Wkly Rep* 56(11):250–253.

Christeff N, Gherbi N, Mammes O, Dalle MT, Gharakhanian S, Lortholary O, Melchior JC, and Nunez EA (1997). Serum cortisol and DHEA concentrations during HIV infection. *Psychoneuroendocrinology* 22(Suppl.1): S11–S18.

Clifford GM, Polesel J, Rickenbach M, Dal Maso L, Keiser O, Kofler A, Rapiti E, Levi F, Jundt G, Fisch T, Bordoni A, De Weck D, Franceschi S; Swiss HIV Cohort (2005). Cancer risk in the Swiss HIV Cohort Study: associations with immunodeficiency, smoking, and highly active antiretroviral therapy. *J Natl Cancer Inst* 97(6):425–432.

Cohen LM, McCue JD, Germain M, Woods A (1997) Denying the dying: advance directives and dialysis discontinuation. *Psychosomatics* 38(1):27–34.

Coldiron BM, Bergstresser PR (1989). Prevalence and clinical spectrum of skin disease in patients infected with human immunodeficiency virus. *Arch Dermatol* 125(3):357–361.

Coleman AE, Norman DJ (1990). OKT3 encephalopathy. *Ann Neurol* 28(6): 837–838.

Collazos J, Ibarra S, Mayo J (2003). Thyroid hormones in HIV-infected persons in the highly active antiretroviral era: evidence of an interrelation between the thyroid axis and the immune system. *AIDS* 17(5):763–765.

Coopman SA, Johnson RA, Platt R, Gazzard BG (1993). Cutaneous disease and drug reactions in HIV infection. *N Engl J Med* 328(23):1670–1674.

Corbett EL, Watt CJ, Walker N, Maher D, Williams BG, Raviglione MC, Dye C (2003). The growing burden of tuberculosis: global trends and interactions with the HIV epidemic. *Arch Intern Med* 163(9):1009–1021.

Cosgrove CJ, Abu-Alfa AK, Perazella MA (2002). Observations on HIV-associated renal disease in the era of highly active antiretroviral therapy. *Am J Med Sci* 323(2):102–106.

Cox DJ, Kiernan BD, Schroeder DB, Cowley M (1998). Psychosocial sequelae of visual loss in diabetes. *Diabetes Educ* 24(4):481–484.

Crum NF, Furtek KJ, Olson PE, Amling CL, Wallace MR (2005). A review of hypogonadism and erectile dysfunction among HIV-infected men during the pre- and post-HAART ears: diagnosis, pathogenesis, and management. *AIDS Patient Care STDS* 19(10):655–671.

D:A:D Study Group, Friis-Moller N, Reiss P, Sabin CA, Weber R, Monforte A, El-Sadr W, Thiebaut R, De Wit S, Kirk O, Fontas E, Law MG, Phillips A,

Lundgren JD (2007). Class of antiretroviral drugs and the risk of myocardial infarction. *N Engl J Med* 356(17):1723–1735.

D:A:D Study Group, Sabin CA, Worm SW, Weber R, Reiss P, El-Sadr W, Dabis F, De Wit S, Law M, D'Arminio Monforte A, Friis-Moller N, Kirk O, Pradier C, Weller I, Phillips AN, Lundgren JD (2008). Use of nucleoside reverse transcriptase inhibitors and risk of myocardial infarction in HIV-infected patients enrolled in the D:A:D study: a multi-cohort collaboration. *Lancet* 371 (9622):1417–1426.

D'Avignon LC, Schofield CM, Hospenthal DR (2008). Pneumocystis pneumonia. *Semin Respir Crit Care Med* 29(2):132–140.

de Moore, GM, Hennessey P, Kunz NM, Ferrando SJ, Rabkin JG (2000). Kaposi's sarcoma: the Scarlet Letter of AIDS: the psychological effects of a skin disease. *Psychosomatics* 41(4):360–363.

Dieperink E, Willenbring M, Ho SB (2000). Neuropsychiatric symptoms associated with hepatitis C and interferon alpha: a review. *Am J Psychiatry* 157 (6):867–875.

DiMartini A, Day N, Dew MA, Lane T, Fitzgerald MG, Magill J, Jain A (2001). Alcohol use following liver transplantation: a comparison of follow-up methods. *Psychosomatics* 42(1):55–62.

DiMartini A, Trzepacz P (2000). Alcoholism and organ transplantation. In P Trzepacz and A DiMartini (eds.), *The Transplant Patient* (pp. 214–238). Cambridge, UK: Cambridge University Press.

Dobs AS, Dempsey MA, Ladenson PW, Polk BF (1988). Endocrine disorders in men infected with human immunodeficiency virus. *Am J Med* 84(3 Pt. 2): 611–616.

Driscoll SD, Meininger GE, Ljungquist K, Hadigan C, Torriani M, Klibanski A, Frontera WR, Grinspoon S (2004). Differential effects of metformin and exercise on muscle adiposity and metabolic indices in human immunodeficiency virus–infected patients. *J Clin Endocrinol Metab* 89(5):2171–2178.

D'Souza G, Wiley DJ, Li X, Chmiel JS, Margolick JB, Cranston RD, Jacobson LP (2008). Incidence and epidemiology of anal cancer in the Multicenter AIDS Cohort Study. *J Acquir Immune Defic Syndr* 48(4):491–499.

Dube MP, Johnson DL, Currier JS, Leedom JM (1997). Protease inhibitor–associated hyperglycaemia. *Lancet* 350(9079):713–714.

Dube MP, Qian D, Edmondson-Melancon H, Sattler FR, Goodwin D, Martinez C, Williams V, Johnson D, Buchanan TA (2002). Prospective, intensive study of metabolic changes associated with 48 weeks of amprenavir-based antiretroviral therapy. *Clin Infect Dis* 35(4):475–481.

Dube MP, Stein JH, Aberg JA, Fichtenbaum CJ, Gerber JG, Tashima KT, Henry WK, Currier JS, Sprecher D, Glesby MJ; Adult AIDS Clinical Trials Group Cardiovascular Subcommittee (2003). Guidelines for the evaluation and management of dyslipidemia in human immunodeficiency virus (HIV)-infected adults receiving antiretroviral therapy: recommendations of the HIV Medicine Association of the Infectious Disease Society of America and the Adult AIDS Clinical Trials Group. *Clin Infect Dis* 37(5):613–627.

Dukers NHTM, Stolte IG, Albrecht N, Coutinho RA, de Wit JBF (2001). The impact of experiencing lipodystrophy on the sexual behavior and well-being among HIV-infected homosexual men. *AIDS* 15(6):812–813.

Dye C, Scheele S, Dolin P, Pathania V, Raviglione MC (1999). Consensus statement. Global burden of tuberculosis: estimated incidence, prevalence, and mortality by country. WHO Global Surveillance and Monitoring Project. *JAMA* 282(7):677–686.

Elewski BE, Sullivan J (1994). Dermatophytes as opportunistic pathogens. *J Am Acad Dermatol* 30(6):1021–1022.

El-Sadr WM, Lundgren JD, Neaton JD, Gordin F, Abrams D, Arduino RC, Babiker A, Burman W, Clumeck N, Cohen CJ, Cohn D, Cooper D, Darbyshire J, Emery S, Fatkenheuer G, Gazzard B, Grund B, Hoy J, Klingman K, Losso M, Markowitz N, Neuhaus J, Phillips A, Rappoport C, Strategies for Management of Antiretroviral Therapy (SMART) Study Group (2006). CD4+ count-guided interruption of antiretroviral treatment. *N Engl J Med* 355(22):2283–2296.

El-Sadr WM, Mullin CM, Carr A, Gibert C, Rappoport C, Visnegarwala, Grunfeld C, Raghavan SS (2005). Effects of HIV disease on lipid, glucose, and insulin levels: results from a large antiretroviral-naive cohort. *HIV Med* 6(2):114–121.

Estol CJ, Lopez O, Brenner RP, Martinez AJ (1989). Seizures after liver transplantation: a clinicopathologic study. *Neurology* 39(10):1297–1301.

Everson GT (2005). Treatment of hepatitis C in patients who have decompensated cirrhosis. *Clin Liver Dis* 9(3):473–486.

Expert Panel on Detection, Evaluation, and Treatment of High Blood Cholesterol in Adults (2001). Executive summary of the third report of the National Cholesterol Education Program (NCEP) Expert Panel on Detection, Evaluation, and Treatment of High Blood Cholesterol in Adults (Adult Treatment Panel III). *JAMA* 285:2486–2497.

Falco V, Rodriguez D, Ribera E, Martinez E, Miro JM, Domingo P, Diazaraque R, Arribas JR, Gonzalez-Garcia JJ, Montero F, Sanchez L, Pahissa A (2002). Severe nucleoside-associated lactic acidosis in human immunodeficiency virus–infected patients: report of 12 cases and review of the literature. *Clin Infect Dis* 34(6):838–846.

Falutz J, Allas S, Blot K, Potvin D, Kotler D, Somero M, Berger D, Brown S, Richmond G, Fessel J, Turner R, Grinspoon S (2007). Metabolic effects of growth hormone–releasing factor in patients with HIV. *N Engl J Med* 357 (23):2359–2370.

Frank TS, LiVolsi VA, Connor AM (1987). Cytomegalovirus infection of the thyroid in immunocompromised adults. *Yale J Biol Med* 60(1):1–8.

Friedman-Kien AE, Laubenstein LJ, Rubinstein P, Buimovici-Klein E, Marmor M, Stahl R, Spigland I, Kim KS, Zolla-Pazner S (1982). Disseminated Kaposi's sarcoma in homosexual men. *Ann Intern Med* 96 (6 Pt 1):693–700.

Frizzera G, Rosai J, Dehner LP, Spector BD, Kersey JH (1980). Lymphoreticular disorders in primary immunodeficiency. New findings based on up-to-date histologic classification of 35 cases. *Cancer* 46(4):692–699.

Gallant JE, Staszewski S, Pozniak AL, DeJesus E, Suleiman JMAH, Miller MD, Coakley DF, Lu B, Toole JJ, Cheng AK (2004). The 903 Study Group: efficacy and safety of tenofovir DF vs. stavudine in combination therapy in antiretroviral-naive patients: a 3-year randomized trial. *JAMA* 292 (2):191–201.

Gardner LI, Holmberg SD, Williamson JM, Szczech LA, Carpenter CC, Rompalo AM, Schuman P, Klein RS; HIV Epidemiology Research Study Group (2003) Development of proteinuria or elevated serum creatinine and mortality in HIV-infected women. *J Acquir Immune Defic Syndr* 32(2):203–209.

Gerard Y, Maulin L, Yazdanpanah Y, de la Tribonniere X, Amiel C, Maurage CA, Robin S, Sablonniere B, Dhennain C, Mouton Y (2000). Symptomatic hyper-lactataemia: an emerging complication of antiretroviral therapy. *AIDS* 14 (17):2723–2730.

Gervasoni C, Ridolfo AL, Vaccarezza M, Fedeli P, Morelli P, Rovati L, Galli M (2004). Long-term efficacy of the surgical treatment of buffalo hump in patients continuing antiretroviral therapy. *AIDS* 18(3):574–576.

Ginsburg IH, Link BG (1993). Psychosocial consequences of rejection and stigma feelings in psoriasis. *Int J Dermatol* 32(8):587–591.

Glasgow BJ, Steinsapir KD, Anders K, Layfield LJ (1985). Adrenal pathology in the acquired immune deficiency syndrome. *Am J Clin Pathol* 84(5):594–597.

Gleason OC, Yates WR (1999). Five cases of interferon alpha induced depression treated with antidepressant therapy. *Psychosomatics* 40(6):510–512.

Gluckstein D, Ruskin J (1995). Rapid oral desensitization to trimethoprim-sulfamethoxazole (TMP-SMZ): use in prophylaxis for *Pneumocystis carinii* pneumonia in patients with AIDS who were previously intolerant to TMP-SMZ. *Clin Infect Dis* 20(4):849–853.

Goldberg DE, Smithen LM, Angelilli A, Freeman WR (2005). HIV-associated retinopathy in the HAART era. *Retina* 25(5):633–649.

Gottlieb MS, Schroff R, Schanker HM, Weisman JD, Fan PT, Wolf RA, Saxon A (1981). *Pneumocystis carinii* pneumonia and mucosal candidiasis in pre-viously healthy homosexual men: evidence of a new acquired cellular immu-nodeficiency. *N Engl J Med* 305(24):1425–1431.

Gruber SA, Doshi MD, Cincotta E, Brown KL, Singh A, Morawski K, Alangaden G, Chandrasekar P, Losanoff JE, West MS, El-Amm JM (2008). Preliminary experience with renal transplantation in HIV+ recipients: low acute rejection and infection rates. *Transplantation* 86(2):269–274.

Grulich AE, Vajdic CM (2005). The epidemiology of non-Hodgkin lymphoma. *Pathology* 37(6):409–419.

Gupta MA, Gupta AK (1998). Depression and suicidal ideation in dermatology patients with acne, alopecia areata, atopic dermatitis, and psoriasis. *Br J Dermatol* 139(5):846–850.

Gupta SK, Mamlin BW, Johnson CS, Dollins MD, Topf JM, Dube MP (2004) Prevalence of proteinuria and the development of chronic kidney disease in HIV-infected patients. *Clin Nephrol* 61(1):1–6.

Guaraldi G, Orlando G, Madeddu G, Vescini F, Ventura P, Campostrini S, Mura MS, Parise N, Caudarella R, Esposito R (2004). Alendronate reduces bone resorption in HIV-associated osteopenia/osteoporosis. *HIV Clin Trials* 5 (5):269–277.

Guttler R, Singer PA, Axline SG, Greaves TS, McGill JJ (1993). *Pneumocystis carinii* thyroiditis. Report of three cases and review of the literature. *Arch Intern Med* 153(3):393–396.

Hadigan C, Corcoran C, Basgoz N, Davis B, Sax P, Grinspoon S (2000). Metformin in the treatment of HIV lipodystrophy syndrome: a randomized controlled trial. *JAMA* 284(4):472–477.

Haenel T, Brunner F, Battegay R (1980). Renal dialysis and suicide: occurrence in Switzerland and in Europe. *Compr Psychiatry* 21(2):140–145.

Hammer SM, Eron JJ Jr, Reiss P, Schooley RT, Thompson MA, Walmsley S, Cahn P, Fischl MA, Gatell JM, Hirsch MS, Jacobsen DM, Montaner JS, Richman DD, Yeni PG, Volberding PA; International AIDS Society–USA (2008). Antiretroviral treatment of adult HIV infection: 2008 recommendations of the International AIDS Society–USA panel. *JAMA* 300(5):555–570.

Heath KV, Hogg RS, Singer J, Chan KJ, O'Shaughnessy MV, Montaner JS (2002). Antiretroviral treatment patterns and incident HIV-associated morphologic and lipid abnormalities in a population-based cohort. *J Acquir Immune Defic Syndr* 30(4):440–447.

Hengge UR, Ruzicka T, Tyring SK, Stuschke M, Roggendorf M, Schwartz RA, Seeber S (2002). Update on Kaposi's sarcoma and other HHV-8 associated diseases. Part 1: Epidemiology, environmental predispositions, clinical manifestations, and therapy. *Lancet Infect Dis* 2(5):281–292.

Hewitt RG (2002). Abacavir hypersensitivity reaction. *Clin Infect Dis* 34(8):1137–1142.

Hill D, Dubey JP (2002). *Toxoplasma gondii*: transmission, diagnosis and prevention. *Clin Microbiol Infect* 8(10):634–640.

Hoffman CJ, Brown TT (2007). Thyroid function abnormalities in HIV-infected persons. *Clin Infect Dis* 45(4):488–494.

Hoffman RG, Cohen MA, Alfonso CA, Weiss JJ, Jones S, Keller M, Condemarin JR, Chiu NM, Jacobsen JM (2003). Treatment of interferon-induced psychosis in patients with comorbid hepatitis C and HIV. *Psychosomatics* 44 (5):417–420.

Holland GN, Pepose JS, Petitt TH, Gottlieb MS, Yee RD, Foos RY (1983). Acquired immune deficiency syndrome: ocular manifestations. *Ophthalmology* 90 (8):859–873.

Hong J, Koo B, Koo J (2008). The psychosocial and occupational impact of chronic skin disease. *Dermatol Ther* 21(1):54–59.

Hoover DR, Saah AJ, Bacellar H, Phair J, Detels R, Anderson R, Kaslow RA (1993). Clinical manifestations of AIDS in the era of pneumocystis prophylaxis. Multicenter AIDS Cohort Study. *N Engl J Med* 329(6):1922–1926.

Hruz PW, Murata H, Qiu H, Mueckler M (2002). Indinavir induces acute and reversible peripheral insulin resistance in rats. *Diabetes* 51(4):937–942.

Hutchinson CM, Hook EW III, Shepherd M, Rompalo AM (1994). Altered clinical presentation and manifestations of early syphilis in patients with human immunodeficiency virus infection. *Ann Intern Med* 121 (2):94–100.

Idemyor V (2007). HIV and tuberculosis coinfection: inextricably linked liaison. *J Natl Med Assoc* 99(12):1414–1419.

Imhof A, Ledergerber B, Gunthard HF, Haupts S, Weber R (2005). Swiss HIV Cohort Study: risk factors for and outcome of hyperlactatemia in HIV-infected persons: is there a need for routine lactate monitoring? *Clin Infect Dis* 41(5):721–728.

Jacobson IM (2001). Managing chronic hepatitis C infection. *Hosp Physician* 37 (1):34–41.

Jacobson MA, Zegans M, Pavan PR, O'Donnell JJ, Sattler F, Rao N, Owens S, Pollard R (1997). Cytomegalovirus retinitis after initiation of highly active antiretroviral therapy. *Lancet* 349(9063):1443–1445.

John M, Moore CB, James IR, Nolan D, Upton RP, McKinnon EJ, Mallal SA (2001). Chronic hyperlactatemia in HIV-infected patients taking antiretroviral therapy. *AIDS* 15(6):717–723.

Jones BE, Young SM, Antoniskis D, Davidson PT, Kramer F, Barnes PF (1993). Relationship of the manifestations of tuberculosis to CD4 cell counts in patients with human immunodeficiency virus infection. *Am Rev Respir Dis* 148(5):1292–1297.

Jones JL, Hanson DL, Dworkin MS, Alderton DL, Fleming PL, Kaplan JE, Ward J (1999). Surveillance for AIDS-defining opportunistic illnesses, 1992–1997. *MMWR CDC Surveill Summ* 48(2):1–22.

Kershner P, Wang-Cheng R (1989). Psychiatric side effects of steroid therapy. *Psychosomatics* 30(2):135–139.

Kestelyn PG, Cunningham ET Jr (2001). HIV/AIDS and blindness. *Bull World Health Organ* 79(3):208–213.

Khanna R, Tachopoulou OA, Fein PA, Chattopadhyay J, Avram MM (2005). Survival experience of peritoneal dialysis patients with human immunodeficiency virus: a 17 year retrospective study. *Adv Perit Dial* 21:159–163.

Klein D, Hurley LB, Quesenberry CP Jr, Sidney S (2002). Do protease inhibitors increase the risk for coronary heart disease in patients with HIV-1 infection? *J Acquir Immune Defic Syndr* 30(5):471–477.

Koch M, Banys P (2001). Liver transplantation in opioid dependence. *JAMA* 285 (8):1056–1058.

Kotler DP, Reka S, Orenstein JM, Fox CH (1992). Chronic idiopathic esophageal ulceration in the acquired immunodeficiency syndrome. Characterization and treatment with corticosteroids. *J Clin Gastroenterol* 15(4):284–290.

Koziel MJ, Peters MG (2007). Viral hepatitis in HIV infection. *N Engl J Med* 356 (14):1445–1454.

Krauth PH, Katz JF (1987). Kaposi's sarcoma involving the thyroid in a patient with AIDS. *Clin Nucl Med* 12(11):848–849.

Laulund S, Visfeldt J, Klinken L (1986). Patho-anatomical studies in patients dying of AIDS. *Acta Pathol Microbiol Immunol Scand A* 94(3):201–221.

Lazarus JV, Olsen M, Ditiu L, Matic S (2008). Tuberculosis–HIV co-infection: policy and epidemiology in 25 countries in the WHO European region. *HIV Med* 9(6):406–414.

Lee GA, Seneviratne T, Noor MA, Lo JC, Schwarz JM, Aweeka FT, Mulligan K, Schambelan M, Grunfeld C (2004). The metabolic effects of lopinavir/ritonavir in HIV-negative women. *AIDS* 18(4):641–649.

Leggat JE, Bloembergen WE, Levine G, Hulbert-Shearon TE, Port FK (1997). An analysis of risk factors for withdrawal from dialysis before death. *J Am Soc Nephrol* 8(11):1755–1763.

Levenson J, Olbrisch M (2000). Psychosocial screening and selection of candidates for organ transplantation. In P Trzepacz and A DiMartini (eds.), *The Transplant Patient* (pp. 21–41). Cambridge, UK: Cambridge University Press.

Levy NB (2000). Psychiatric considerations in primary medical care of the patient in renal failure. *Adv Ren Replace Ther* 7(3):231–238.

Lewden C, May T, Rosenthal E, Burty C, Bonnet F, Costagliola D, Jougla E, Semaille C, Morlat P, Salmon D, Cacoub P, Chene G, on behalf of the ANRS EN19 Mortalite Study Group and Mortavic (2008). Changes in causes of death among adults infected by HIV between 2000 and 2005: the "Mortalite 2000 and 2005" surveys (ANRS EN19 and Mortavic). *J Acquir Immune Defic Syndr* 48(5):590–598.

Lo J, You SM, Canavan B, Liebau J, Beltrani G, Koutkia P, Hemphill L, Lee H, Grinspoon S (2008). Low-dose physiological growth hormone in patients with HIV and abdominal fat accumulation. *JAMA* 300 (5):509–519.

Loftis JM, Hauser P (2003). Comanagement of depression and HCV treatment. *Psychiatr Ann* 33(6):385–391.

Long JL, Engels EA, Moore RD, Gebo KA (2008). Incidence and outcomes of malignancy in the HAART era in an urban cohort of HIV-infected individuals. *AIDS* 22(4):489–496.Lustman PJ, Anderson RJ, Freedland KE, de Groot M, Carney RM, Clouse RE (2000). Depression and poor glycemic control: a meta-analytic review of the literature. *Diabetes Care* 23(7):934–942.

MacDonald JC, Karavellas MP, Torriani FJ, Morse LS, Smith IL, Reed JB, Freeman WR (2000). Highly active antiretroviral therapy–related immune recovery in AIDS patients with cytomegalovirus retinitis. *Ophthalmology* 107(5):877–883.

Mallal S, Phillips E, Carosi G, Molina JM, Workman C, Tomazic J, Jagel-Guedes E, Rugina S, Kozyrev O, Cid JF, Hay P, Nolan D, Hughes S, Hughes A, Ryan S, Fitch N, Thorborn D, Benbow A, for the PREDICT-1 Study Team (2008). HLA-B*5701 screening for hypersensitivity to abacavir. *N Engl J Med* 358 (6):568–579.

Marik PE, Kiminoyo K, Zaloga GP (2002). Adrenal insufficiency in critically ill patients with human immunodeficiency virus. *Crit Care Med* 30 (6):1267–1273.

Martinez E, Conget I, Lozano L, Casamitjana R, Gatell JM (1999). Reversion of metabolic abnormalities after switching from HIV-1 protease inhibitors to nevirapine. *AIDS* 13(7):805–810.

Mary-Krause M, Cotte L, Simon A, Partisani M, Costagliola D (2003). Clinical Epidemiology Group from the French Hospital Database: increased risk of myocardial infarction with duration of protease inhibitor therapy in HIV-infected men. *AIDS* 17(17):2479–2486.

Masur H, Kovacs JA (1998). Treatment and prophylaxis of *Pneumocystis carinii* pneumonia. *Infect Dis Clin North Am* 2(2):419–28.

Masur H, Michelis MA, Greene JB, Onorato I, Stouwe RA, Holzman RS, Wormser G, Brettman L, Lange M, Murray HW, Cunningham-Rundles S (1981). An outbreak of community-acquired *Pneumocystis carinii* pneumonia: initial manifestation of cellular immune dysfunction. *N Engl J Med* 305(24):1431–1438.

McCarty M, Coker R, Claydon E (1992). Case report: disseminated *Pneumocystis carinii* infection in a patient with the acquired immune deficiency syndrome causing thyroid gland calcification and hypothyroidism. *Clin Radiol* 45 (3):209–210.

McComsey GA, Kendall MA, Tebas P, Swindells S, Hogg E, Alston-Smith B, Suckow C, Gopalakrishnan G, Benson C, Wohl DA (2007). Alendronate with calcium and vitamin D supplementation is safe and effective for the treatment of decreased bone mineral density in HIV. *AIDS* 2007 21 (18):2473–2482.

McComsey G, Lonergan JT (2004). Mitochondrial dysfunction: patient monitoring and toxicity management. *J Acquir Immune Defic Syndr* 37(Suppl 1): S30–S35.

McComsey GA, Ward DJ, Hessenthaler SM, Sension MG, Shalit P, Lonergan JT, Fisher RL, Williams VC, Hernandez JE (2004). Trial to Assess the Regression of Hyperlactatemia and to Evaluate the Regression of Established Lipodystrophy in HIV-1-Positive Subjects (TARHEEL; ESS40010) Study Team: improvement in lipoatrophy associated with highly active antiretroviral therapy in human immunodeficiency virus–infected patients switched from stavudine to abacavir or zidovudine: the results of the TARHEEL study. *Clin Infect Dis* 38(2):263–270.

Melendez MM, McNurlan MA, Mynarcik DC, Khan S, Gelato MC (2008). Endothelial adhesion molecules are associated with inflammation in subjects with HIV disease. *Clin Infect Dis* 46(5):775–780.Milazzo F, Piconi S, Trabottoni D, Magni C, Coen M, Capetti A, Fusi ML, Parravicini C, Clerici M (1999). Intractable pruritus in HIV infection; immunology and characterization. *Allergy* 54(3):266–272.

Miller K, Corcoran C, Armstrong C, Caramelli K, Anderson E, Cotton D, Basgoz N, Hirschhorn L, Tuomala R, Schoenfeld D, Daugherty C, Mazer N, Grinspoon S (1998). Transdermal testosterone administration in women with acquired immunodeficiency syndrome wasting: a pilot study. *J Clin Endocrinol Metab* 83(8):2717–2725.

Miranda A, Morgan M, Jamal L, Laserson K, Barreira D, Silva G, Santos J, Wells C, Paine P, Garrett D (2007). Impact of antiretroviral therapy on the incidence of tuberculosis: the Brazilian experience, 1995–2001. *PLoS ONE* 2 (9):e826.

Mollison LC, Mijch A, McBride G, Dwyer B (1991). Hypothyroidism due to destruction of the thyroid by Kaposi's sarcoma. *Rev Infect Dis* 13(5):826–827.

Monkemuller KE, Wilcox CM (2000a). Diagnosis and treatment of esophagitis in AIDS. *Compr Ther* 26(3):163–168.

Monkemuller KE, Wilcox CM (2000b). Investigation of diarrhea in AIDS. *Can J Gastroenterol* 14(11):933–940.

Moraes HV (2002). Ocular manifestations of HIV/AIDS. *Curr Opin Ophthalmol* 13(6):397–403.

Moyle GJ, Sabin CA, Cartledge J, Johnson M, Wilkins E, Churchill D, Hay P, Fakoya A, Murphy M, Scullard G, Leen C, Reilly G; for the RAVE (Randomized Abacavir versus Viread Evaluation) group UK (2006). A randomized comparative trial of tenofovir DF or abacavir as replacement for a thymidine analogue in persons with lipoatrophy. *AIDS* 20(16):2043–2050.

Musselman DL, Lawson DH, Gumnick JF, Manatunga AK, Penna S, Goodkin RS, Greiner K, Nemeroff CB, Miller AH (2001). Paroxetine for the prevention of depression induced by high-dose interferon alfa. *N Engl J Med* 344 (13):961–966.

Mylonakis E, Koutkia P, Grinspoon S (2001). Diagnosis and treatment of androgen deficiency in human immunodeficiency virus–infected men and women. *Clin Infect Dis* 33(6):857–864.

Navin TR, Weber R, Vugia DJ, Rimland D, Roberts JM, Addiss DG, Visvesvara GS, Wahlquist SP, Hogan SE, Gallagher LE, Juranek DD, Schwartz DA, Wilcox CM, Stewart JM, Thompson SE 3rd, Bryan RT (1999). Declining CD4+ T-lymphocyte counts are associated with increased risk of enteric parasitosis and chronic diarrhea: results of a 3-year longitudinal study. *J Acquir Immune Defic Syndr Hum Retrovirol* 20(2):154–159.

Negredo E, Martinez-Lopez E, Paredes R, Rosales J, Perez-Alvarez N, Holgado S, Gel S, del Rio L, Tena X, Rey-Joly C, Clotet B (2005). Reversal of HIV-1-associated osteoporosis with once-weekly alendronate. *AIDS* 19(3):343–345.

Negredo E, Ribalta J, Paredes R, Ferre R, Sirera G, Ruiz L, Salazar J, Reiss P, Masana L, Clotet B (2002). Reversal of atherogenic lipoprotein profile in HIV-1 infected patients with lipodystrophy after replacing protease inhibitors by nevirapine. *AIDS* 16(10):1383–1389.

Ng CW, Lam MS, Paton NI (2000). Cryptococcal meningitis resulting in irreversible visual impairment in AIDS patients: a report of two cases. *Singapore Med J* 41(2):80–82.

Noor MA, Seneviratne T, Aweeka FT, Lo JC, Schwarz JM, Mulligan K, Schambelan M, Grunfeld C (2002). Indinavir acutely inhibits insulin-stimulated glucose disposal in humans: a randomized, placebo-controlled study. *AIDS* 16(5):F1–F8.

O'Donnell K, Chung JY (1997). The diagnosis of major depression in end-stage renal disease. *Psychother Psychosom* 66(1):38–43.

Oette M, Hemker J, Feldt T, Sagir A, Best J, Haussinger D (2005). Acute syphilitic blindness in an HIV-positive patient. *AIDS Patient Care STDS* 19 (4):209–211.

Ognibene FP, Shelhamer J, Gill V, Macher AM, Loew D, Parker MM, Gelmann E, Fauci AS, Parrillo JE, Masur H (1984). The diagnosis of *Pneumocystis carinii* pneumonia in patients with the acquired immunodeficiency syndrome using subsegmental bronchoalveolar lavage. *Am Rev Respir Dis* 129(6):929–932.

Onyike CU, Bonner JO, Lyketsos CG, Treisman GJ (2004). Mania during treatment of chronic hepatitis C with pegylated interferon and ribavarin. *Am J Psychiatry* 161(3):429–435.

Palacios R, Santos J, Ruiz J, Gonzalez M, Marquez M (2003). Factors associated with the development of diabetes mellitus in HIV-infected patients on antiretroviral therapy: a case–control study. *AIDS* 17(6):933–935.

Palella FJ Jr, Delaney KM, Moorman AC, Loveless MO, Fuhrer J, Satten GA, Aschman DJ, Holmberg SD (1998). Declining morbidity and mortality among patients with advanced human immunodeficiency virus infection. HIV Outpatient Study Investigators. *N Engl J Med* 338(13):853–860.

Pappas PG, Pottage JC, Powderly WG, Fraser VJ, Stratton CW, McKenzie S, Tapper ML, Chmel H, Bonebrake FC, Blum R (1992). Blastomycosis in patients with the acquired immunodeficiency syndrome. *Ann Intern Med* 116(10):847–853.

Pazianas M, Miller P, Blumentals WA, Bernal M, Kothawala P (2007). A review of the literature on osteonecrosis of the jaw in patients with osteoporosis treated with oral bisphosphonates: prevalence, risk factors, and clinical characteristics. *Clin Ther* 29(8):1548–1558.

Pedrazzoni M, Vescovi PP, Maninetti L, Michelini M, Zaniboni G, Pioli G, Costi D, Alfano FS, Passeri M (1993). Effects of chronic heroin abuse on bone and mineral metabolism. *Acta Endocrinol (Copenh)* 129(1):42–45.

Penn I (1975). The incidence of malignancies in transplant recipients. *Transplant Proc* 7(2):323–326.

Perkocha LA, Geaghan SM, Yen TS, Nishimura SL, Chan SP, Garcia-Kennedy R, Honda G, Stoloff AC, Klein HZ, Goldman RL, et al. (1990). Clinical and pathological features of bacillary peliosis hepatis in association with human immunodeficiency virus infection. *N Engl J Med* 323(23):1581–1586.

Pessanha TM, Campos JM, Barros AC, Pone MV, Garrido JR, Pone SM (2007). Iatrogenic Cushing's syndrome in an adolescent with AIDS on ritonavir and inhaled fluticasone. Case report and literature review. *AIDS* 21(4):529–532.

Petrosillo N, Nicastri E, Viale P (2005). Nosocomial pulmonary infections in HIV-positive patients. *Curr Opin Pulm Med* 11(3):231–235.

Polesel J, Clifford GM, Rickenbach M, Dal Maso L, Battegay M, Bouchardy C, Furrer H, Hasse B, Levi F, Probst-Hensch NM, Schmid P, Franceschi S; the Swiss HIV Cohort Study (2008). Non-Hodgkin's lymphoma incidence in the Swiss HIV Cohort Study before and after highly active antiretroviral therapy. *AIDS* 22(2):301–306.

Portu JJ, Santamaria JM, Zubero Z, Almeida-Llamas MV, Aldamiz-Etxebarria San Sebastian M, Gutierrez AR (1996). Atypical scabies in HIV-positive patients. *J Am Acad Dermatol* 34(5 Pt.2):915–917.

Power R, Tate HL, McGill SM, Taylor C (2003). A qualitative study of the psychosocial implications of lipodystrophy syndrome on HIV positive individuals. *Sex Transm Infect* 79(2):137–141.

Pulakhandam U, Dincsoy HP (1990). Cytomegaloviral adrenalitis and adrenal insufficiency in AIDS. *Am J Clin Pathol* 93(5):651–656.

Qiu J, Terasaki PI, Waki K, Cai J, Gjertson DW (2006). HIV-positive renal recipients can achieve survival rates similar to those of HIV-negative patients. *Transplantation* 81(12):1658–1661.

Ragni MV, Dekker A, DeRubertis FR, Watson CG, Skolnick ML, Goold SD, Finikiotis MW, Doshi S, Myers DJ (1991). *Pneumocystis carinii* infection presenting as necrotizing thyroiditis and hypothyroidism. *Am J Clin Pathol* 95(4):489–493.

Raison CL, Borisov AS, Broadwell SD, Capuron L, Woolwine BJ, Jacobson IM, Nemeroff CB, Miller AH (2005). Depression during pegylated interferon-alpha plus ribavirin therapy: prevalence and prediction. *J Clin Psychiatry* 66 (1):41–48.

Rajagopalan R, Laitinen D, Dietz B (2008). Impact of lipoatrophy on quality of life in HIV patients receiving anti-retroviral therapy. *AIDS Care* 20 (10):1197–1201.

Raviglione MC, Snider DE Jr, Kochi A (1995). Global epidemiology of tuberculosis. Morbidity and mortality of a worldwide epidemic. *JAMA* 273 (3):220–226.

Reichsman F, Levy NB (1972): Adaptation to hemodialysis. A four-year study of 25 patients. *Arch Intern Med* 130(6):859–865.

Remick S (1996). Non-AIDS defining cancers. *Hematol Oncol Clin North Am* 10 (5):1203–1213.

Riddler SA, Smit E, Cole SR, Li R, Chmiel JS, Dobs A, Palella F, Visscher B, Evans R, Kingsley LA (2003). Impact of HIV infection and HAART on serum lipids in men. *JAMA* 289(22):2978–2982.

Rigopoulos D, Paparizos V, Katsambas A (2004). Cutaneous markers of HIV infection. *Clin Dermatol* 22(6):487–498.

Roland ME, Stock PG (2006). Liver transplantation in HIV-infected recipients. *Semin Liver Dis* 26(3):273–284.

Rolfs RT, Joesoef MR, Hendershot EF, Rompalo AM, Augenbraun MH, Chiu M, Bolan G, Johnson SC, French P, Steen E, Radolf JD, Larsen S (1997). A randomized trial of enhanced therapy for early syphilis in patients with and without human immunodeficiency virus infection. The Syphilis and HIV Study Group. *N Engl J Med* 337(5):307–314.

Ross, MJ, Klotman PE (2004). HIV-associated nephropathy. *AIDS* 18(8):1089–1099.

Samaras K, Pett S, Gowers A, McMurchie M, Cooper DA (2005). Iatrogenic Cushing's syndrome with osteoporosis and secondary adrenal failure in human immunodeficiency virus–infected persons receiving inhaled corticosteroids and ritonavir-boosted protease inhibitors: six cases (2005). *J Clin Endocrinol Metab* 90(7):4394–4398.

Schambelan M, Benson CA, Carr A, Currier JS, Dube MP, Gerber JG, Grinspoon SK, Grunfeld C, Kotler DP, Mulligan K, Powderly WG, Saag MS (2002). Management of metabolic complications associated with antiretroviral therapy for HIV–1 infection: recommendations of an International AIDS Society–USA panel. *J Acquir Immune Defic Syndr* 31(3):257–275.

Schambelan M, Mulligan K, Grunfeld C, Daar ES, LaMarca A, Kotler DP, Wang J, Bozzette SA, Breitmeyer JB (1996). Recombinant human growth hormone in patients with HIV-associated wasting. A randomized, placebo-controlled trial. Serostim Study Group. *Ann Intern Med* 125(11):873–882.

Schild AF, Prieto J, Glenn M, Livingstone J, Alfieri K, Raines J (2004). Maturation and failure rates in a large series of arteriovenous dialysis access fistulas. *Vasc Endovascular Surg* 38(5):449–453.

Sellmeyer DE, Grunfeld C (1996). Endocrine and metabolic disturbances in human immunodeficiency virus infection and the acquired immune deficiency syndrome. *Endocr Rev* 17(5):518–532.

Shah M, Tierney K, Adams-Huet B, Boonyavarakul A, Jacob K, Quittner C, Dinges WL, Peterson D, Garg A (2005). The role of diet, exercise, and smoking in dyslipidaemia in HIV-infected patients with lipodystrophy. *HIV Med* 6(4):291–298.

Shapiro P, Williams DL, Foray AT, Gelman IS, Wukich N, Sciacca R (1995). Psychosocial evaluation and prediction of compliance problems and morbidity after heart transplantation. *Transplantation* 60(12):1462–1466.

Smith PD, Quinn TC, Strober W, Janoff EN, Masur H. NIH conference (1992). Gastrointestinal infections in AIDS. *Ann Intern Med* 116(1):63–77.

Soriano V, Garcia-Gasco P, Vispo E, Ruiz-Sancho A, Blanco F, Martin-Carbonero L, Rodriguez-Novoa S, Morello J, de Mendoza C, Rivas P, Barreiro P, Gonzalez-Lahoz J (2008). Efficacy and safety of replacing lopinavir with atazanavir in HIV-infected patients with undetectable plasma viraemia: final results of the SLOAT trial. *J Antimicrob Chemother* 61(1):200–205.

Soriano V, Puoti M, Sulkowski M, Mauss S, Cacoub P, Cargnel A, Dieterich D, Hatzakis A, Rockstroh J (2004). Care of patients with hepatitis C and HIV co-infection. *AIDS* 18(1):1–12.

Spitzer RD, Chan JC, Marks JB, Valme BR, McKenzie JM (1991). Case report: hypothyroidism due to *Pneumocystis carinii* thyroiditis in a patient with acquired immunodeficiency syndrome. *Am J Med Sci* 302(2):98–100.

Stanley TL, Grinspoon SK (2008). GH/GHRH axis in HIV lipodystrophy. *Pituitary* 12:143–152.

Starkman MN (2003). Psychiatric manifestations of hyperadrenocorticism and hypoadrenocorticism (Cushing's and Addison's diseases). In OM Wolkowitz and AJ Rothschild (eds.), *Psychoneuroendocrinology: The Scientific Basis of Clinical Practice* (pp. 165–188). Arlington VA: American Psychiatric Publishing.

Statistics, N.C.f.H. (2005). Health, United States, 2005, with Chartbook on Trends on the Health of Americans. 2005, Hyattsville, MD: U.S. Government Printing Office.

Staubach P, Eckhardt-Henn A, Dechene M, Vonend A, Metz M, Magerl M, Breuer P, Maurer M (2006). Quality of life in patients with chronic urticaria is differentially impaired and determined by psychiatric comorbidity. *Br J Dermatol* 154(2):294–298.

Szczech LA, Edwards LJ, Sanders LL, van der Horst C, Bartlet JA, Heald AE, Svetkey LP (2002). Protease inhibitors are associated with a slowed progression of HIV-related renal diseases. *Clin Nephrol* 57(5):336–341.

Szczech LA, Hoover DR, Feldman JG, Cohen MH, Gange SJ, Gooze L, Rubin NR, Young MA, Cai X, Shi Q, Gao W, Anastos K (2004). Association between renal disease and outcomes among HIV-infected women receiving or not receiving antiretroviral therapy. *Clin Infect Dis* 39(8):1199–1206.

Tappero JW, Perkins BA, Wenger JD, Berger TG (1995). Cutaneous manifestations of opportunistic infections in patients infected with human immunodeficiency virus. *Clin Microbiol Rev* 8(3):440–450.

Trask P, Esper P, Riba M, Redman B (2000). Psychiatric side effects of interferon therapy: prevalence, proposed mechanisms, and future directions. *Clin Oncol* 18(11):2316–2326.

U.S. Renal Data System (2005). *USRDS 2005 Annual Data Report: Atlas of End-Stage Renal Disease in the United States.* Bethesda, MD: National Institutes of Health, National Institute of Diabetes and Digestive and Kidney Diseases.

Villette JM, Bourin P, Doinel C, Mansour I, Fiet J, Boudou P, Dreux C, Roue R, Debord M, Levi F (1990). Circadian variations in plasma levels of hypophyseal, adrenocortical and testicular hormones in men infected with human immunodeficiency. *J Endocrinol Metab* 70(3):572–577.

Vos F, Pieters G, Keuter M, van Der Ven A (2006). Graves' disease during immune reconstitution in HIV-infected patients treated with HAART. *Scand J Infect Dis* 38(2):124–126.

Wagner GJ, Ryan GW (2005). Hepatitis C virus treatment decision-making in the context of HIV co-infection: the role of medical, behavioral and mental health factors in assessing treatment readiness. *AIDS* 19(S3):S190–S198.

Wali RK, Drachenberg CI, Papadimitriou JC, Keay S, Ramos E (1998). HIV-1-associated nephropathy and response to highly active antiretroviral therapy. *Lancet* 352(9130):783–784.

Wallace MR, Brann OS (2000). Gastrointestinal manifestations of HIV infection. *Curr Gastroenterol Rep* 2(4):283–293.

Welch K, Finkbeiner W, Alpers CE, Blumenfeld W, Davis RL, Smuckler EA, Beckstead JH (1984). Autopsy findings in the acquired immune deficiency syndrome. *JAMA* 252(9):1152–1159.

Wells CD, Cegielski JP, Nelson LJ, Laserson KF, Holtz TH, Finlay A, Castro KG, Weyer K (2007). HIV infection and multidrug-resistant tuberculosis: the perfect storm. *J Infect Dis* 196 (Suppl.1):S86–107.

Wijdicks EF (2001). Neurotoxicity of immunosuppressive drugs. *Liver Transplant* 7(11):937–942.

Wilcox CM (1993). Serious gastrointestinal disorders associated with human immunodeficiency virus infection. *Crit Care Clin* 9(1):73–88.

Williams G, Alarcon E, Jittimanee S, Walusimbi M, Sebek M, Berga E, Villa TS (2008). HIV testing and care of the patient co-infected with tuberculosis and HIV. *Int J Tuberc Lung Dis* 12(8):889–894.

Winston JA, Bruggeman LA, Ross MD, Jacobsen J, Ross L, D'Agati VD, Klotman PE, Klotman ME (2001). Nephropathy and establishment of a renal reservoir of HIV type 1 during primary infection. *N Engl J Med* 344 (26):1979–1984.

Wolff AJ, O'Donnell AE (2001). Pulmonary manifestations of HIV infection in the era of highly active antiretroviral therapy. *Chest* 120(6):1888–1893.

Woo SB, Hellstein JW, Kalmar JR (2006). Systematic review: bisphosphonates and osteonecrosis of the jaws. *Ann Intern Med* 144(10):753–761.

Wood C, Harrington W Jr (2005). AIDS and associated malignancies. *Cell Res* 15(11-12):947–952.

Wood R, Phanuphak P, Cahn P, Pokrovskiy V, Rozenbaum W, Pantaleo G, Sension M, Murphy R, Mancini M, Kelleher T, Giordano M (2004) Long-term efficacy and safety of atazanavir with stavudine and lamivudine in patients previously treated with nelfinavir or atazanavir. *J Acquir Immune Defic Syndr* 36(2):684–692.

Wunder DM, Bersinger NA, Fux CA, Mueller NJ, Hirschel B, Cavassini M, Elzi L, Schmid P, Bernasconi E, Mueller B, Furrer H; Swiss HIV Cohort Study (2007). Hypogonadism in HIV-1-infected men is common and does not resolve during antiretroviral therapy. *Antivir Ther* 1(2):261–265.

Yusuf TE, Baron TH (2004). AIDS cholangiopathy. *Curr Treat Options Gastroenterol* 7(2):111–117.

Zonis De Zukerfeld R, Ingratta R, Sanchez Negrete G, Matusevich A, Intebi C (2003–2004). Psychosocial aspects in osteoporosis [in Spanish]. *Vertex* 14 (54):253–259.

11

A BIOPSYCHOSOCIAL APPROACH TO TREATMENT

Mary Ann Cohen and Harold W. Goforth

Know syphilis in all its manifestations and relations, and all other things clinical will be added unto you.

Sir William Osler (Bean WB, 1968)

The care of persons with HIV and AIDS presents clinicians, caregivers, families, and loved ones with special biopsychosocial challenges posed by the infectious nature of HIV, the specific modes of HIV transmission, the particular way HIV affects the brain, the age of onset, and the complex stigma of HIV. These challenges differentiate AIDS from other severe and complex illnesses, causes, have significant clinical and public health implications, and necessitate early recognition and treatment. The multifactorial nature of these challenges is summarized in Table 11.1, and some unique aspects of AIDS are briefly summarized in Table 11.2.

AIDS psychiatrists, psychosomatic medicine psychiatrists, physicians trained in both medicine and psychiatry, and other mental health clinicians can play a vital role the care of persons with HIV and AIDS, in the prevention of HIV transmission, and in training of other clinicians to alleviate distress, reduce ongoing high-risk behavior and nonadherence, provide support for patients and families, and improve patients' quality of life. In this chapter, we will review the biopsychosocial aspects of AIDS and suggest strategies to address the unique challenges of this devastating and complex illness.

TABLE 11.1 A Biopsychosocial Approach to HIV and AIDS

Biological	Psychological	Social
Opportunistic Infections (Most Common)	Diagnoses (Most Common)	Social Stressors (Most Common)
Protozoal	**Mood disorders**	Alienation
		Stigma
Pnuemocystis jeroveki pneumonia	Major depressive disorder	Poverty
Toxoplasma gondii encephalitis	Mood disorder due to medical condition with depression	Job loss
Bacterial		Rejection
Mycobacterium avium intracellulare	Mood disorder due to medical condition with mania	Eviction
Viral	Bipolar disorder	**Losses**
Cytomegalovirus disease	**Cognitive disorders**	Disparities
Fungal	HIV-associated dementia	AIDSism
Cryptococcal meningitis	Delirium	Racism
Esophageal candidiasis	**Substance use disorders**	Ageism
Opportunistic Cancers	Adjustment disorders	
Kaposi's sarcoma	**Anxiety disorders**	
	Posttraumatic stress disorder	
	Bereavement	
Multimorbid Medical Illnesses (Most Common)	Symptoms	
Chronic hepatitis C and cirrhosis	Depression	
Cancers	Anxiety	
Cardiac disease	Confusion	
Cerebrovascular disease	Psychosis	
Diabetes mellitus	Suicidality	
Lung disease	Existential anxiety	
Clostridium difficile colitis	Grief	
Neuropathy and myelopathy	Demoralization	
Renal disease		
Symptoms		
Pain		
Insomnia		
Fatigue		
Nausea		
Vomiting		

Diarrhea
Wasting
Pruritus
Hiccups
Incontinence
Weakness
Paresis and paralysis

TABLE 11.2 How AIDS Differs from Most Other Severe and Complex Medical Illnesses

- Infectious etiology
- Modes of transmission: unsafe sex, sharing of needles in injecting drug use, perinatal
- AIDS is preventable.
- Disinhibition can lead to HIV, HBV, HCV, and STD transmission.
- Stigma
- Age of onset from birth to old age
- Treatment, stabilization, or prevention with antiretrovirals is possible.
- Exacerbation by treatment with antiretrovirals can occur.
- Multiple infections and complex medical comorbidities
- High prevalence of psychiatric disorders, including substance use and its consequences
- High prevalence of delirium due to respiratory, cardiac, and metabolic illnesses
- High prevalence of delirium due to end-stage renal and liver disease
- High prevalence of HIV-associated dementia
- Unique neurological deficits, paresis, paralysis, and pain
- Unique behavioral manifestations

HBV, hepatitis B virus; HCV, hepatitis C virus; STD, sexually transmitted disease.

HISTORY OF AIDS PSYCHIATRY

Although the AIDS epidemic was first described in the medical literature in 1981, it was not until 1983 that the first articles were published about the psychosocial or psychiatric aspects of AIDS. The first article was not written by a psychiatrist. This article, written by Holtz and colleagues (1983), was essentially a plea for attention to the psychosocial aspects of AIDS. They stated that "noticeably absent in the flurry of publications about the current epidemic of acquired immune deficiency syndrome (AIDS) is reference to the psychosocial impact of this devastating new syndrome." The authors deplored ostracism of persons with AIDS by both their families and their medical systems of care. These authors were the first to describe the profound withdrawal from human contact as the "sheet sign" observed when a person with AIDS drew a bed sheet over his or her face and head, essentially withdrawing and hiding from visitors.

The first psychiatrist to make use of the literature to address these issues was Stuart E. Nichols (1983). In his article in *Psychosomatics*, Nichols described the need for compassion, support, and understanding to address the fear, depression, and alienation experienced by patients. He also made recommendations for use of psychotherapy and group therapy as well as antidepressant medications to help persons with AIDS cope with intense feelings about this new illness that was still of undetermined etiology. Nichols stated: "Since AIDS apparently is a new disease, there is no specific psychiatric literature to which one can refer for guidance. One must be willing to attempt to provide competent and compassionate care in an area with more questions than answers." The earliest articles published in the first decade of AIDS psychiatry, from 1983 to 1993, were primarily descriptive observations, case reports, case series, and documentation and prevalence of psychiatric diagnoses associated with AIDS. They were written by sensitive and compassionate clinicians, some of whom openly expressed their outrage at ostracism and rejection of persons with HIV and AIDS by not only the community at large but also by the medical community. These clinicians also emphasized the need for compassion and for competent medical and psychiatric care. These early articles are summarized in Table 11.3.

In the 26 years (1983–2009) since AIDS psychiatry references first appeared in the medical literature, there have been 14,830 articles written (according to PubMed, accessed on September 24, 2009), in addition to two textbooks (Fernandez and Ruiz, 2006; Cohen and Gorman, 2008), other books (Treisman and Angelino, 2004), and numerous chapters. Most of the

TABLE 11.3 Early Literature of AIDS Psychiatry*

Year	Issues Addressed, Comments
1983	Psychosocial impact of AIDS—ostracism, the "sheet sign," and the need for psychiatric literature about AIDS (Holtz et al.) Psychiatric aspects of AIDS—need for psychiatric consultations and for group therapy; first article by a psychiatrist about AIDS psychiatry (Nichols)
1984	Psychiatric implications of AIDS—the first book about AIDS psychiatry (Nichols and Ostrow) Psychosocial aspects of AIDS—the first description of the biopsychosocial approach applied in the general care setting by Cohen (Deuchar) AIDS anxiety in the "worried well" (Forstein, 1984a) Psychosocial impact of AIDS (Forstein, 1984b) Case reports and treatment recommendations for persons with AIDS seen in psychiatric consultation (Barbuto) Psychiatric complications of AIDS (Nurnberg et al.) Neuropsychiatric complications of AIDS (Hoffman) Cryptococcal meningitis presenting as mania in AIDS (Thienhaus and Khosla) Description of a support group for persons with AIDS (Nichols) Psychiatric problems in patients with AIDS at New York Hospital (Perry and Tross)

1985   Findings in 13 of 40 persons with AIDS seen in psychiatric consultation (Dilley et al.)
Description of psychiatric and psychosocial aspects of AIDS (Holland and Tross)

1986   A biopsychosocial approach to AIDS (Cohen and Weisman)
Neuropsychiatric aspects of AIDS (Price and Forejt)

1987   Psychiatric aspects of AIDS (Faulstich)
Dementia as the presenting or sole manifestation of HIV infection (Navia and Price)
Psychiatric aspects of AIDS: a biopsychosocial approach—comprehensive chapter (Cohen)
Stigmatization of AIDS patients by physicians (Kelly et al.)

1988   Discrimination against people with AIDS (Blendon and Donelan)
First article on high prevalence of suicide among persons with AIDS (Marzuk et al.)

1989   AIDSism, a new form of discrimination (Cohen)
Anxiety and stigmatizing aspects of HIV infection (Fullilove)

1990   Firesetting and HIV-associated dementia (Cohen et al.)
Suicidality and HIV testing (Perry et al.)

1992   A biopsychosocial approach to the HIV epidemic (Cohen)
Suicidality and HIV status (McKegney and O'Dowd)

1993   Manic syndrome early and late in the course of HIV (Lyketsos et al.)

*Listed here are descriptions of psychosocial and psychiatric aspects of AIDS, with emphasis on discrimination. Only a sample of articles, chapters, and books published in the first decade of AIDS psychiatry (1983–1993) is provided.

articles reflect a growing body of research in the area and the beginnings of an evidence base for the practice of AIDS psychiatry. Some of these articles provide evidence for the need for a comprehensive biopsychosocial approach to the care of persons with HIV and AIDS.

A Biopsychosocial Approach to HIV and AIDS and AIDSism

In 1981, one of the authors (Cohen, 2008) responded to her first psychiatric consultation request to evaluate a 29-year-old man with AIDS and depression who was hospitalized on a general medical care inpatient unit of an urban academic medical center. There was a tray of food on the floor outside his room. When she knocked on his door, received a response, and entered his room, she discovered that the floor of the room was very sticky and her shoes stuck to it and made strange noises as she approached the bedside. The patient's head was covered with a sheet. When she introduced herself and began to speak to the patient, he gradually removed the sheet from his head. He was extremely cachectic, almost skeletal, and appeared much older than his stated age of 29 years. He spoke slowly and softly and related well. He had evidence of cognitive impairment, depression, and substance use disorder as well as multiple and complex medical illnesses. He was alienated from his family.

The "sticky-floor syndrome" joined the "sheet sign" as one of the early unique responses to the AIDS pandemic. The sticky floor was the result of an accumulation of spilled food and beverages as well as the patient's body fluids that went unattended by fearful hospital maintenance staff. Because the patient was weak and had difficulty grasping and holding onto objects there were frequent spills. Ambulation was slow and difficult for him and he did not always make it to the bathroom in time. It was readily apparent that a hospital-wide, multidisciplinary program and education of every level of staff on all shifts were needed to improve the care of persons with AIDS, diminish stigma and discrimination, and help to alleviate fear, anxiety, and stigma in caregivers.

In 1983, the infectious disease director, a social worker, and Cohen developed a multidisciplinary AIDS program at the hospital to provide coordinated and comprehensive care for persons with AIDS and to provide education for hospital staff and medical students and their faculty. This program was the first to be described in the literature as a response to the epidemic (Deuchar, 1984; Cohen and Weisman, 1986). The comprehensive program was described as a means of coordinating care and communication among the multiple specialties and across disciplines involved in the care of persons with AIDS. This program had a biopsychosocial approach with the perspective that each individual is a member of a family and community and deserves a coordinated approach to medical care and treatment with dignity. The program included the development of a multidisciplinary treatment team, provision of ongoing psychological support for patients and families, and education and support for hospital staff.

As the scenario described above illustrates, many persons with AIDS were treated as lepers in the early years of the epidemic. Some found that they were shunned and ostracized. In some areas of the world, persons with AIDS were quarantined because of the irrational fears, discrimination, and stigma associated with this pandemic. Initially, in the United States, some persons who were diagnosed with AIDS were rejected by not only their communities but also their families and friends. Some persons with AIDS lost their homes, some children and adolescents were excluded from classrooms, and some lost their jobs. In the early 1980s, a diagnosis of AIDS led to rejection by shelters for the homeless, nursing homes, long-term care facilities, and facilities for the terminally ill. The attitudes of families, houses of worship, prison guards, employers, teachers, hospital staff, and funeral directors led to catastrophic stigma and discrimination. Persons with AIDS had difficulty finding support, obtaining health care, keeping a job, finding a home, and finding a chronic-care facility or even a place to die.

Discrimination against persons with AIDS was described (Cohen, 1989) as a new form of discrimination called "AIDSism." AIDSism is built on a foundation of homophobia, misogyny, racism, addictophobia, and fears of contagion and death. Discrimination and stigma were recognized early in the AIDS psychiatry literature as contributing to psychological distress (Holtz et al., 1983; Nichols, 1983, 1984; Deuchar, 1984; Holland and Tross, 1985; Cohen and Weisman, 1986; Blendon and Donelan, 1988; Cohen, 1989; Fullilove, 1989; Chesney and Smith, 1992) and have been explored subsequently following the introduction of potent antiretroviral therapy (Herek et al., 2002; Parker and Aggleton, 2003; Brown et al., 2003; Kaplan et al., 2005; Cohen, 2008).

Early in the epidemic, many physicians surveyed had negative attitudes toward persons with HIV and AIDS (Kelly et al., 1987; Thompson, 1987; Wormser and Joline, 1989). Although the medical profession has made great strides against discrimination and stigma and most physicians are "accustomed to caring for HIV-infected patients with concern and compassion" (Gottlieb, 2001), society as a whole has not kept up—not only globally but also in the United States—and AIDSism still exists both outside and inside the medical profession. As recently as June 2006, a full quarter-century since the epidemic was first described, a child with AIDS was initially excluded from attending a New York sleep-away camp until his parents threatened legal action. In February 2009, a dermatologist refused to biopsy a facial lesion because the patient was HIV positive. The patient consulted a second dermatologist, who was comfortable with and experienced in the care of persons with HIV and AIDS, and had the lesion biopsied. On May 12, 2009, Lambda Legal filed suit in U.S. federal court on behalf of a 75-year-old university provost who fulfilled all criteria for admission to an Arkansas assisted living facility but was forced to leave it on the day after arrival when detailed review of his medical records indicated HIV seropositivity (Lambda Legal, 2009; see also Chapter 4 of this handbook). AIDS stigma and AIDSism have implications not only for the individuals who experience the anguish of stigma but also for public health. Stigma and AIDSism present a barrier to getting tested for HIV, to obtaining test results, to disclosing serostatus to intimate partners, to obtaining optimal medical care in a timely manner, and to engaging in safer sex practices.

Psychosomatic medicine psychiatrists who specialize in AIDS psychiatry as well as general psychiatrists and other mental health clinicians are in a unique position to work with primary HIV clinicians, infectious disease specialists, and other physicians and health professionals to combat AIDS stigma and AIDSism.

AIDS Psychiatry: Paradigm and Paradox

AIDS paradigms

For psychiatrists who work in psychosomatic medicine, AIDS and other manifestations of HIV infection may be thought of as a paradigm of a medical illness. AIDS is an illness similar to the other complex and severe medicalillnesses that define the subspecialty. *Psychosomatic medicine*, the psychiatric aspects of complex and severe medical illness, was previously called "consultation-liaison psychiatry" and became a subspecialty of psychiatry in 2003. AIDS is a paradigm of psychosomatic medicine because it has elements of nearly every illness described in the *American Psychiatric Publishing Textbook of Psychosomatic Medicine* (Levenson, 2005). Persons with HIV and AIDS are also vulnerable to other multimorbid complex and severe medical illnesses, including those related and unrelated to HIV infection. The concept of AIDS as paradigm is illustrated in Figure 11.1.

Particularly for persons with psychiatric disorders, access to care may be compromised, because severe mental illness is associated with nonadherence to care. Untreated depression, substance dependence, cognitive impairment, posttraumatic stress disorder, or psychosis can impede the ability to adhere to care. Persons with severe mental illness may have difficulty getting to medical appointments, taking medications regularly, or obtaining

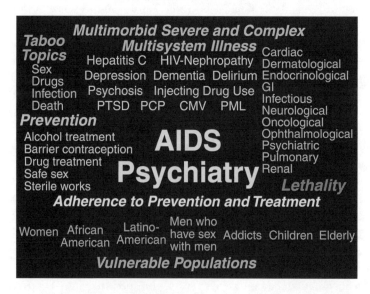

Figure 11.1 AIDS psychiatry: a paradigm for psychosomatic medicine and a biopsychosocial approach. CMV, cytomegalovirus; GI, gastrointestinal; PCP, *Pneumocystis* pneumonia; PML, progressive multifocal leukoencephalopathy; PTSD, posttraumatic stress disorder.

laboratory tests and follow-up care. As a result, persons with AIDS and untreated psychiatric disorders may present with AIDS-related illnesses not usually encountered in developed countries since the advent of antiretroviral therapy (ART). Since the development of such therapies, the life expectancy of persons with HIV has increased, and for persons who are adherent to care, the incidence of the opportunistic infections and cancers previously associated with AIDS has decreased (Huang et al., 2006).

At the same time, however, among those persons who are adherent to care there has been an increase in the prevalence of endocrine, pulmonary, cardiac, gastrointestinal, renal, and metabolic disorders. Some of these disorders may be comorbid and unrelated to HIV and AIDS, while others may be related to HIV and AIDS or to its treatments. The life expectancy of persons with HIV and AIDS who are treated with antiretroviral therapy is now similar to that of the general population (Manfredi 2004a, 2004b). Among the 68,669 persons with AIDS who died in New York City from 1999 to 2004, the percentage of deaths from non-HIV-related causes increased significantly from 19.8% to 26.3% (Sackoff et al., 2006). Of these non-HIV-related deaths, 76% were related to substance use, cardiovascular disease, and cancer. Other causes of death included diabetes, suicide, homicide, and chronic renal disease.

Sackoff and colleagues (2006) and Aberg (2006) recommend a paradigm shift in the care of persons with AIDS from a primary focus on HIV prevention and care to a more comprehensive approach to medical and mental health. The complexity and severity of the multiple medical and psychiatric illnesses prevalent in persons with HIV and AIDS are important in the psychiatric assessment and substantiate the need for a comprehensive and compassionate biopsychosocial approach that takes into account the full range of medical, psychiatric, social, and cultural factors and their synergistic implications relevant to patient care (Deuchar, 1984; Cohen and Weisman, 1986, 1988; Cohen, 1987, 1992, 2008; Cohen and Alfonso, 2004).

Biopsychosocial aspects of HIV and AIDS treatment

AIDS is a severe, chronic, multiorgan, multisystem illness with many severe multimorbid psychiatric and other medical illnesses. AIDS is also a prevalent illness that presents with psychiatric responses to illness, is associated with psychiatric illness because of the affinity of HIV for brain and neural tissue, and occurs with comorbid psychiatric illness as well as other medical illnesses. Thus a biopsychosocial approach to the care of persons with HIV and AIDS is needed.

Psychiatrists make ideal AIDS educators. General psychiatrists who work in the areas of inpatient and outpatient psychiatry settings, private offices, addiction psychiatry, geriatric psychiatry, child and adolescent psychiatry, correctional facilities, and long-term care facilities are all in a prime position to provide education, help prevent transmission of HIV, suggest or provide condoms and information about safe sex, and suggest or offer HIV testing that can lead to early diagnosis and treatment. Most psychiatrists take detailed sexual and drug histories and work with patients to help them change behaviors. The significance of taking a detailed sexual history was especially evident in a population-based study of men in New York City. This study revealed discordance between sexual behavior and self-reported sexual identity: nearly 10% of straight-identified men reported at least one sexual encounter with another man in the previous year (Pathela et al., 2006). Most psychiatrists form long-term, ongoing relationships with their patients and work with patients toward achieving gratification in long-term, intimate-partner relationships. All of these characteristics can be of major importance in primary prevention and early diagnosis and treatment of HIV infection.

HIV and AIDS also present us with paradoxes. Although the use of available antiretroviral therapies has resulted in the transformation of AIDS from being a death sentence to being a chronic illness, one of the most tragic paradoxes of HIV is the disparity in access to such care as a result of racial, political, spiritual, and economic factors. Unfortunately, this paradox is present in many areas of the world, in certain areas of the United States, and in other industrialized nations. Another tragic situation is the lack of access to care among persons with psychiatric illness. In addition, age, intelligence, and level of education do not necessarily correlate with ability to adhere to risk reduction, safe sexual behavior, and medical care (Cochran and Mays, 1990; De Buono et al., 1990; MacDonald et al., 1990; Reinisch and Beasley, 1990). Among adolescents who say, "I can use a condom, I just don't" (Mustanski et al., 2006), and the elderly (Goodkin et al., 2003; Stoff, 2004; Karpiak et al., 2006), who may not feel a need for barrier contraception to prevent pregnancy and whose physicians may be uncomfortable discussing sexual activity, there are high rates of HIV infection. The process of care for persons with AIDS at the end of life is also paradoxical in that there is a clear need for provision of care along a continuum that includes both palliative and curative care, but such care appears hard to implement, even though its concept has been proposed. The need to overcome the "false dichotomy of curative vs. palliative care for late stage AIDS" has been suggested (Selwyn and Forstein, 2003).

AIDSISM AND THE MULTIPLE DISPARITIES OF HIV AND AIDS

AIDSism results from a multiplicity of prejudicial and discriminatory factors and is built on a foundation of racism, homophobia, ageism, addictophobia, misogyny, and discomfort with mental and medical illness, poverty, sexuality, infection, and death in many communities throughout the world. AIDSism has clearly contributed to disparities in the care of persons with HIV and AIDS.

Racial, ethnic, and socioeconomic disparities

Racial, ethnic, and socioeconomic disparities have been observed and documented in all aspects of the U.S. health-care system (Agency for Health Care Research and Quality, 2005a). The overall HIV death rate of African Americans was found to be 10.95 times higher than that of whites (Agency for Health Care Research and Quality, 2005b), and racial disparities have been shown to contribute to increased HIV incidence and inadequate access to medical and psychiatric care (CDC, 2006a). U.S. correctional facilities and urban drug epicenters may be seen as microcosms of discrimination. Correctional facilities may also be instrumental in perpetuating the HIV epidemic both inside and outside of prison walls (Hammett et al., 2002; Blankenship et al., 2005; Golembeski and Fullilove, 2005; CDC, 2006b).

It would be difficult to measure the true impact of these disparities on persons with HIV and AIDS. In addition to the incalculable distress, suffering, and anguish of the illness and its stigma (Cohen et al., 2002), persons with AIDS have multimorbid medical and psychiatric illnesses, all of which are found among those who also experience disparities in care (Cohen et al., 1991; Cohen, 1996; Kolb et al., 2006).

Psychiatric disparities

Psychiatric factors take on new relevance and meaning as we approach the end of the third decade of the AIDS pandemic. Persons with AIDS are living longer and healthier lives as a result of appropriate medical care and advances in antiretroviral therapy. However, in the United States and throughout the world, some men, women, and children with AIDS are unable to benefit from medical progress. Inadequate access to care results from a multiplicity of barriers, including psychiatric ones. Psychiatric disorders and distress also play a significant role in the transmission of, exposure to, and infection with HIV (Cohen and Alfonso, 1994, 1998; Blank et al., 2002). They are relevant to prevention, clinical care, and adherence throughout every aspect of illness, from the initial risk behavior to death, and they result in considerable suffering, from diagnosis to end-stage illness (Cohen and Alfonso, 2004). Untreated psychiatric disorders can be exacerbated by HIV stigma, making persons with HIV and AIDS especially vulnerable to suicide (Marzuk et al., 1988; Perry et al., 1990; McKegney and O'Dowd, 1992; Alfonso and Cohen, 1997). Psychiatric treatment with individual (Cohen and Weisman, 1986; Cohen, 1987; Cohen and Alfonso, 1998, 2004), group (Alfonso and Cohen, 1997), and family therapy can help alleviate suffering, improve adherence, and prevent suicide.

A Biopsychosocial Approach to Maintaining Health

Maintaining medical wellness

Persons with AIDS need general medical care as well as specialty care from HIV clinicians. Many HIV specialists may not feel entirely comfortable providing ongoing medical care for patients; yet children, adolescents, adults, and older persons with HIV and AIDS all need comprehensive medical care. It is important to recognize that the intense and frequent care provided by HIV clinicians may not address the total care needs of patients. The high prevalence of multimorbid diabetes mellitus, cancer, hypertension, hyperlipidemia, hepatitis C and cirrhosis, endocrine disorders, HIV nephropathy and other renal disorders, neuropathy, myelopathy, HIV-associated dementia, and coronary artery disease in adults with HIV necessitates referrals to not only subspecialists but also primary care internists and geriatricians. By maintaining wellness, persons with HIV and AIDS can live healthier, longer, independent lives and maximize their life potential. In addition to medical care, wellness includes attending to nutrition, sexual health, exercise, and stress reduction as well as evaluation and treatment of alcohol, nicotine, and other substance use and misuse.

Nutrition

Suggested menus for a balanced diet consisting of healthful, nutritious, and appetizing foods need to be tailored to not only the individual's medical requirements but also their cultural and ethnic preferences. Drug–food interactions need to be considered as well. The nutritional aspects of HIV wellness are summarized in Table 11.4.

Exercise

Regular exercise is recommended for all persons with HIV and AIDS. Again, this should be tailored to each individual's medical and physical needs as well as to past and current exercise patterns. For those persons who exercise regularly, clinicians may wish to explore the nature and frequency of exercise in order to express interest and encouragement. Some persons with HIV and AIDS may not be aware that there are

TABLE 11.4 Nutritional Aspects of HIV Wellness

- Balanced meals
- Nutritious, healthful, appetizing foods
- Tailored to medical needs
- Mindful of ethnic, religious, and cultural considerations
- Avoidance of drug–food interactions, such as with grapefruit and cruciferous vegetables
- Avoidance of fatty and fried foods, except where necessary for antiretroviral medications

many no-cost or low-cost gyms, health clubs, and exercise programs available in some areas of the United States and other parts of the world, so it is important to note local resources of this type to patients. It is helpful for clinicians to be prepared with a list of these options to help persons with HIV and AIDS access services (see Chapter 14 for further details on resources). Many of the suggested exercises in Table 11.5 can be done without a special facility or equipment and can be enjoyable. Some exercises require that another person stand by to provide support and encouragement. All exercise is more enjoyable when done to music, especially music that encourages movement and is chosen by the individual in accordance with their preferences.

TABLE 11.5 Suggested Exercise Guidelines for HIV Wellness

- Aerobic exercise for healthy individuals can consist of walking, jogging, swimming, water aerobics, or riding a recumbent bicycle starting at 5 minutes per day and working up to 40 minutes, if tolerated, about 3 to 4 times per week.
- Aerobic exercise for medically ill persons may consist of walking throughout a room, apartment, or home for 5 minutes to 20 minutes per day, if tolerated.
- Balance exercises: standing on two feet without support
- Standing on one foot while holding onto the back of a sturdy chair if someone else is present and gradually learning to stand on one foot for 10 seconds at a time
- Getting up from a firm seat using two legs with and without use of hands and arms for support; repeating this from 5 repetitions to 20 repetitions, if tolerated
- Sitting down on the floor and getting up using legs and arms and pushing off from the floor
- Strength training: rising from sitting to standing is helpful for maintaining quadriceps strength as well as balance
- Light weights from 1 to 5 pounds can be used for biceps curls and triceps extensions; a plastic 12 or 16 ounce water bottle is ideal if no weights are available.
- Movement therapy: moving in time to music can be done in bed, in a wheelchair, or with a walker

TABLE 11.6 Relaxation Response

This should be done from one to three times a day for 1 minute or more if tolerated.
• Sit or lie down in a comfortable position.
• Breathe in and out as you would normally breathe.
• Become aware of your breathing.
• Concentrate on breathing in and breathing out.
• As you breathe out, say the word "one" to yourself.
• Breathe in and then say the word "one" to yourself as you breathe out.
• Concentrate on breathing in and saying the word "one" to yourself as you breathe out.
• Disregard all other thoughts that come to mind.

Adapted from Benson H (2000). *The Relaxation Response*. New York: Harper Collins.

Stress reduction

Yoga, relaxation response, progressive relaxation, deep-breathing exercises, meditation, and massage therapy can be invaluable. The relaxation response is described in Table 11.6.

Other outlets for stress can include writing a diary, memoir, or a life narrative; reading; knitting; and artwork. Listening to music can be extremely relaxing as well.

Substance use treatment

Smoking cessation. As HIV moves from an acute life-threatening condition to one of chronic care, more attention has been devoted to providing patients with preventative primary care services. Rates of smoking in patients with HIV have been estimated to be as high as 75%, and smoking remains one of the leading causes of death in the world (Burns et al., 1996; Niaura et al., 2000). Tobacco use places HIV-infected patients at increased risk of pulmonary infections, orpharyngeal carcinomas, and AIDS-defining malignancies (Miguez-Burbano et al., 2003; Shiboski et al., 1999; Castle et al., 2002). Prevention in the form of addressing ongoing tobacco use is increasingly important in this population, as life expectancies are now not appreciably different from those for individuals with other chronically ill disease states.

Currently, three specific products are FDA approved for smoking cessation, and all are potentially useful in the goal of tobacco cessation. Nicotine replacement therapy (NRT) in the form of patches, gum, and inhaled products serves as the mainstay of therapy. It is important to gather an accurate smoking history and to not underprescribe these products, as cravings will continue with doses that are too low. It is also important that the product not be tapered too quickly, as rebound craving can result. Typically, nicotine patches are provided as background therapy, starting with a 21 mg/day patch for patients smoking 1.5 pack per day or more, and decreasing the patch by 7 mg every 2 weeks until therapy is completed. A typical taper lasts 3 weeks. During this time, nicotine gum or inhaled products can also be prescribed on an as-needed basis to control any nicotine breakthrough cravings that may result. These as-needed NRT products can also be continued after completion of the patch taper in the event of occasional nicotine cravings that may potentially lead to relapse.

Bupropion is also approved for smoking cessation and works in a manner distinct from nicotine replacement therapy. It has been shown to reduce nicotine cravings and nicotine withdrawal symptoms, and its efficacy appears to be similar to that of nicotine replacement therapy, approximately doubling the rate of being a nonsmoker after 3 months. One study showed prolonged benefit with its use; after 1 year, patients on bupropion had a 50% increased rate of nicotine abstinence. Current data from medically ill patients also support bupropion's combined use with nicotine replacement therapy in both improving abstinence rates (odds ratio 2.57) over those with nicotine replacement alone and lengthening the median time to relapse (65 days versus 23 days) (Steinberg et al., 2009). One of the authors (HWG) routinely uses combined NRT and bupropion extended release for initial smoking cessation therapy and has found that most patients tolerate the combination well.

Varenicline (Chantix) is the third medication that has received FDA approval for nicotine cessation. It has demonstrated superior efficacy over that of bupropion in one head-to-head comparison trial. Rates of continuous nicotine abstinence at 1 year were placebo, 10%; bupropion, 15%; and varenicline, 23% (Jorenby et al., 2006). However, varenicline has also been noted to be associated with increased rates of serious neuropsychiatric adverse events, which precludes its recommendation as first-line use in patients with current psychiatric illness without careful consideration of potential risks and benefits to the patient (U.S. FDA Public Health Advisory on Chantix, 2008).

Substance abuse. Patients abusing substances such as opiates, cocaine, and alcohol have a high comorbid prevalence of psychiatric disorders—especially mood disorders. Importantly, mood disorders in HIV-seropositive populations have strong associations with ART nonadherence and an increased willingness to share needles, syringes, and other drug paraphernalia (Abbott et al., 1994; Stein et al., 2003; Braine et al., 2005). Any patient presenting with a substance abuse disorder should be screened carefully for the presence of other comorbid psychiatric disorders. An in-depth social history targeting a history of abuse should also be taken. Childhood sexual experiences are strongly predictive of substance abuse and HIV transmission through high-risk sexual practices (Kalichman et al., 2004; Arreola et al., 2008). Failure to identify these risk factors can thwart other potentially successful treatments for HIV, including antiretroviral therapy. The reader is referred to a recent review of at-risk practices within the triply diagnosed community—HIV, substance abuse, and mental illness—for further information (Goforth and Fernandez, 2009).

Opiate replacement therapy remains a prominent treatment in HIV psychiatry and has elements of both preventive therapy and active treatment. Preventive goals in the treatment of opiate addiction are to prevent HIV transmission, minimize HIV strain contamination, diminish emergence of multidrug-resistant HIV viral strains, prevent HCV and HBV infection, and prevent the myriad other medical complications of opiate addiction, including other types of infection. Because opiate addiction places a high social burden on persons with HIV and AIDS and on their families, another goal of treatment is reduce this burden. For a more in-depth discussion of the pharmacology of methadone and buprenorphine treatment programs, please see Chapter 7.

However, opiate replacement therapy cannot occur in a vacuum; psychosocial interventions designed to bolster opiate abstinence remain important. Encouragingly, HIV patients with concurrent mood disorders who receive psychiatric treatment appear more likely than others to seek and receive antiretroviral therapy for their HIV disease. Antidepressant therapy also appears to point toward a reduction in overall health expenditures in this population (Sambamoorthi et al., 2000).

In addition to antidepressant therapy, other psychosocial intervention measures also show promise in this population. One study examining a 3-month nursing intervention in patients previously lost to follow-up showed improved access and adherence to and retention in HIV therapy. Interventions included home visits, accompanying women to the initial visit, and assisting with integrating care among mental heath, substance abuse, and HIV providers (Andersen et al., 2005). Similarly, data from an intensive outpatient cocaine treatment program designed in part to bolster psychosocial coping factors showed that risky behavior decreased significantly over a 9-month period among those participating in the treatment program (Gottheil et al., 1998).

In a dually diagnosed, substance-abusing cohort, the impact of a biopsychosocial approach to the treatment of patients with HIV cannot be underestimated. While methadone maintenance programs and buprenorphine programs remain cornerstones of treatment, additional interventions from a psychosocial standpoint have shown hope in reducing risk behavior and improving access and adherence to care. Community services should be enlisted to bolster these patients' success and reinforce adherence to treatment (see Chapter 14 for a list of community resources).

Conclusion

AIDSism, stigma, discrimination, and fear, in conjunction with denial, omnipotence, and lack of awareness, complicate and perpetuate the HIV pandemic. The creation of supportive, nurturing, nonjudgmental health-care environments along with programs to maintain health can help combat AIDSism and provide comprehensive and compassionate care. AIDS psychiatrists and other mental health professionals need to be integrated closely into clinical, academic, and research aspects of HIV prevention and treatment. In order for persons with HIV and AIDS to live longer, healthier, and more comfortable lives, with preservation of independence and dignity, it is important to establish special nurturing, supportive, and loving health-care environments and wellness programs. Such environments and programs can enable persons with AIDS, their loved ones, and caregivers to meet the challenges of AIDS with optimism and dignity (Cohen and Alfonso, 2004).

References

Abbott PJ, Weller SB, Walker SR (1994). Psychiatric disorders of opioid addicts entering treatment: preliminary data. *J Addict Dis.* 13: 1–11

Aberg JA (2006). The changing face of HIV care: common things really are common. *Ann Intern Med* 145:463–465.

Agency for Health Care Research and Quality (2005a). *National Healthcare Disparities Report, 2005.* Retrieved March 20, 2007, from http://www.ahrq.gov/qual/nhdr05/nhdr05.htm

Agency for Healthcare Research and Quality (2005b). *National Healthcare Disparities Report, 2005.* Appendix D: Data Tables. Retrieved March 20, 2007, from http://www.ahrq.gov/qual/nhdr05/nhdr05.htm

Alfonso CA, Cohen MAA (1997). The role of group psychotherapy in the care of persons with AIDS. *J Am Acad Psychoanal* 25:623–638.

Andersen M, Tinsley J, Milfort D, Wilcox R, Smereck G, Pfoutz S, Creech S, Mood D, Smith T, Adams L, Thomas R, Connelly C. (2005) HIV health care access issues for women living with HIV, mental illness, and substance abuse. *AIDS Patient Care STDS* 19:449–459.

Arreola S, Neilands T, Pollack L, Paul J, Catania J (2008). Childhood sexual experiences and adult health sequelae among gay and bisexual men: defining childhood sexual abuse. *J Sex Res* 45:246–252.

Barbuto J (1984). Psychiatric care of seriously ill patients with acquired immune deficiency syndrome. In SE Nichols and DG Ostrow (eds.), *Psychiatric Implications of Acquired Immune Deficiency Syndrome.* Washington, DC: American Psychiatric Press.

Bean WB (1968). *Sir William Osler: Aphorisms from His Bedside Teachings and Writings.* Springfield, IL: Charles C. Thomas.

Benson H (2000). *The Relaxation Response.* New York: Harper Collins.

Blank MB, Mandell DS, Aiken L, Hadley TR. (2002). Co-occurrence of HIV and serious mental illness among Medicaid recipients. *Psychiatr Serv* 53:868–873.

Blankenship KM, Smoyer AB, Bray SJ, Mattocks K (2005). Black–white disparities in HIV/AIDS: the role of drug policy in the corrections system. *J Health Care Poor Underserved* 16:140–156.

Blendon RJ, Donelan K (1988). Discrimination against people with AIDS: the public's perspective. *N Engl J Med* 319:1022–1026.

Braine N, Des Jarlais DC, Goldblatt C, Zadoretzky C, Turner C (2005). HIV risk behavior among amphetamine injectors at U.S. syringe exchange programs. *AIDS Educ Prev* 17:515–524.

Brown L, Macintyre K, Trujillo L (2003). Interventions to reduce HIV/AIDS stigma: what have we learned? *AIDS Educ Prev* 15:49–69.

Burns DN, Hillman D, Neaton JD, Sherer R, Mitchell T, Capps L, Vallier WG, Thurnherr MD, Gordin FM (1996). Cigarette smoking, bacterial pneumonia, and other clinical outcomes in HIV-1 infection. Terry Beirn Community Programs for Clinical Research on AIDS. *J Acquir Immune Defic Syndr Hum Retrovirol* 13:374–383.

Castle PE, Wacholder S, Lorincz AT, Scott DR, Sherman ME, Glass AG, Rush BB, Schussler JE, Schiffman M (2002). A prospective study of high-grade cervical neoplasia risk among human papillomavirus–infected women. *J Natl Cancer Inst* 94:406–1414.

[CDC] Centers for Disease Control and Prevention (1983). Immunodeficiency in female partners of males with acquired immune deficiency syndrome (AIDS)—New York. *MMWR Morb Mortal Wkly Rep* 31: 697–698.

[CDC] Centers for Disease Control and Prevention (2006a). Racial/ethnic disparities in diagnoses of HIV/AIDS—33 states, 2001–2004. *MMWR Morb Mortal Wkly Rep* 55:121–125.

[CDC] Centers for Disease Control and Prevention (2006b). HIV transmission among male inmates in a state prison system—Georgia, 1992–2005. *MMWR Morb Mortal Wkly Rep* 55:421–426.

Chesney MA, Smith AW (1992). Critical delays in HIV testing and care: the potential role of stigma. *Am Behav Sci* 42:1162–1174.

Cochran SD, Mays VM (1990). Sex, lies and HIV. *N Engl J Med* 22:774–775.

Cohen MA (1987). Psychiatric aspects of AIDS: A biopsychosocial approach. In GP Wormser, RE Stahl, and EJ Bottone (eds.), *AIDS Acquired Immune Deficiency Syndrome and Other Manifestations of HIV Infection*. Park Ridge, NJ: Noyes Publishers.

Cohen MA (1989). AIDSism, a new form of discrimination. *Am Med News*, January 20, 32:43.

Cohen MA (1992). Biopsychosocial aspects of the HIV epidemic. In GP Wormser (ed.), *AIDS and Other Manifestations of HIV Infection*, second edition (pp. 349–371). New York: Raven Press.

Cohen MAA (1996). Creating health care environments to meet patients' needs. *Curr Issues Public Health* 2:232–240.

Cohen MA (2008). History of AIDS psychiatry—a biopsychosocial approach—paradigm and paradox. In MA Cohen and JM Gorman (eds.),

Comprehensive Textbook of AIDS Psychiatry (pp. 3–14). New York: Oxford University Press.

Cohen MA, Aladjem AD, Brenin D, Ghazi M (1990). Firesetting by patients with the acquired immunodeficiency syndrome (AIDS). *Ann Intern Med* 112:386–387.

Cohen MAA, Aladjem AD, Horton A, Lima J, Palacios A, Hernandez L, Mehta P (1991). How can we combat excess mortality in Harlem? A one-day survey of adult general care. *Int J Psychiatry Med* 21:369–378.

Cohen MAA, Alfonso CA (1994). Dissemination of HIV: how serious is it for women, medically and psychologically? *Ann N Y Acad Sci* 736:114–121.

Cohen MA, Alfonso CA (1998). Psychiatric care and pain management in persons with HIV infection. In GP Wormser (ed.), *AIDS and Other Manifestations of HIV Infection*, third edition. Philadelphia: Lippincott-Raven.

Cohen MA, Alfonso CA (2004). AIDS psychiatry: psychiatric and palliative care, and pain management. In GP Wormser (ed.), *AIDS and Other Manifestations of HIV Infection*, fourth edition (pp. 537–576). San Diego: Elsevier Academic Press.

Cohen MA, Gorman JM (2008). *Comprehensive Textbook of AIDS Psychiatry*. New York: Oxford University Press.

Cohen MA, Hoffman RG, Cromwell C, Schmeidler J, Ebrahim F, Carrera G, Endorf F, Alfonso CA, Jacobson JM (2002). The prevalence of distress in persons with human immunodeficiency virus infection. *Psychosomatics* 43:10–15.

Cohen MA, Weisman H (1986). A biopsychosocial approach to AIDS. *Psychosomatics* 27:245–249.

Cohen MA, Weisman HW (1988). A biopsychosocial approach to AIDS. In RP Galea, BF Lewis, and LA Baker (eds.), *AIDS and IV Drug Abusers*. Owings Mills, MD: National Health Publishing.

De Buono BA, Zinner SH, Daamen M, McCormack WM (1990). Sexual behavior of college women in 1975, 1986 and 1989. *N Engl J Med* 322:821–825.

Deuchar N (1984). AIDS in New York City with particular reference to the psychosocial aspects. *Br J Psychiatry* 145:612–619.

Dilley JW, Ochitill HN, Perl M, Volberding PA (1985). Findings in psychiatric consultation with patients with acquired immune deficiency syndrome. *Am J Psychiatry* 142:82–86.

Faulstich ME (1987). Psychiatric aspects of AIDS. *Am J Psychiatry* 144:551–556.

Fernandez F, Ruiz P (2006). *Psychiatric Aspects of HIV/AIDS* (pp. 39–47). Philadelphia: Lippincott Williams & Wilkins.

Forstein M (1984a). AIDS anxiety in the worried well. In SE Nichols and DG Ostrow (eds.), *Psychiatric Implications of Acquired Immune Deficiency Syndrome* (pp. 77–82). Washington, DC: American Psychiatric Press.

Forstein M (1984b). The psychosocial impact of the acquired immunodeficiency syndrome. *Semin Oncol* 11:77–82.

Fullilove MT (1989). Anxiety and stigmatizing aspects of HIV infection. *J Clin Psychiatry* 50(Suppl.):5–8.

Goforth HW, Fernandez F (2009). The triple threat: mental illness, substance abuse, and human immunodeficiency virus. In B Johnson (ed.), *Addiction Medicine: Science and Practice*. New York: Springer Publishers.

Golembeski C, Fullilove RE (2005). Criminal (in)justice in the city and its associated health consequences. *Am J Public Health* 95:1701–1706.

Goodkin K, Heckman T, Siegel K, Linsk N, Khamis I, Lee D, Lecusay R, Poindexter CC, Mason SJ, Suarez P, Eisdorfer C (2003). "Putting a face" on HIV infection/AIDS in older adults: a psychosocial context. *J Aquir Immune Defic Syndr* 33(Suppl. 2):S171–S184.

Gottheil E, Lundy A, Weinstein SP, Sterling RC (1998). Does intensive outpatient cocaine treatment reduce AIDS risky behaviors? *J Addict Dis* 17:61–69.

Gottlieb MS (2001). AIDS—past and future. *N Engl J Med* 344:1788–1791.

Gottlieb MS, Schroff R, Schanker HM, Weisman JD, Fan PT, Wolf RA, Saxon A (1981). *Pneumocystis carinii* pneumonia and mucosal candidiasis in previously healthy homosexual men: evidence of a new acquired cellular immunodeficiency. *N Engl J Med* 305:1425–1431.

Hammett TM, Harmon MP, Rhodes W (2002). The burden of infectious disease among inmates of and releasees from US correctional facilities 1997. *Am J Public Health* 92:1789–1794.

Herek GM, Capitanio JP, Widaman KF (2002). HIV-related stigma and knowledge in the United States: prevalence and trends, 1991–1999. *Am J Public Health* 92:371–377.

Hoffman RS (1984). Neuropsychiatric complications of AIDS. *Psychosomatics* 25:393–340.

Holland JC, Tross S (1985). Psychosocial and neuropsychiatric sequelae of the acquired immunodeficiency syndrome and related disorders. *Ann Intern Med* 103:760–764.

Holtz H, Dobro J, Kapila R, Palinkas R, Oleske J (1983). Psychosocial impact of acquired immunodeficiency syndrome. *JAMA* 250:167.

Huang L, Quartin A, Jones D, Havlir DV (2006). Intensive care of patients with HIV infection. *N Engl J Med* 355:173–181.

Jorenby DE, Hays JT, Rigotti NA, Azoulay S, Watsky EJ, Williams KE, Billing CB, Gong J, Reeves KR (2006). Varenicline Phase 3 Study Group. Efficacy of varenicline, an $\alpha_4\beta_2$ nicotinic acetylcholine receptor partial agonist, vs. placebo or sustained-release bupropion for smoking cessation: a randomized controlled trial. *JAMA* 296:56–63.

Kalichman SC, Gore-Felton C, Benotsch E, Cage M, Rompa D (2004). Trauma symptoms, sexual behaviors, and substance abuse: correlates of childhood sexual abuse and HIV risks among men who have sex with men. *J Child Sex Abuse* 13:1–15.

Kaplan AH, Scheyett A, Golin CE (2005). HIV and stigma: analysis and research program. *Curr HIV/AIDS Rep* 2:184–188.

Karpiak SE, Shippy RA, Cantor MH (2006). *Research on Older Adults with HIV*. New York: AIDS Community Research Initiative of America.

Kelly JA, St. Lawrence JS, Smith S Jr, Hood HV, Cook DJ (1987). Stigmatization of AIDS patients by physicians. *Am J Public Health* 77:789–791.

Kolb B, Wallace AM, Hill D, Royce M (2006). Disparities in cancer care among racial and ethnic minorities. *Oncology* 20:1256–1261.

Lambda Legal (2009). Protecting our seniors. Retrieved September 24, 2009, from http://www.lambdalegal.org/publications/articles/protecting-our-seniors.html

Levenson JL (2005). *American Psychiatric Publishing Textbook of Psychosomatic Medicine* (pp. 3–14). Washington, DC: American Psychiatric Publishing.

Lyketsos CG, Hanson AL, Fishman M, Rosenblatt A, McHugh PR, Treisman GJ (1993). Manic syndrome early and late in the course of HIV. *Am J Psychiatry* 150(2):326–327.

MacDonald NE, Wells GA, Fisher WA, Warren WK, King MA, Doherty JA, Bowie WR (1990). High-risk STD/HIV behavior among college students. *JAMA* 263:3155–3159.

Manfredi R (2004a). HIV infection and advanced age: emerging epidemiological, clinical and management issues. *Ageing Res Rev* 3:31–54.

Manfredi R (2004b). Impact of HIV infection and antiretroviral therapy in the older patient. *Expert Rev Anti Infect Ther* 2:821–824.

Marzuk PM, Tierney H, Tardiff K, Gross EM, Morgan EB, Hsu MA, Mann JJ (1988). Increased risk of suicide in persons with AIDS. *JAMA* 259:1333–1337.

McKegney FP, O'Dowd MA (1982). Suicidality and HIV status. *Am J Psychiatry* 149:396–398.

Miguez-Burbano MJ, Burbano X, Ashkin D, Pitchenik A, Allan R, Pineda L, Rodriguez N, Shor-Posner G (2003). Impact of tobacco use on the development of opportunistic respiratory infections in HIV seropositive patients on antiretroviral therapy. *Addict Biol* 8:39–43.

Mustanski B, Donenberg G, Emerson E (2006). I can use a condom, I just don't: the importance of motivation to prevent HIV in adolescent seeking psychiatric care. *AIDS Behav* 10:753–762.

Navia BA, Price RW (1987). The acquired immunodeficiency syndrome dementia as the presenting or sole manifestation of human immunodeficiency virus infection. *Arch Neurol* 44:65–69.

Niaura R, Shadel WG, Morrow K, Tashima K, Flanigan T, Abrams DB (2000). Human immunodeficiency virus infection, AIDS, and smoking cessation: the time is now. *Clin Infect Dis* 31:808–812.

Nichols SE (1983). Psychiatric aspects of AIDS. *Psychosomatics* 24:1083–1089.

Nichols SE (1984). Social and support groups for patients with acquired immune deficiency syndrome. In SE Nichols and DG Ostrow (eds.), *Psychiatric Implications of Acquired Immune Deficiency Syndrome* (pp. 77–82). Washington, DC: American Psychiatric Press.

Nichols SE, Ostrow DG (eds.) (1984). *Psychiatric Implications of Acquired Immune Deficiency Syndrome.* Washington, DC: American Psychiatric Press.

Nurnberg HG, Prudic J, Fiori M, Freedman EP (1984). Psychopathology complicating acquired immune deficiency syndrome. *Am J Psychiatry* 141:95–96.

Parker R, Aggleton P (2003). HIV and AIDS-related stigma and discrimination: a conceptual framework and implications for action. *Soc Sci Med* 57:13–24.

Pathela P, Hajat A, Schillinger J, Blank S, Sell R, Mostashari F (2006). Discordance between sexual behavior and self-reported sexual identity: a population-based survey of New York City men. *Ann Intern Med* 145:416–425.

Perry SW, Tross S (1984). Psychiatric problems of AIDS inpatients at the New York Hospital: preliminary report. *Public Health Rep* 99:200–205.

Perry S, Jacobsberg L, Fishman B (1990). Suicidal ideation and HIV testing. *JAMA* 263:679–682.

Price WA, Forejt J (1986). Neuropsychiatric aspects of AIDS: a case report. *Gen Hosp Psychiatry* 8:7–10.

Reinisch JM, Beasley R (1990). America fails sex information test. In *The Kinsey Institute New Report on Sex: What You Must Know to Be Sexually Literate* (pp. 1–26). New York: St. Martin's Press.

Sackoff JE, Hanna DB, Pfeiffer MR, Torian LV (2006). Causes of death among persons with AIDS in the era of highly active antiretroviral therapy: New York City. *Ann Intern Med* 145:397–406.

Sambamoorthi U, Walkup J, Olfson M, Crystal S (2000). Antidepressant treatment and health services utilization among HIV-infected Medicaid patients diagnosed with depression. *J Gen Intern Med* 15:311–320.

Selwyn PA, Forstein M (2003). Overcoming the false dichotomy of curative vs. palliative care for late-stage AIDS. "Let me live the way I want to live until I can't." *JAMA* 290:806–814.

Shiboski CH, Neuhaus JM, Greenspan D, Greenspan JS (1999). Effect of receptive oral sex and smoking on the incidence of hairy leukoplakia in HIV-positive gay men. *J Acquir Immune Defic Syndr* 21:236–242.

Stein MD, Solomon DA, Herman DS, Anderson BJ, Miller I (2003). Depression severity and drug injection HIV risk behaviors. *Am J Psychiatry* 160:1659–1662.

Steinberg MB, Greenhaus S, Schmelzer AC, Bover MT, Foulds J, Hoover DR, Carson JL (2009). Triple combination pharmacotherapy for medically ill smokers: a randomized trial. *Ann Intern Med* 150:447–454.

Stoff DM (2004). Mental health research in HIV/AIDS and aging: problems and prospects. *AIDS* 18(Suppl. 1):S3–S10.

Thienhaus OJ, Khosla N (1984). Meningeal cryptococcosis misdiagnosed as a manic episode. *Am J Psychiatry* 141:1459–1460.

Thompson LM (1987). Dealing with AIDS and fear: would you accept cookies from an AIDS patient? *South Med J* 80:228–232.

Treisman GJ, Angelino AF (2004). *The Psychiatry of AIDS: A Guide to Diagnosis and Treatment*. Baltimore: Johns Hopkins University Press.

U.S. FDA Public Health Advisory on Chantix (2008). http://www.fda.gov/bbs/topics/NEWS/2008/NEW01788.html. Accessed 19 April 2009

Wormser GP, Joline C (1989). Would you eat cookies prepared by an AIDS patient? Survey reveals harmful attitudes among professionals. *Postgrad Med* Postgrad Med 86:174–184.

12

PALLIATIVE AND SPIRITUAL CARE OF PERSONS WITH HIV AND AIDS

Mary Ann Cohen, Joseph Z. Lux, Harold W. Goforth, and Sami Khalife

Palliative care of persons with HIV and AIDS has changed over the course of the first three decades of the pandemic. The most radical shifts occurred in the second decade with the introduction of combination antiretroviral therapy and other advances in HIV care. In the United States and throughout the world, progress in prevention of HIV transmission has not kept pace with progress in treatment, thus the population of persons living with AIDS continues to grow. Furthermore, economic, psychiatric, social, and political barriers leave many persons without access to adequate HIV care. As a result, persons who lack access to care may need palliative care for late-stage AIDS while persons with access to AIDS treatments are more likely to need palliative care for multimorbid medical illnesses such as cardiovascular disease, cancer, pulmonary disease, and renal disease. Palliative care of persons with HIV and AIDS cannot be confined to the end of life. We present palliative care on a continuum as part of an effort to alleviate suffering and attend to pain, emotional distress, and existential anxiety during the course of the illness. We will provide guidelines for psychiatric and palliative care and pain management to help persons with AIDS cope better with their illnesses and live their lives to the fullest extent, and minimize pain and suffering for them and their loved ones.

This chapter reviews basic concepts and definitions of palliative and spiritual care, as well as the distinct challenges facing clinicians involved in HIV palliative care. Finally, issues such as bereavement, cultural sensitivity, communication, and psychiatric contributions to common physical symptom control are reviewed.

303

Defining Palliative Care

The terms *palliative care* and *palliative medicine* are often used interchangeably. Modern palliative care has evolved from the hospice movement into a more expansive network of clinical care delivery systems with components of home care and hospital-based services (Butler et al., 1996; Stjernsward and Papallona, 1998). Palliative care must meet the needs of the "whole person," including the physical, psychological, social, and spiritual aspects of suffering (World Health Organization, 1990). The nature and focus of palliative care have evolved over the century, expanding beyond the concept of comfort care only for the dying. This care may begin with the onset of a life-threatening illness and proceed beyond death to include bereavement interventions for family and others. Indeed, for persons with HIV/AIDS, many aspects of palliative care are applicable at every stage of illness, from initial diagnosis to the end of life (Cohen and Alfonso, 2004). Although palliative care does not merely consist of providing comfort at the end of life, comfort does take on greater importance when cure becomes less feasible. Ideally, as illness proceeds, gradual movement from curative approaches to palliation takes place along a smooth continuum (Cohen and Alfonso, 2004). Table 12.1 summarizes the comprehensive, biopsychosocial approach recommended for AIDS palliative care.

The definition of palliative care set forth by the World Health Organization is one that encompasses the requirements of body, mind, and spirit. This definition and the associated goals of care are summarized in Table 12.2.

Table 12.1 AIDS Palliative Care: A Biopsychosocial Approach

Biological	Psychological	Social
Pain	Depression	Alienation
Dyspnea	Anxiety	Social isolation
Insomnia	Confusion	Stigma
Fatigue	Psychosis	Spirituality
Nausea	Mania	Financial loss
Vomiting	Withdrawal	Job loss
Diarrhea	Intoxication	Loss of key roles
Blindness	Substance dependence	Loss of independence
Paralysis	Existential anxiety	Loss of friends
Weakness	Death anxiety	Loss of partners
Cachexia	Suicidality	Loss of home
Incontinence	Bereavement	Loss of health
Pruritus	Dementia	Disfigurement from illness
Hiccups	Delirium	Disfigurement from antiretrovirals

Source: Adapted and modified from Cohen MA, Alfonso CA (2004). AIDS psychiatry: psychiatric and palliative care, and pain management. In GP Wormser (ed.), *AIDS and Other Manifestations of HIV Infection*, fourth edition (pp. 537–576). Copyright 2004, with permission from Elsevier.

TABLE 12.2 Definition and Goals of Palliative Care

1. Affirms life and regards dying as a normal process
2. Views the dying process as a valuable experience
3. Neither hastens nor postpones death
4. Provides relief from pain and other symptoms
5. Integrates psychological and spiritual care
6. Offers a support system to help patients live as actively as possible until death
7. Helps family cope with illness and bereavement
8. Is multidisciplinary and includes a caregiver team of physicians, nurses, mental health professionals, clergy, and volunteers

Source: World Health Organization (1990, 1998).

Similarly, the Canadian Palliative Care Association (1995) states that palliative care must strive to meet the physical, psychological, social, and spiritual expectations and needs of patients, while also remaining sensitive to personal, cultural, and religious values, beliefs, and practices. Thus, the goal of palliative care is to alleviate suffering and maximize quality of life for patients and their families.

PALLIATIVE CARE ISSUES AND CHALLENGES IN AIDS

AIDS is a chronic illness with exacerbations and remissions, a growing disease burden, medical and psychological comorbidities, and toxic side effects from treatment (Selwyn and Forstein, 2003). For persons with AIDS, the World Health Organization's definition of palliative care as "active total care" includes use of antiretroviral therapy, prevention and management of opportunistic infections, and a palliative approach comprised of offering symptomatic and supportive care at all stages of illness (Foley and Flannery, 1995; Stephenson et al., 2000; Cohen and Alfonso, 2004).

Pain and symptom management

Throughout the HIV illness trajectory, there is a high prevalence of pain, side effects related to antiretroviral therapy, and other symptoms that may be underrecognized and undertreated (Moss, 1990; O'Neill and Sherrard, 1993; Singer et al., 1993; Filbet and Marceron, 1994; Foley, 1994; LaRue et al., 1994; Breitbart et al., 1996c, 1998, 1999; Fantoni et al., 1997; Kelleher et al., 1997; LaRue and Colleau, 1997; Wood et al., 1997; Fontaine et al., 1999; Vogl et al., 1999; Mathews et al., 2000; Selwyn and Rivard, 2002; Selwyn et al., 2003).

Pain management

The deleterious effect of uncontrolled pain on a patient's psychological state is often intuitively understood and recognized. Yet pain is dramatically undertreated in persons with HIV (Schofferman, 1988; Breitbart et al., 1992; Rosenfeld et al., 1997) and other disorders. The World Health Organization (1986) recommends a stepwise process for the pharmacological treatment of pain related to cancer; this model has been adopted by clinicians treating AIDS patients with pain (Newshan and Wainapel, 1993; Reiter and Kudler, 1996). The stepwise progression of pain control consists of (1) nonopioid prescription, with or without an adjuvant; (2) prescription of a weak opioid, with or without and adjuvant; and (3) prescription of a strong opioid, with or without a nonopioid with or without an adjuvant. Adjuvants may include nonsteroidal anti-inflammatory drugs (NSAIDs) such as acetaminophen (APAP). This analgesic "ladder" is more effective for the treatment of nociceptive than for neuropathic pain (Cohen and Alfonso, 2004). Neuropathic pain related to HIV can be treated with adjuvant or coanalgesic agents, such as tricyclic antidepressants and anticonvulsants (Cornblath and McArthur, 1988; Newshan and Wainapel, 1993; Reiter and Kudler, 1996), with reasonable expectation of improved control, although likely not elimination of the neuropathic pain syndrome.

Currently, the best data are for the use of moderate- to high-dose gabapentin (1500–3600 mg/total daily dose) (Hahn et al., 2004). Gabapentin is especially advantageous because it is not metabolized in the body at all and does not pose a risk of drug–drug interactions. However, since it is excreted by the kidneys, doses of gabapentin may need to be adjusted in accordance with renal function and glomerular filtration rates in persons with HIV and chronic renal insufficiency. High-quality data supporting tricyclics are very limited. Early results suggesting a role for lamotrigine in the management of HIV distal neuropathy were flawed by a small study size and have yet to be replicated in a sample of adequate size and power (Simpson et al., 2003; Silver et al., 2007). Acute and chronic pain is best treated on a round-the-clock schedule (Goldberg, 1993; Newshan and Wainapel, 1993) to provide adequate background analgesia, with an as-needed (prn) medication available for breakthrough pain, rather than solely on a prn basis, regardless of the etiology of pain. This regimen eliminates the humiliating anguish of patients begging for pain medications and reduces the actual total amount of pain medication required, since pain is never permitted to crescendo.

The medications recommended for management of pain in persons with AIDS are summarized in Table 12.3. The drug–drug interactions of pain medications and antiretroviral medications are presented in Table 12.4.

TABLE 12.3 Suggested Pain Medications and Dosages

Neuropathic Pain	Nociceptive Pain (Narcotics Oral Dosing)
Gabapentin, 900–3600 mg/day in three divided doses	Propoxyphene—not recommended
Pregabalin, 25–300 mg/day in one or two total doses	Meperidine—not recommended
Nortriptyline, 10–50 mg/night	Codeine—not recommended
Lamotrigine, 25–200 mg/day—can be given in single daily dose	Hydrocodone, 5–15 mg every 4–6 hours *Often combined with APAP*—do not exceed 4000 mg/day with APAP. Also, APAP-containing preparations not recommended for those with comorbid liver dysfunction
Duloxetine, 60–120 mg/day—can be given in single daily dose	Oxycodone, 5–10 mg every 4–6 hours to start—can titrate to effective dose *Often combined with APAP*—do not exceed 4000 mg/day with APAP. Also, APAP-containing preparations not recommended for those with comorbid liver dysfunction
Narcotics—see next column	Oxycodone (slow release), begin 20 mg po every 12 hours, and titrate to effect
Nonopiate Nociceptive Pain	Morphine, 5–10 mg every 4–6 hours to start—titrate to effective dose
NSAIDs Ibuprofen, 400–800 mg every 8 hours	Morphine (slow release), 15 mg every 12 hours to start—titrate to effective dose
Naproxen, 375–500 mg every 8 hours	
Etodolac, 400 mg every 12 hours	
Acetominophen (APAP), 500–1000 mg po every 6 hours	
Psychostimulants May be used to counteract sedating features of opiates and to reduce overall opiate dose. Dose twice daily— upon arising and in early afternoon to spare iatrogenic insomnia	Hydromorphone, 2 mg every 4–6 hours— titrate to effective dose
Dextroamphetamine, 5–10 mg po daily—long half-life allows once-daily dosing	
Methylphenidate, 5–20 mg po twice daily in morning and early afternoon	
Neuroleptics May assist with hyperlimbic component of pain and reduce amount of needed narcotic	Fentanyl transdermal application system: begin with 25 mcg patch and change patch every 72 hours

(continued)

TABLE 12.3 (Continued)

Neuropathic Pain	Nociceptive Pain (Narcotics Oral Dosing)
Haloperidol, 0.5–1 mg po every 6–12 hours	**CAUTION:** Do NOT use for acute pain, and do NOT use in opiate naïve individuals even at lowest dosage.
Risperidone, 0.25–1 mg po every 8–12 hours	
Other Adjuvant Pain Control Techniques	Methadone, 5 mg every 8 hours—titrate to effective dose
Lidocaine patch	**CAUTION:** There are no commonly accepted conversion formulas from other opiates to methadone, so be very cautious when converting to methadone even in opiate-experienced individuals.
Capsaicin cream	
EMLA cream	
Clonidine	
Benzodiazepines/muscle relaxants	

TABLE 12.4 Narcotic Drug–Drug Interactions and Metabolism

Pain Medication	Metabolism	Interactions with Antiretroviral Medications
Hydrocodone	P450 2D6 to hydromorphone and 3A4 to norhydrocodone	Ritonavir and other PIs that inhibit 2D6/3A4 may reduce efficacy by preventing transformation into active metabolite. May also extend half-life of primary substance
Oxycodone	2D6 to oxymorphone and 3A4 to noroxycodone	Ritonavir and other PIs that inhibit 2D6/3A4 may extend half-life and create toxicity
Morphine	Chiefly metabolized through glucuronidation (UGT 2B7 and UGT 1A3)	Unlikely
Hydromorphone	Chiefly metabolized through glucuronidation (UGT 2B7 and UGT 1A3) Also, ketone reductase	Unlikely
Oxymorphone	Chiefly metabolized through glucuronidation (UGT 2B7 and UGT 1A3)	Unlikely
Fentanyl	P450 3A4	Use of ritonavir and other PIs increases half-life—may produce toxicity
Methadone	P450 3A4	Use of ritonavir and other PIs increases half-life—may produce toxicity

PI, protease inhibitor; UGT, UGT, uridine 5′-diphosphate glucuronosyltransferase.
Source: Data from Olkkola et al. (1999); Armstrong and Cozza (2003a, 2003b).

Most pain syndromes associated with AIDS respond to pharma-cotherapy (Cohen and Alfonso, 2004). Nonetheless, nonpharmacologic analgesic modalities such as surgical procedures, radiation therapy, and neurological stimulatory approaches can provide effective adjuvant therapy (Carmichael, 1991; Geara et al., 1991; Jonsson et al., 1992; Tosches et al., 1992; Newshan and Wainapel, 1993; Portenoy, 1993; Jacox et al., 1994). International guidelines also suggest the importance of incorporating psychosocial and behavioral approaches into an opioid management plan (Maddox et al., 1997; Ontario Workplace Safety and Insurance Board, 2000; Kalso et al., 2003; Pain Society and Royal Colleges of Anaesthetists, 2004). Behavioral interventions such as hypnosis, bio-feedback, and multicomponent cognitive-behavioral interventions have been shown to be effective in the management of acute, procedurally related cancer pain (Hilgard and LeBaron, 1982; Kellerman et al., 1983; Jay et al., 1986) as well as non-cancer pain (Morley et al., 1999; Guzman et al., 2001; Adams et al., 2006). Typically, behavioral interventions used in the management of pain employ the basic elements of relaxation and distraction or diversion of attention. We have found these techniques amenable to group model intervention, which also provides an element of support for participants. A review by Breitbart and colleagues (2004) addresses in detail the use of behavioral, psychotherapeutic, and psycho-pharmacologic interventions in pain control.

Management of other physical symptoms

Physical symptoms other than pain can often go undetected and cause significant emotional distress. Many of the more common symptoms are addressed systematically in Chapter 9 in this handbook. Aggressive treat-ment of troublesome physical symptoms is necessary to enhance the patient's quality of life (Bruera et al., 1990; Harding et al., 2005), and in many cases improvement in depression and anxiety may depend on control of disabling physical symptoms. In addition to providing physical, psycho-logical, and emotional comfort for the patient, symptom management may also improve adherence to antiretroviral therapy (Selwyn and Forstein, 2003). The treatment of distressing physical symptoms is summarized in Table 12.5. The practitioner is urged to begin with lower dosages than these suggested ranges, as HIV patients have demonstrated more susceptibility to side effects than that of other patients.

A comprehensive review of pharmacologic and nonpharmacologic inter-ventions for common physical symptoms encountered in the terminally ill can be found in the *Oxford Textbook of Palliative Medicine*, third edition (Doyle et al., 2003) and the *Handbook of Psychiatry and Palliative Medicine* (Chochinov and Breitbart, 2000).

TABLE 12.5 Palliative Care and Symptom Management

Symptom	Treatment
Intractable hiccups	Chlorpromazine, 25 mg; olanzapine, 2.5–5 mg
Dyspnea	Oxygen; morphine; fan; relaxation; mirtazapine; very low–dose neuroleptics
Nausea	Ondansetron, 4–8 mg po/IV q6h; olanzapine, 2.5–5 mg po qhs; mirtazapine: 7.5–30 mg po qhs
Pruritus	Doxepin—topical and oral formulations, 10–25 mg po q6h
Pain (nociceptive)	Strong opioid analgesics, e.g., fentanyl, hydromorphone, methadone, oxycodone, morphine sulfate; see Table 12.3
Pain (neuropathic)	Adjuvant analgesics, e.g., antidepressants, anticonvulsants, stimulants, antihistamines; see Table 12.3

Source: Cohen MA, Alfonso CA (2004). AIDS psychiatry: psychiatric and palliative care, and pain management. In GP Wormser (ed.), *AIDS and Other Manifestations of HIV Infection,* fourth edition (pp. 537–576). Copyright 2004, with permission from Elsevier.

Management of behavioral symptoms

Violent behavior

Terminally ill patients may become combative or violent. In these circumstances, likely psychiatric etiologies are delirium or dementia (Cohen, 1998; Roger, 2006), or delirium superimposed on underlying dementia, although other psychiatric disorders with associated violence and poor impulse control should not be overlooked. The diagnosis and management of these psychiatric conditions are discussed in more detail in Chapters 6, 7, and 8 in this handbook. The general management of violence in HIV-infected palliative care patients includes identification and treatment of underlying causes, attention to patient and staff safety, avoidance of restraints whenever possible, use of a calming demeanor with environmental orientation, and often pharmacotherapy.

Delirium is particularly common in patients needing palliative care, with a reported prevalence ranging from 28% to 88% of patients just prior to death (Massie et al., 1983; Minagawa et al., 1996; Caraceni et al., 2000; Lawlor et al., 2000). Palliative care patients with an agitated delirium may become confused and violent, place themselves and those around them at risk, and intensify the psychological distress of themselves, family members, and health-care staff. There are few drug trials for the management of delirium in terminally ill (Jackson and Lipman, 2004) or AIDS patients (Breibart et al., 1996). A recent review of neuroleptic trials for delirium in varied study populations reported improvement with haloperidol and with atypical neuroleptics, including risperidone, olanzapine, and quetiapine (Seitz et al., 2007).

One important consideration is that persons with HIV are at increased risk of developing extrapyramidal symptoms (EPS) with neuroleptic use (Ramachandran et al., 1997). The authors have had good experience particularly with the use of olanzapine and quetiapine in HIV-infected persons, using the lowest required dose to minimize EPS. The risk of EPS may be especially great in patients with comorbid methamphetamine abuse because of their increased basal ganglia abnormalities (Meltzer et al., 1998; Nath et al., 2001; Chang et al., 2005). A benzodiazepine may be combined with a neuroleptic in cases of more severe agitation (Casarett and Inouye, 2001). However, benzodiazepines should be avoided as monotherapy, with the exception of use in alcohol or sedative-hypnotic withdrawal, as this may exacerbate symptoms of delirium (Breitbart et al., 1996a).

The use of neuroleptics remains the standard of care for delirium, with data increasing on the use of atypicals for delirium (Sasaki et al., 2003; Parellada et al., 2004). Recent studies have suggested a dose-dependent relationship between the use of neuroleptics (typicals and atypicals) and increased rates of cerebrovascular events and death in patients with dementia of the predominant Alzheimer's and vascular varieties who received neuroleptics for agitated behavior (Gill et al., 2007; Rochon et al., 2008). While such adverse events may translate into similar findings in other disease states (e.g., AIDS dementia), it is important to interpret these results cautiously as the findings were based on retrospective or post-hoc analyses in aged groups with advanced dementia and little cognitive reserve. Prospective studies of delirium in both elderly nondemented surgical populations and elderly institutionalized patients with dementia have not documented an increased risk for adverse events when neuroleptics are administered (Kalisvaart et al., 2005; Raivio et al., 2007).

Also, the importance of screening and treating delirium appropriately cannot be overemphasized. Delirium has been noted across multiple studies to be a strong and independent predictor for prolonged length of hospital or ICU stay, reintubation, higher mortality, and cost of care (van Zyl and Seitz, 2006; Pun and Ely, 2007). Agitation can lead to patient and provider injuries, and the affective states of fear and paranoia that often accompany delirium need to be treated to prevent agitation and reduce patient suffering. Use of neuroleptics to control delirium must be assessed on an individual basis and the risks and benefits of each situation weighed when using this class of medication. In today's clinical environment, documentation of such considerations and the rationale for their use being beneficial are mandatory.

In the last days of life, patients may develop terminal delirium, often characterized by extreme restlessness despite treatment with neuroleptics. This is often distressing for the patient's family (Morita et al., 2004a, 2007; Namba et al., 2007), and a decision is sometimes made between the palliative care clinicians and family to maintain a state of terminal sedation with lorazepam, midazolam, or propofol infusions (Casarett and Inouye, 2001). Family members may experience distress and ambivalence about the use of terminal sedation, thus ongoing communication and support for the family is an essential component of end-of-life palliative care (Morita et al., 2004b).

Suicidal ideation

The rate of suicidal behavior is higher in patients with AIDS than in the general population, although the relative risk varies widely in different studies (Starace and Sherr, 1998). Persons with HIV or AIDS may also express a desire for a hastened death, physician assisted-suicide, or euthanasia. In the United States, euthanasia is illegal, and physician-assisted suicide is legal only in the state of Oregon. In Europe, physician-assisted suicide and euthanasia are legal in The Netherlands, Belgium, and Luxembourg; physician-assisted suicide is legal in Switzerland. Despite this legal landscape, a 1995 study of physicians in the San Francisco Bay area, where physician-assisted suicide has not been decriminalized, found that a majority of physicians providing care for HIV-infected patients reported having granted a request for physician-assisted suicide at least once (Slome et al., 1997).

A limited evidence base has clarified the importance of these issues for HIV-positive persons. In a European survey of HIV-positive outpatients, 78% supported legalizing euthanasia for cases of severe physical suffering, and 47% supported it for cases of severe psychological suffering. Half of the study participants reported that the possibility of euthanasia would reduce their anxiety (Andraghetti et al., 2001). In a study of HIV-infected outpatients in New York City, 55% of patients said they would consider physician-assisted suicide, and these individuals reported more depression, suicidal ideation, hopelessness, and psychological distress. Pain-related variables were not directly associated with an interest in physician-assisted suicide in this HIV-positive population (Breitbart et al., 1996b). In comparison to these HIV-infected patients, patients with more advanced HIV disease may actually be less likely to express an interest in a desire for hastened death. In a study of HIV patients admitted to a New York City palliative care facility, the prevalence of a high desire for a hastened death ranged from 4.4% to 8.3%, depending on the study instruments used (Rosenfeld et al., 2006). Studies employing in-depth interviews to explore HIV-positive patients' motivations for euthanasia or physician-assisted suicide have found associations with fears of loss of independence, dignity, and control (Green, 1995) as well as social isolation (Lavery et al., 2001).

The arguments for and against physician-assisted suicide and euthanasia will continue to debated by clinicians, ethicists, and policy makers. Whatever the outcome of this debate, HIV-infected patients expressing a desire for hastened death, physician-assisted suicide, or euthanasia require a multidisciplinary approach with an emphasis on understanding and addressing their distressing physical, psychological, and social concerns. Palliative care providers should focus on treatment options for uncontrolled physical symptoms. A mental health team should explore the areas of potential psychiatric, psychological, and social distress such as depression, suicidality, hopelessness, social isolation, and loss of dignity, autonomy, and control, and offer patients targeted interventions.

Treatment failure

Despite the promise of new antiretroviral regimens, viral suppression with antiretroviral therapy (ART) may not be feasible because of drug–drug interactions resulting in suboptimal drug levels, poor adherence, preexisting drug resistance, or a combination of these factors (Easterbrook and Meadway, 2001). Debate over the viral fitness of HIV and the possible benefit of continued ART despite high viral load continues (Deeks et al., 2001; Frenkel and Mullins, 2001). The risks and benefits of ART in late-stage AIDS are summarized in Table 12.6.

No guidelines currently exist for the cessation of ART after treatment failure; this is an important consideration for clinical trials and for the

TABLE 12.6 Potential Benefits and Risks of Antiretroviral Treatment in Late-Stage HIV Disease

---

*Potential Benefits**

- Selection for less fit virus (i.e., less pathogenic than wild type), even in the presence of elevated viral loads
- Protection against HIV encephalopathy or dementia
- Relief or easing of symptoms possibly associated with high viral loads (e.g., constitutional symptoms)
- Continued therapeutic effect, albeit attenuated
- Psychological and emotional benefits of continued disease-combating therapy

Potential Risks

- Cumulative and multiple drug toxic effects in the setting of therapeutic futility (including certain rare, potentially life-threatening toxic effects)
- Diminished quality of life from demands of treatment regimen
- Therapeutic confusion (i.e., use of future-directed, disease-modifying therapy in a dying patient)
- Distraction from end-of-life and advance-care planning issues, with narrow focus on medication adherence and monitoring

---

*Evidence is lacking for some of these potential benefits, although they are commonly considered in clinical decision making.
Source: From Selwyn PA, Forstein M (2003). Overcoming the false dichotomy of curative vs. palliative care for late-stage HIV/AIDS: "Let me live the way I want to live, until I can't." *JAMA* 290:806–814. Copyright (2003), with permission from JAMA/Archives Journals.

development of the best practices for advanced HIV disease (Selwyn and Forstein, 2003). Failure to cure should not cause the physician to withdraw emotionally because of a perceived or unconscious sense of futility; rather, it is a signal to reiterate commitment to the patient and to stay with him or her throughout the course of illness (Selwyn and Forstein, 2003).

Multiple medical problems and coexisting diagnoses

Although ART has increased the life expectancy of patients with HIV and reduced the incidence of AIDS-related illnesses (Huang et al., 2006), the frequency of pulmonary, cardiac, gastrointestinal, and renal diseases that are often not directly related to underlying HIV disease has increased (Morris et al., 2002; Casalino et al., 2004; Narasimhan et al., 2004; Vincent et al., 2004). A substantial number of persons with AIDS have comorbidities that may complicate their management. Hepatitis B and C, for example, are common in individuals who become infected with HIV via intravenous drug use. Coinfection with HIV is a strong risk factor for progression to end-stage liver disease (Easterbrook and Meadway, 2001). Multimorbid medical conditions are discussed further in Chapter 10 of this handbook.

Fluctuation in condition and difficulty determining terminal stage

Determining the prognosis of patients with advanced HIV disease can be difficult, as responses to therapy are often unpredictable. Identification of the predictors of mortality and prognostic variables for patients with advanced illness in the era of ART can help inform planning and coordination of care (Shen et al., 2005).

In 1996, short-term mortality predictors promulgated by the National Hospice Organization included CD4 cell count, viral load, and certain opportunistic infections (National Hospice Organization, 1996). These traditional HIV prognostic markers, however, no longer accurately predict death in late-stage patients because of the impact of ART. Instead, Shen and colleagues (2005) predict survival, the only significant predictors of mortality being age greater than 65 years and number of impairments in activities of daily living or Karnofsky performance score. Thus, as previously suggested by Justice et al. (1996), functional status may be a more useful means of predicting mortality in AIDS patients than biological markers (Sansone and Frengley, 2000; Selwyn et al., 2000; Puoti et al., 2001; Valdez et al., 2001; Welch and Morse, 2002).

COMMUNICATION ABOUT END-OF-LIFE ISSUES

Because of the nonlinear progression of late-stage AIDS, advance care planning and goals of care should be addressed repeatedly during the course of illness (Selwyn and Forstein, 2003). AIDS patients in particular are less likely than other patient populations to discuss advance directives and life-limiting interventions (Curtis and Patrick, 1997; Mouton et al., 1997; Wenger et al., 2001). Persons with AIDS may also experience doubt and ambivalence as their clinical condition fluctuates; this demands flexibility, patience, and tolerance on the part of the clinician. Regular and direct inquiry into how patients are handling the uncertainty of their lives provides support and indicates that the clinician is ready to hear the patient's concerns (Selwyn and Forstein, 2003). Possible barriers to discussions about end-of-life issues include physicians' reluctance to discuss death (Curtis and Patrick, 1997) and cross-cultural concerns. See Chapter 13 of this handbook for a review of end-of-life issues, ethical issues, advance directives, and surrogate decision-making.

Cross-cultural issues in the care of the dying

Ethnicity and culture strongly influence a person's attitude toward death and dying. Although there is a "universal fear of cancer [and other terminal diseases] that results from its [cancer's] association with images of extreme debility and pain and the fear of death" (Butow et al., 1997, p. 320), individuals from Western cultures use different coping strategies to deal with serious illness than those of individuals from non-Western cultures (Barg and Gullate, 2001).

Studies on cultural and ethnic differences in the face of life-threatening illness indicate that patients' cultural beliefs should be considered when disclosing the diagnosis and prognosis of a terminal illness, during evaluation of the patient, and during intervention. The "ABCDE" model (Koenig and Gates-William, 1995) provides a framework for a culturally sensitive evaluation (see Table 12.7).

Doctor–patient communication

Doctor–patient communication is an essential component of caring for a dying patient (Buckman 1993, 1998; Smith, 2000; Baile and Beale, 2001; Parker et al., 2001; Fallowfield, 2004). Despite the recognized importance of caregiver–patient communication, many physicians are not adequately trained in communication skills (Fallowfield et al., 1998).

Buckman (1998) and Baile and Beale (2001) have promoted what is commonly referred to as the six-step protocol for breaking bad news (see

TABLE 12.7 "ABCDE" Model for Culturally Sensitive Evaluation

Attitudes about illness, family and related responsibilities
Beliefs about religion and spirituality, with special sensitivity to potential
    expectations of "miracles"
Cultural context in which both the patient and their family operate
Decision-making style and how cultural beliefs and practices might affect it
Environment and any key features of it that may impact the patient during the
    course of their illness

Source: Koenig BA, Gates-William J (1995). Understanding cultural difference in caring for dying patients. *West J Med* 163:244–249, Copyright (1995), with permission from BMJ Publishing Group.

TABLE 12.8 Six-Step Protocol for Breaking Bad News

1. Getting the physical context right
2. Finding out how much the patient knows
3. Finding out how much the patient wants to know
4. Sharing information (aligning and educating)
5. Responding to the patient's feelings
6. Planning and following through

Source: Baile W, Beale E (2001). Giving bad news to cancer patients: matching process and content. *J Clin Oncol* 19(9):2575–2577; Buckman R (1998). Communication in palliative care: a practical guide. In D Doyle, GWC Hanks, and N MacDonald (eds.), *Oxford Textbook of Palliative Medicine*, second edition (pp. 141–156). Copyright (1998), with permission from Oxford University Press.

Table 12.8). This protocol is easy to follow and can be used by clinicians of all specialties.

PROGRAMS AND MODELS OF HIV PALLIATIVE CARE DELIVERY

Even end-stage AIDS patients can be restored to independence and good quality of life (Rackstraw et al., 2000; Stephenson et al., 2000). Fully developed, ideal palliative care programs offer control of symptoms and provision of support to those living with chronic, life-threatening illnesses such as AIDS. Such programs optimally include all of the following components: (1) a home care program (e.g., hospice program); (2) a hospital-based palliative care consultation service; (3) a day care program or ambulatory care clinic; (4) palliative care inpatient unit (or dedicated palliative care beds in hospital); (5) a bereavement program; (6) training and research programs; and (7) Internet-based services.

The merits of specialized hospices versus nonspecialized hospices for the delivery of HIV palliative care have been reviewed (Schofferman, 1987; Mansfield et al., 1992). Staff at specialized hospices become more experienced in the management of HIV-related problems and, as a result, are particularly sensitive to the social and psychological issues associated with HIV illness. Moreover, the environment of the specialized hospice provides patients with the opportunity to meet and gain encouragement from other patients in similar settings (Easterbrook and Meadway, 2001). Patients in the later stages of AIDS commonly express the desire to die at home (Easterbrook and Meadway, 2001). Where available, hospital support teams and community HIV nurse specialists can be helpful in carrying out this wish. For further review of special settings such as psychiatric facilities, nursing homes, correctional facilities, and homeless outreach, please see Chapter 1 of this handbook.

Spiritual Care

Puchalski and Romer (2000) define *spirituality* as that which allows a person to experience transcendent meaning in life. Karasu (1999) views spirituality as a construct that involves concepts of faith and/or meaning. *Faith* is a belief in a higher transcendent power, not necessarily identified as God. It need not involve participation in the rituals or beliefs of a specific organized religion. Indeed, the transcendent power may be identified as external to the human psyche or internalized; it is the relationship and connectedness to this power, or spirit that is an essential component of the spiritual experience and is related to the concept of meaning.

Meaning, or having a sense that one's life has meaning, involves the conviction that one is fulfilling a unique role and purpose in a life that is a gift—a life that comes with a responsibility to live to one's full potential as a human being. In so doing, one is able to achieve a sense of peace, contentment, or even transcendence through connectedness with something greater than oneself (Frankl, 1959). The "faith" component of spirituality is most often associated with religion and religious belief, whereas the "meaning" component of spirituality appears to be a more universal concept that can exist in individuals who do, or do not, identify themselves as being religious.

The FACIT Spiritual Well-Being Scale, or FACITSWBS (Peterman et al., 1996), is a widely used measure of spiritual well-being that consists of both a faith and meaning component of spirituality. The FACITSWBS generates a total score as well as two subscale scores: one corresponding to "Faith," and a second corresponding to "Meaning/Peace." Other measures commonly used to measure aspects of spirituality include the Daily Spiritual Experiences Scale, or DSES (Underwood and Teresi, 2002), and the Spiritual Beliefs Inventory, or SBI-15 (Baider et al., 2001).

Assessing spirituality

A spiritual history should be taken as early in the treatment as possible, as it provides an opportunity to give more comprehensive care and serves in building a relationship with a patient. Several general communication strategies should help to elicit patient concerns around spiritual concerns. These include the use of open-ended questions, asking patients follow-up questions to elicit more detail about their concerns, acknowledging and normalizing patient apprehension and distress, the use of empathetic comments in response to patient concerns, and inquiring about patient's emotions around these issues (Lo et al., 2003).

There are several methods of taking a spiritual history. Puchalski and Romer (2000) recommend the acronym *FICA* to structure a spiritual history: Faith and belief, Importance, Community, and Address. A good spiritual assessment should include the questions outlined in Table 12.9 (Koenig, 2002; Pulchalski and Romer, 2000).

In addition to these more open-ended questions, several formal assessment tools exist for the assessment of spirituality (Maugans, 1996). Most importantly, a detailed spiritual assessment should not be regarded as a one-time discussion but rather as the beginning of a dialogue that continues throughout a patient's care. This type of assessment should serve to let the patient know that the provider is open to these discussions and that the patient's concerns regarding spiritual issues will be met in a supportive and respectful manner (Post et al., 2000). Simply being present, actively listening, offering empathetic responses, and trying to understand the patient's point of view will foster a productive dialogue and offer great comfort to the patient.

TABLE 12.9 Questions to Ask When Performing a Spiritual Assessment

1. Do you consider yourself a spiritual or religious person?
2. What gives your life meaning?
3. Do the religious or spiritual beliefs provide comfort and support or cause stress?
4. What importance do these beliefs have in your life?
5. Could these beliefs influence your medical decisions?
6. Do you have beliefs that might conflict with your medical care?
7. Are you part of a spiritual or religious community? Are they important to you or a source of support?
8. What are your spiritual needs that someone should address? How would you like these needs to be addressed as part of your health care?

Sources: Koenig HG (2002). Religion, spirituality, and medicine: how are they related and what does it mean? *Mayo Clin Proc* 12:1189–1191; Puchalski C, Romer AL (2000). Taking a spiritual history allows clinicians to understand patients more fully. *J Palliat Med* 3:129–137. Copyright (2000), with permission from Mary Ann Liebert, Inc.

Treatment of spiritual suffering

Rousseau (2000) has developed an approach to the treatment of spiritual suffering that centers on (1) controlling physical symptoms; (2) providing a supportive presence; (3) encouraging life review to assist in recognizing purpose value and meaning; (4) exploring guilt, remorse, forgiveness, and reconciliation; (5) facilitating religious expression; (6) reframing goals; (7) encouraging meditative practices; and (8) focusing on healing rather than cure. This approach to spiritual suffering encompasses a blend of several basic psychotherapeutic principles common to different psychotherapies. It should be noted that this intervention contains a heavy emphasis on facilitating religious expression and confession that may be extremely useful to many patients, but not all patients or clinicians will feel comfortable with this approach.

Meaning-centered interventions

In contrast, Breitbart and colleagues (Greenstein and Breitbart, 2000; Breitbart, 2002; Breitbart and Heller, 2003; Gibson and Breitbart, 2004) have attempted to apply the work of Viktor Frankl and his concepts of meaning-based psychotherapy (Frankl, 1955) to address spiritual suffering. While Frankl's logotherapy was not designed for the treatment of patients with life-threatening illness, his concepts of meaning and spirituality clearly have applications in psychotherapeutic work with patients at advanced stages of their illness. Many of these patients seek guidance and help in dealing with issues of sustaining meaning, hope, and understanding in the face of their illness while avoiding overt religious emphasis. This "meaning-centered group psychotherapy" (Greenstein and Breitbart, 2000) uses a mixture of didactics, discussion, and experiential exercises that focus on particular themes related to meaning and advanced cancer. It is designed to help patients with advanced cancer sustain or enhance a sense of meaning, peace, and purpose in their lives, even as they approach the end of life. Gibson and Breitbart (2004) have developed a manual for an individual form of this therapy and are currently conducting outcome studies to determine the feasibility and efficacy of both the group and individual forms of this therapy.

Treatment of demoralization

Kissane and colleagues (2001) have described a syndrome of "demoralization" in the terminally ill, which is distinct from depression. Demoralization syndrome consists of a triad of hopelessness, loss of meaning, and existential distress expressed as a desire for death. It is associated with life-threatening medical illness, disability, bodily disfigurement, fear, loss of dignity, social

Table 12.10 Multidisciplinary Model for Treatment of Demoralization Syndrome

1. Ensure continuity of care and active symptom management
2. Ensure dignity in the dying process
3a. Use various types of psychotherapy to help sustain a sense of meaning
3b. Limit cognitive distortions and maintain family relationships (i.e., via meaning-based, cognitive-behavioral, interpersonal, and family psychotherapy interventions)
4. Use life review and narrative, giving attention to spiritual issues
5. Use pharmacotherapy for comorbid anxiety, depression, or delirium

Source: Kissane D, Clarke DM, Street AF (2001). Demoralization syndrome: a relevant psychiatric diagnosis for palliative care. *J Palliat Care* 17:12–21. Copyright (2001), with permission from Mary Ann Liebert, Inc.

isolation, and feelings of being a burden. Because of the sense of impotence and hopelessness, those with the syndrome predictably progress to a desire to die or commit suicide. Kissane and colleagues (2001) have formulated a treatment approach for demoralization syndrome (see Table 12.10).

Dignity-conserving care

Finally, ensuring dignity in the dying process is a critical goal of palliative care. Despite use of the term *dignity* in arguments for and against a patient's self-governance in matters pertaining to death, there is little empirical research on how this term has been used by patients who are nearing death.

Chochinov and colleagues (2002a, 2002b) examined how dying patients understand and define the term *dignity* to develop a model of dignity in the terminally ill. A semistructured interview was designed to explore how patients cope with their illness and their perceptions of dignity. Three major categories emerged: (1) illness-related concerns (those that derive from or are related to the illness itself and threaten to or actually do impinge on the patient's sense of dignity); (2) dignity-conserving repertoire (internally held qualities or personal approaches or techniques that patients use to bolster or maintain their sense of dignity); and (3) social dignity inventory (social concerns or relationship dynamics that enhance or detract from a patient's sense of dignity). These broad categories and their carefully defined themes and sub-themes form the foundation for an emerging model of dignity among the dying. The concept of dignity and the notion of dignity-conserving care offer a way of understanding how patients face advancing terminal illness. They also present an approach that clinicians can use to explicitly target the maintenance of dignity as a therapeutic objective. Accordingly, Chochinov and colleagues (2002a) have developed a short-term dignity therapy for palliative patients that incorporates those facets from this model that are most likely to bolster the dying patient's will to live, lessen the desire for death or lessen overall level of distress, and improve quality of life.

Communicating about spiritual issues

Communicating about spirituality with patients effectively requires comfort in several domains: (1) a basic knowledge of common spiritual concerns and sources of spiritual pain for patients; (2) the principles and beliefs of the major religions common to the patient populations one treats; (3) basic clinical communication skills, such as active and empathetic listening, with an ability to identify and highlight spiritually relevant issues; and (4) the ability to remain present while patients struggle with spiritual issues in light of their mortality (Storey and Knight, 2001). This final domain is often the most trying, especially for clinicians early in their career.

The American Academy of Hospice and Palliative Medicine offers the following guidelines for clinicians when communicating about spiritual issues (Doyle, 1992; Hay, 1996; Storey and Knight, 2001). First, it is important to recognize that every patient is an individual and has a unique belief system that should be honored and respected. A patient's spiritual views may or may not incorporate religious beliefs, as spirituality is considered the more inclusive category. Therefore, initial discussions should focus on broad spiritual issues and then, when appropriate, on more specific religious beliefs. Caregivers should maintain appropriate boundaries and avoid discussions of their own religious beliefs, as it is usually not relevant. Finally, fostering hope and integrating meaning into a patient's life is often a more important aspect of providing spiritual healing than any adherence to a particular belief system or religious affiliation.

Role of the Psychiatrist and Other Clinicians at Time of Death and Afterward

Grief and bereavement

Bereavement care is an integral dimension of palliative care. Knowledge of and competence in assessing grief is essential to recognizing the 20% of the bereaved who need additional assistance. Routine assessment of the bereaved for risk factors associated with complicated grief provides a method by which psychosomatic medicine specialists can preventatively intervene to reduce unnecessary morbidity. Effective therapies are available to assist in the management of complicated grief (Kissane, 2004). Grief is an inevitable dimension of our humanity, an adaptive adjustment process, and one that, with adequate support, can eventually be traversed.

Although words such as *grief, mourning*, and *bereavement* are commonly used interchangeably, the following definitions may be helpful:

- *Bereavement* is the state of loss resulting from death (Parkes, 1998).
- *Grief* is the emotional response associated with loss (Stroebe et al., 1993).
- *Mourning* is the process of adaptation, including the cultural and social rituals prescribed as accompaniments (Raphael, 1983).
- *Anticipatory grief* precedes the death and results from the expectation of that event (Raphael, 1983).
- *Complicated grief* represents a pathological outcome involving psychological, social, or physical morbidity (Rando, 1983).
- *Disenfranchised grief* represents the hidden sorrow of the marginalized, where there is less social permission to express many dimensions of loss (Doka, 1989).

Anticipatory grief

As the patient and family journey through palliative care, the clinical phases of grief progress from anticipatory grief through to the immediate news of the death, to the stages of acute grief and, potentially for some, the complications of bereavement. Anticipatory grief generally draws the supportive family into a configuration of mutual comfort and greater closeness as the news of the illness and its proposed management is tackled. For a time, this perturbation advantages the care of the sick, until the pressures of daily life draw the family back toward their prior constellation. Movement back and forth is evident thereafter, as news of illness progression unfolds. Periods of grief can become interspersed with phases of contentment and happiness. When the family is engaged in home care of their dying member, their cohesion may increase as they share their fears, hopes, joy, and distress. In some families, the stress of loss may result in further divisiveness and the accentuation of previously contentious dynamics.

Difficulties can emerge for some families as they express their anticipatory grief. Impaired coping manifests itself via protective avoidance, denial of the seriousness of the threat, anger, or withdrawal from involvement. Sometimes family dysfunction is glaring. More commonly, however, subthreshold or mild depressive or anxiety disorders develop gradually as individuals struggle to adapt to unwelcome changes. While anticipatory grief was historically suggested to reduce postmortem grief (Parkes, 1975), intense distress is now well recognized as a marker of risk for complicated grief. During this phase of anticipatory grief, clinicians can help the family that is capable of effective communication by encouraging them to openly share their feelings as they go about the instrumental care of their dying family member or friend. Saying goodbye is a process that evolves over time, with opportunities for reminiscence, celebration of the life and contributions of the dying person, expressions of gratitude, and completion of any unfinished business (Meares, 1981). These tasks have the potential to generate creative and positive emotions out of what is otherwise a sad time for all.

Acute grief and time course of bereavement

The bereaved move through sequences of phases over time; these phases are never rigidly demarcated but rather merge gradually one into the other (Raphael, 1983; Parkes, 1998). The time course of mourning is shaped by the nature of the loss, the context in which the loss took place, and a multitude of factors ranging from personal resilience to cultural, social, and ethnic affiliations. There is no sharply defined end point to grief. The clinical task is to differentiate those expressions of grief that remain with the spectrum of normalcy from those that cross the threshold of complicated grief.

Complicated grief

Normal and abnormal responses to bereavement span a broad spectrum. Intensity of reaction, presence of a range of related grief behaviors, and time course all factor into the differentiation between normal and abnormal grief. Common psychiatric disorders resulting from grief include clinical depression, anxiety disorders, alcohol abuse or other substance abuse and dependence, and, less commonly, psychotic disorders and posttraumatic stress disorder. When frank psychiatric disorders complicate bereavement, their recognition and management is straightforward. Subthreshold states, however, present a greater clinical challenge.

Grief therapies

Because loss is so ubiquitous in the palliative care setting, psychosomatic medicine clinicians need skill in the application of grief therapies. For most of the bereaved, personal resilience ensures normal adaptation in the face of their painful situation. As such, there is no justification for routine intervention, as grief is not a disease. Those considered at risk of maladaptive outcome, however, can be treated preventatively. Those who later develop complicated bereavement need active treatments.

The spectrum of interventions spans individual, group, and family-oriented therapies, and encompasses all schools of psychotherapy as well as appropriately indicated pharmacotherapies. Adoption of any model or parts thereof is based on the clinical issues and their associated circumstances. Thus, variation will be influenced by age, perception of support, the nature of the death, the personal health of the bereaved, and the presence of comorbid states. Most interventions consist of six to eight sessions over several months. In this sense, grief therapy is focused and time limited. Multimodal therapies, however, are commonplace. Thus, group and individual therapies better support the lonely so that socialization interpersonally complements any intrapersonal support.

A family approach to grief intervention is exemplified by family-focused grief therapy (FFGT), developed by Kissane and Bloch (2002). Such a model aims to improve family functioning while also supporting the expression of grief. This approach can be applied preventatively to those families judged through screening to be at high risk of complicated outcomes (Kissane and Bloch, 2002). Thus, FFGT commences during palliative care and includes the ill family member. It continues throughout the early phases of bereavement until there is confidence that morbidity has been prevented or appropriately treated. This approach invites the family to identify and work on aspects of family life that they specifically recognize as a cause of concern. Through enhancing cohesion, promoting open communication of thoughts and feelings, and teaching effective problem solving, conflict is reduced and tolerance of different opinions is optimized. The improved functioning of the family as a unit becomes the means to accomplish adaptive mourning.

CONCLUSION

Palliative care for patients with advanced AIDS requires a biopsychosocial approach consistent with the patient's expressed goals of care. As the possibility of a cure or prolongation of life becomes less remote in the care of the person with advanced AIDS, the focus of treatment shifts to symptom control and enhanced quality of life. Patients are uniquely vulnerable to both physical and psychiatric complications. The role of the psychiatrist in the care of the terminally ill or dying AIDS patient is critical to both adequate symptom control and integration of the medical, psychological, and spiritual dimensions of human experience in the last weeks of life. To be most effective in this role, the psychiatrist must have specialized knowledge of not only the psychiatric complications of terminal illness and the existential issues confronting those at the end of life but also the common physical symptoms that plague persons with advanced AIDS and contribute so dramatically to their suffering.

REFERENCES

Adams N, Poole H, Richardson C (2006). Psychological approaches to chronic pain management: part 1. *J Clin Nurs* 15:290–300.

Andraghetti R, Foran S, Colebunders R, Tomlinson D, Vyras P, Borleffs CJ, Fleerackers Y, Schrooten W, Borchert M (2001). Euthanasia: from the perspective of HIV infected persons in Europe. *HIV Med* 2:3–10.

Armstrong SC, Cozza KL (2003a). Pharmacokinetic drug interactions of morphine, codeine, and their derivatives: theory and clinical reality, part I. *Psychosomatics* 44(2):167–172.

Armstrong SC, Cozza KL (2003b). Pharmacokinetic drug interactions of morphine, codeine, and their derivatives: theory and clinical reality, part II. *Psychosomatics* 44(6):515–520.

Baider L, Holland JC, Russak SM, Kaplan De-Nour A (2001). The system of belief inventory (SBI-15). *Psycho-Oncology* 10:534–540.

Baile W, Beale E (2001). Giving bad news to cancer patients: matching process and content. *J Clin Oncol* 19:2575–2577.

Barg FK, Gullate MM (2001). Cancer support groups: meeting the needs of African Americans with cancer. *Semin Oncol Nurs* 17:171–178.

Breitbart W (2002). Spirituality and meaning in supportive care: spirituality and meaning-centered group psychotherapy interventions in advanced cancer. *Support Care Cancer* 10(4):272–280.

Breitbart W, Heller KS (2003). Reframing hope: meaning-centered care for patients near the end-of-life. *J Palliat Med* 6:979–988.

Breitbart W, Kaim M, Rosenfeld B (1999). Clinicians' perceptions of barriers to pain management in AIDS. *J Pain Symptom Manage* 18:203–212.

Breitbart W, Marotta R, Platt MM, Weisman H, Derevenco M, Grau C, Corbera K, Raymond S, Lund S, Jacobsen P (1996a). A double-blind trial of haloperidol, chlorpromazine, and lorazepam in the treatment of delirium in hospitalized AIDS patients. *Am J Psychiatry* 153(2):231–237.

Breitbart W, McDonald MV, Rosenfeld B, Monkman ND, Passik S (1998). Fatigue in ambulatory AIDS patients. *J Pain Symptom Manage* 15:159–167.

Breitbart WS, Passik S, Eller KC, Sison A (1992). Suicidal ideation in AIDS: the role of pain and mood [NR 267 (abstract)]. Presented at the 145th Annual Meeting of the American Psychiatric Association, Washington, DC.

Breitbart W, Payne D, Passik S (2004). Psychological and psychiatric interventions in pain control. In D Doyle, G Hanks, N Cherny, and K Calman (eds.), *Oxford Textbook of Palliative Medicine*, third edition (pp. 424–437). New York: Oxford University Press.

Breitbart W, Rosenfeld BD, Passik SD (1996b). Interest in physician-assisted suicide among ambulatory HIV-infected patients. *Am J Psychiatry* 153 (2):238–242.

Breitbart W, Rosenfeld B, Passik SD, McDonald MV, Thaler H, Portenoy RK (1996c). The undertreatment of pain in ambulatory AIDS patients. *Pain* 65:243–249.

Bruera E, MacMillan K, Pither J, MacDonald RN (1990). Effects of morphine on the dyspnea of the terminal cancer patients. *J Pain Symptom Manage* 5:1–5.

Buckman R (1993). *How to Break Bad News: A Guide for Healthcare Professionals.* London: Macmillan Medical.

Buckman R (1998). Communication in palliative care: a practical guide. In D Doyle, GWC Hanks, and N MacDonald (eds.), *Oxford Textbook of Palliative Medicine*, second edition (pp. 141–156). New York: Oxford University Press.

Butler RN, Burt R, Foley KM, Morris J, Morrison RS (1996). Palliative medicine: providing care when cure is not possible. A roundtable discussion: Part I. *Geriatrics* 51:33–36.

Butow P, Tattersall M, Goldstein D (1997). Communication with cancer patients in culturally diverse societies. *Ann N Y Acad Sci* 809:317–329.

Canadian Palliative Care Association (1995). *Palliative Care. Towards a Consensus in Standardized Principles of Practice*. Ottawa, ON: Canadian Palliative Care Association.

Caraceni A, Nanni O, Maltoni M, Piva L, Indelli M, Arnoldi E, Monti M, Montanari L, Amadori D, De Conno F (2000). Impact of delirium on the short-term prognosis of advanced cancer patients. *Cancer* 89(5):1145–1149.

Carmichael JK (1991). Treatment of herpes zoster and postherpetic neuralgia. *Am Fam Physician* 44:203–210.

Casalino E, Wolff M, Ravaud P, Choquet C, Bruneel F, Regnier B (2004). Impact of HAART advent on admission patterns and survival in HIV-infected patients admitted to an intensive care unit. *AIDS* 18:1429–1433.

Casarett DJ, Inouye SK (2001). American College of Physicians–American Society of Internal Medicine End-of-Life Care Consensus Panel: Diagnosis and management of delirium near the end of life. *Ann Intern Med* 135(1):32–40.

Chang L, Ernst T, Speck O, Grob CS (2005). Additive effects of HIV and chronic methamphetamine use on brain metabolite abnormalities. *Am J Psychiatry* 162:361–369.

Chochinov HM, Breitbart W (eds.) (2000). *Handbook of Psychiatry and Palliative Medicine*. New York: Oxford University Press.

Chochinov HM, Hack T, Hassard T, Kristjanson LJ, McClement S, Harlos M (2002a). Dignity in the terminally ill: a cross-sectional, cohort study. *Lancet* 360:2026–2030.

Chochinov HM, Hack T, McClement S, Harlos M, and Kristjanson L (2002b). Dignity in the terminally ill: an empirical model. *Soc Sci Med* 54:433–443.

Cohen MA (1998). Psychiatric care in an AIDS nursing home. *Psychosomatics* 39 (2):154–161.

Cohen MA, Alfonso CA (2004). AIDS psychiatry: psychiatric and palliative care, and pain management. In GP Wormser (ed.), *AIDS and Other Manifestations of HIV Infection*, fourth edition (pp. 537–576). San Diego: Elsevier Academic Press.

Cornblath DR, McArthur JC (1988). Predominantly sensory neuropathy in patients with AIDS and AIDS-related complex. *Neurology* 38:794–796.

Curtis JR, Patrick DL (1997). Barriers to communication about end-of-life care in AIDS patients. *J Gen Intern Med* 12:736–741.

Deeks S, Wrin T, Liegler T, Hoh R, Hayden M, Barbour JD, Hellmann NS, Petropoulos CJ, McCune JM (2001). Virologic and immunologic consequences of discontinuing combination antitretroviral-drug therapy in HIV-infected patients with detectable viremia. *N Engl J Med* 344:472–480.

Doka K (1989). Disenfranchised grief. In K Doka (ed.), *Disenfranchised Grief: Recognizing Hidden Sorrow* (pp. 3–11). Lexington, MA: Lexington Books.

Doyle D (1992). Have we looked beyond the physical and psychosocial? *J Pain Symptom Manage* 7(5):302–311.

Doyle D, Hanks G, Cherny N, Calman K (eds.) (2003). *Oxford Textbook of Palliative Medicine*, third edition. New York: Oxford University Press.

Easterbrook P, Meadway J (2001). The changing epidemiology of HIV infection: new challenges for HIV palliative care. *J R Soc Med* 94(9):442–448.

Fallowfield L (2004). Communication and palliative medicine. In D Doyle, G Hanks, N Cherny, and K Calman (eds.), *Oxford Textbook of Palliative Medicine*, third edition (pp. 101–107). New York: Oxford University Press.

Fallowfield L, Lipkin M, Hall A (1998). Teaching senior oncologists communication skills: results from phase I of a comprehensive longitudinal program in the United Kingdom. *J Clin Oncol* 16:1961–1968.

Fantoni M, Ricci F, Del Borgo C, Izzi I, Damiano F, Moscati AM, Marasca G, Bevilacqua N, Del Forna A (1997). Multicentre study on the prevalence of symptoms and symptomatic treatment in HIV infection. *J Palliat Care* 13:9–13.

Filbet M, Marceron V (1994). A retrospective study of symptoms in 193 terminal inpatients with AIDS [abstract]. *J Palliat Care* 10:92.

Foley F (1994). AIDS palliative care [abstract]. *J Palliat Care* 10:132.

Foley F, Flannery S (1995). AIDS palliative care: challenging the palliative paradigm. *J Palliat Care* 11:34–37.

Fontaine A, LaRue F, Lassauniere JM (1999). Physicians' recognition of the symptoms experienced by HIV patients: how reliable? *J Pain Symptom Manage* 18:263–270.

Frankl VF (1955). *The Doctor and the Soul*. New York: Random House.

Frankl VF (1959). *Man's Search for Meaning*, fourth edition. Boston: Beacon Press.

Frenkel L, Mullins J (2001). Should patients with drug-resistant HIV-1 continue to receive antiretroviral therapy? *N Engl J Med* 344:520–522.

Geara F, Le Bourgeois JP, Piedbois P, Pavlovitch JM, Mazeron JJ (1991). Radiotherapy in the management of cutaneous epidemic Kaposi's sarcoma. *Int J Radiat Oncol Biol Phys* 21:1517–1522.

Gibson CA, Breitbart W (2004). Individual meaning-centered psychotherapy treatment manual. Unpublished.

Gill SS, Bronskill SE, Normand SL, Anderson GN, Sykora K, Lam K, Bell CM, Lee PE, Fisher HD, Hermann N, Gurwitz JH, Rochon PA (2007). Antipsychotic drug use and mortality in older adults with dementia. *Ann Intern Med* 146(11):775–786.

Goldberg RJ (1993). Acute pain management. In A Stoudemire and BS Fogel (eds.), *Psychiatric Care of the Medical Patient* (pp. 323–340). New York: Oxford University Press.

Green G (1995). AIDS and euthanasia. *AIDS Care* 7 (Suppl. 2):S169–S173.

Greenstein M, Breitbart W (2000). Cancer and the experience of meaning: a group psychotherapy program for people with cancer. *Am J Psychother* 54:486–500.

Guzman J, Esmail R, Karjalainen K, Malmivaara A, Irvin E, Bombardier C (2001). Multidisciplinary rehabilitation for chronic low back pain: systematic review. *BMJ* 322:1511–1516.

Hahn K, Arendt G, Braun JS, von Giesen HJ, Husstedt IW, Maschke M, Straube ME, Schielke E; German Neuro-AIDS Working Group (2004). A placebo-controlled trial of gabapentin for painful HIV-associated sensory neuropathies. *J Neurol* 251(10):1260–1266.

Harding R, Easterbrook P, Higginson IJ, Karus D, Raveis VH, Marconi K (2005). Access and equity in HIV/AIDS palliative care: a review of the evidence and responses. *Palliat Med* 19(3):251–258.

Hay MW (1996). Developing guidelines for spiritual caregivers in hospice: principles for spiritual assessment. Presented at the National Hospice Organization Annual Sympsium and Exposition, November 6–9, Chicago, IL.

Hilgard E, LeBaron S (1982). Relief of anxiety and pain in children and adolescents with cancer: quantitative measures and clinical observations. *Int J Clin Exp Hypn* 30:417–442.

Huang L, Quartin A, Jones D, Havlir DV (2006). Intensive care of patients with HIV infection. *N Engl J Med* 355:173–181.

Jackson KC, Lipman AG (2004). Drug therapy for delirium in terminally ill patients. *Cochrane Database Syst Rev* 2:CD004770.

Jacox AJ, Carr DB, Payne R (1994). New clinical-practice guidelines for the management of pain in patients with cancer. *N Engl J Med* 330:651.

Jay SM, Elliott C, Varni JW (1986). Acute and chronic pain in adults and children with cancer. *J Consult Clin Psychol* 54:601–607.

Jonsson E, Coombs DW, Hunstad D, Richardson JR Jr, von Reyn CF, Saunders RL, Heaney JA (1992). Continuous infusion of intrathecal morphine to control acquired immunodeficiency syndrome–associated bladder pain. *J Urol* 147:687–689.

Justice AC, Aiken LH, Smith HL, Turner BJ (1996). The role of functional status in predicting inpatient mortality with AIDS: a comparison with current predictors. *J Clin Epidemiol* 49:193–201.

Kalisvaart KJ, de Jonghe JF, Bogaards MJ, Vreeswijk R, Egberts TC, Burger BJ, Eikelenboom P, van Gool WA (2005). Haloperidol prophylaxis for elderly hip-surgery patients at risk for delirium: a randomized placebo-controlled study. *J Am Geriatr Soc* 53(10):1658–1666.

Kalso E, Allan L, Dellemijn PL, Faura CC, Ilias WK, Jensen TS, Perrot S, Plaghki LH, Zenz M (2003). Recommendations for using opioids in chronic non-cancer pain. *Eur J Pain* 7:381–386.

Karasu BT (1999). Spiritual psychotherapy. *Am J Psychother* 53:143–162.

Kelleher P, Cox S, McKeogh M (1997). HIV infection: the spectrum of symptoms and disease in male and female patients attending a London hospice. *Palliat Med* 11:152–158.

Kellerman J, Zeltzer L, Ellenberg L, Dash J (1983). Adolescents with cancer: hypnosis for the reduction of acute pain and anxiety associated with medical procedures. *J Adolesc Health Care* 4:85–90.

Kissane DW (2004). Bereavement. In D Doyle, G Hanks, N Cherny, and K Calman (eds.), *Oxford Textbook of Palliative Medicine*, third edition (pp. 1135–1154). New York: Oxford University Press.

Kissane D, Bloch S (2002). *Family Focus Grief Therapy: A Model of Family-centered Care during Palliative Care and Bereavement*. Buckingham: Open University Press.

Kissane D, Clarke DM, Street AF (2001). Demoralization syndrome: a relevant psychiatric diagnosis for palliative care. *J Palliat Care* 17:12–21.

Koenig BA, Gates-William J (1995). Understanding cultural difference in caring for dying patients. *West J Med* 163:244–249.

Koenig HG (2002). Religion, spirituality, and medicine: how are they related and what does it mean? *Mayo Clinic Proc* 12:1189–1191.

LaRue F, Brasseur L, Musseault P, Demeulemeester R, Bonifassi L, Bez G (1994). Pain and symptoms in HIV disease: a national survey in France [abstract]. *J Palliat Care* 10:95.

LaRue F, Colleau SM (1997). Underestimation and undertreatment of pain in HIV disease: multicentre study. *BMJ* 314:23–28.

Lavery JV, Boyle J, Dickens BM, Maclean H, Singer PA (2001). Origins of the desire for euthanasia and assisted suicide in people with HIV-1 or AIDS: a qualitative study. *Lancet* 358:362–367.

Lawlor PG, Gagnon B, Mancini IL, Pereira JL, Hanson J, Suarez-Almazor ME, Bruera ED (2000). Occurrence, causes, and outcome of delirium in patients with advanced cancer: a prospective study. *Arch Inter Med* 160 (6):786–794.

Lo B, Kates LW, Ruston D, Arnold RM, Cohen CB, Puchalski CM, Pantilat SZ, Rabow MW, Schreiber RS, Tulsky JA (2003). Responding to requests regarding prayer and religious ceremonies by patients near the end-of-life and their families. *J Palliat Med* 3:409–415.

Maddox JD, Joranson D, Angarola RT (1997). The use of opioids for the treatment of chronic pain (position statement). *Clin J Pain* 167:30–34.

Mansfield S, Barter G, Singh S (1992). AIDS and palliative care. *Int J STD AIDS* 3:248–50.

Massie MJ, Holland J, Glass E (1983). Delirium in terminally ill cancer patients. *Am J Psychiatry* 140(8):1048–1050.

Mathews WC, McCutcheon JA, Asch S, Turner BJ, Gifford AL, Kuromiya K, Brown J, Shapiro MF, Bozzette SA (2000). National estimates of HIV-related symptom prevalence from the HIV Cost and Services Utilization Study. *Med Care* 38:750–762.

Maugans TA (1996). The SPIRITual history. *Arch Fam Med* 5:11–16.

Meares R (1981). On saying goodbye before death. *JAMA* 246:1227–1229.

Meltzer C, Wells S, Becher M, Flanigan K, Oyler G, Lee R (1998). AIDS-related MR hyperintensity of the basal ganglia. *Am J Neuroradiol* 19:83089.

Minagawa H, Uchitomi Y, Yamawaki S, Ishitani K (1996). Psychiatric morbidity in terminally ill cancer patients: a prospective study. *Cancer* 78(5):1131–1137.

Morita T, Akechi T, Ikenaga M, Inoue S, Kohara H, Matsubara T, Matsuo N, Namba M, Shinjo T, Tani K, Uchitomi Y (2007). Terminal delirium: recommendations from bereaved families' experiences. *J Pain Symptom Manage* 34 (6):579–589.

Morita T, Hirai K, Sakaguchi Y, Tsuneto S, Shima Y (2004a). Family-perceived distress from delirium-related symptoms of terminally ill cancer patients. *Psychosomatics* 45(2):107–113.

Morita T, Ikenaga M, Adachi I, Narabayashi I, Kizawa Y, Honke Y, Kohara H, Mukaiyama T, Akechi T, Uchitomi Y (2004b). Japan Pain, Rehabilitation, Palliative Medicine, and Psycho-Oncology (J-PRPP) Study Group: family experience with palliative sedation therapy for terminally ill cancer patients. *J Pain Symptom Manage* 28(6):557–565.

Morley S, Eccleston C, Williams A (1999). Systematic review and meta-analysis of randomized controlled trials of cognitive behaviour therapy for chronic pain in adults, excluding headache. *Pain* 80:1–13.

Morris A, Creasman J, Turner J, Luce JM, Wachter RM, Huang L (2002). Intensive care of human immunodeficiency virus–infected patients during the era of highly active antiretroviral therapy. *Am J Respir Crit Care Med* 166:262–267.

Moss V (1990). Palliative care in advanced HIV disease: presentation, problems, and palliation. *AIDS* 4(Suppl. 1):S235–S242.

Mouton C, Teno JM, Mor V, Piette J (1997). Communications of preferences for care among human immunodeficiency virus–infected patients: barriers to informed decisions? *Arch Fam Med* 6:342–347.

Namba M, Morita T, Imura C, Kiyohara E, Ishikawa S, Hirai K (2007). Terminal delirium: families' experience. *Palliat Med* 21(7):587–594.

Narasimhan M, Posner AJ, DePalo VA, Mayo PH, Rosen MJ (2004). Intensive care in patients with HIV infection in the era of highly active antiretroviral therapy. *Chest* 125:1800–1804.

Nath A, Maragos WF, Avison MJ, Schmitt FA, Berger JR (2001). Acceleration of HIV dementia with methamphetamine and cocaine. *J Neurovirol* 7:66–71.

National Hospice Organization (1996). *Guidelines for Determining Prognosis for Selected Non-Cancer Diagnoses.* Alexandria, VA: National Hospice Organization.

Newshan GT, Wainapel SF (1993). Pain characteristics and their management in persons with AIDS. *J Assoc Nurses AIDS Care* 4:53–59.

Olkkola KT, Palkama VJ, Neuvonen PJ (1999). Ritonavir's role in reducing fentanyl clearance and prolonging its half-life. *Anesthesiology* 91 (3):681–685.

O'Neill W, Sherrard J (1993). Pain in human immunodeficiency virus disease: a review. *Pain* 54:3–14.

Ontario Workplace Safety and Insurance Board (2000). Report of the Chronic Pain Expert Advisory Panel. Ontario: Ontario Workplace Safety and Insurance Board.

Pain Society and Royal Colleges of Anaesthetists (2004). Consensus Statement from the Pain Society and Royal Colleges of Anaesthetists. General Practitioners and Psychiatrists: Recommendations. London: The Royal College of Anaesthetists.

Parellada E, Baeza I, de Pablo J, Martinez G (2004). Risperidone in the treatment of patients with delirium. *J Clin Psychiatry* 65(3):348–353.

Parker B, Baile W, deMoor C, et al. (2001). Breaking bad news about cancer: patients' preferences for communication. *J Clin Oncol* 19 (7):2049–2056.

Parkes C (1975). Determinants of outcome following bereavement. *Omega* 6:303–323.

Parkes C (1998). *Bereavement: Studies of Grief in Adult Life*, third edition. Madison, WI: International Universities Press.

Peterman AH, Fitchett G, Cella DF (1996). Modeling the relationship between quality of life dimensions and an overall sense of well-being. Presented at the Third World Congress of Psycho-Oncology, New York, NY.

Portenoy RK (1993). Chronic pain management. In A Stoudemire and BS Fogel (eds.), Psychiatric Care of the Medical Patient. New York: Oxford University Press.

Post SG, Puchalski CM, Larson DB (2000). Physicians and patient spirituality: professional boundaries, competency, and ethics. *Ann Intern Med* 132:578–583.

Puchalski C, Romer AL (2000). Taking a spiritual history allows clinicians to understand patients more fully. *J Palliat Med* 3:129–137.

Pun BT, Ely EW (2007). The importance of diagnosing and managing ICU delirium. *Chest* 132(2):624–636.

Puoti M, Spinetti A, Ghezzi A, et al. (2001). Mortality from liver disease in patients with HIV infection: a cohort study. *J Acquir Immune Defic Syndr* 24:211–217.

Rackstraw S, Conley A, Meadway J (2000). Recovery from progressive multi-focal leukoencephalopathy following directly observed highly active antiretroviral therapy (HAART) in a specialized brain impairment unit. *AIDS* 14 (Suppl. 4):S129.

Raivio MM, Laurila JV, Strandberg TE, Tilvis RS, Pitkala KH (2007). Neither atypical nor conventional antipsychotics increase mortality or hospital admissions among elderly patients with dementia: a two-year prospective study. *Am J Geriatr Psychiatry* 15(5):416–424.

Ramachandran G, Glickman L, Levenson J, Rao C (1997). Incidence of extra-pyramidal syndromes in AIDS patients and a comparison group of medically ill patients. *J Neuropsychiatry Clin Neurosci* 9(4):579–583.

Rando T (1983). *Treatment of Complicated Mourning*. Champaign, IL: Research Press.

Raphael B (1983). *The Anatomy of Bereavement*. London: Hutchinson.

Reiter GS, Kudler NR (1996). Palliative care and HIV: systemic manifestations and late-stage issues. *AIDS Clin Care* 8:27–36.

Rochon PA, Normand SL, Gomes T, Gill SS, Anderson GM, Melo M, Sykora K, Lipscombe L, Bell CM, Gurwitz JH (2008). Antipsychotic therapy and short-term serious events in older adults with dementia. *Arch Intern Med* 168 (10):1090–1096.

Roger KS (2006). A literature review of palliative care, end of life, and dementia. *Palliat Support Care* 4(3):295–303.

Rosenfeld B, Breitbart W, Gibson C, Kramer M, Tomarken A, Nelson C, Pessin H, Esch J, Galietta M, Garcia N, Brechtl J, Schuster M (2006). Desire for hastened death among patients with advanced AIDS. *Psychosomatics* 47 (6):504–512.

Rosenfeld B, Breitbart W, McDonald MV, Passik SD, Thaler H, Portenoy RK (1997). Pain in ambulatory AIDS patients: impact of pain on physiological functioning and quality of life. *Pain* 68:323–328.

Rousseau P (2000). Spirituality and the dying patient. *J Clin Oncol* 18:2000–2002.

Sansone RG, Frengley JD (2000). Impact of HAART on causes of death of persons with late-stage AIDS. *J Urban Health* 77:165–175.

Sasaki Y, Matsuyama T, Inoue S, Sunami T, Inoue T, Denda K, Koyama T (2003). Prospective, open-label, flexible-dose study of quetiapine in the treatment of delirium. *J Clin Psychiatry* 64(11):1316–1321.

Schofferman J (1987). Hospice care of the patient with AIDS. *J Hospice* 3:51–74.

Schofferman J (1988). Pain: diagnosis and management in the palliative care of AIDS. *J Palliat Care* 4:46–49.

Seitz DP, Gill SS, van Zyl LT (2007). Antipsychotics in the treatment of delirium: a systematic review. *J Clin Psychiatry* 68(1):11–21.

Selwyn PA, Forstein M (2003). Overcoming the false dichotomy of curative vs. palliative care for late-stage HIV/AIDS: "Let me live the way I want to live, until I can't." *JAMA* 290:806–814.

Selwyn PA, Goulet JL, Molde S, Constantino J, Fennie KP, Wetherill P, Gaughan DM, Brett-Smith H, Kennedy C (2000). HIV as a chronic disease: long-term care for patients with HIV at a dedicated skilled nursing facility. *J Urban Health* 77:187–203.

Selwyn PA, Rivard M (2002). Palliative care for AIDS: challenges and opportunities in the era of highly active anti-retroviral therapy. *Innovations in End-of-Life Care* 4(3). Retrieved April 6, 2007, from www.edc.org/lastacts

Selwyn PA, Rivard M, Kapell D, Goeren B, LaFosse H, Schwartz C, Caraballo R, Luciano D, Post LF (2003). Palliative care for AIDS at a large urban teaching hospital: program description and preliminary outcomes. *J Palliat Med* 6 (3):461–474.

Shen JM, Blank A, Selwyn PA (2005). Predictors of mortality for patients with advanced disease in an HIV palliative care program. *J Acquir Immune Defic Syndr* 40(4):445–447.

Silver M, Blum D, Grainger J, Hammer AE, Quessy S (2007). Double-blind, placebo-controlled trial of lamotrigine in combination with other medications for neuropathic pain. *J Pain Symptom Manage* 34(4):446–454.

Simpson DM, McArthur JC, Olney R, Clifford D, So Y, Ross D, Baird BJ, Barrett P, Hammer AE; Lamotrigine HIV Neuropathy Study Team (2003). Lamotrigine for HIV-associated painful sensory neuropathies: a placebo-controlled trial. *Neurology* 60(9):1508–1514.

Singer JE, Fahy-Chandon B, Chi S, Syndulko K, Tourtellotte WW (1993). Painful symptoms reported by ambulatory HIV-infected men in a longitudinal study. *Pain* 54:15–19.

Slome LR, Mitchell TF, Charlebois E, Benevedes JM, Abrams DI (1997). Physician-assisted suicide and patients with human immunodeficiency virus disease. *N Engl J Med* 336(6):417–421.

Smith TJ (2000). Tell it like it is. *J Clin Oncol* 18:3441–3445.

Starace F, Sherr L (1998). Suicidal behaviors, euthanasia, and AIDS. *AIDS* 12 (4):339–347.

Stephenson J, Woods S, Scott B, Meadway J (2000). HIV-related brain impairment: from palliative care to rehabilitation. *Int J Palliat Nurs* 6:6–11.

Stjernsward J, Papallona S (1998). Palliative medicine: a global perspective. In D Doyle, GWC Hanks, and N MacDonald (eds.), *Oxford Textbook of Palliative Medicine*, second edition (pp. 1227–1245). New York: Oxford University Press.

Storey P, Knight C (2001). *American Academy of Hospice and Palliative Medicine UNIPAC Two: Alleviating Psychological and Spiritual Pain in the Terminally Ill*. Larchmont, NY: Mary Ann Liebert.

Stroebe M, Stroebe W, Hansson R (eds.) (1993). *Handbook of Bereavement*. Cambridge, UK: Cambridge University Press.

Tosches WA, Cohen CJ, Day JM (1992). A pilot study of acupuncture for the symptomatic treatment of HIV-associated peripheral neuropathy [8:14 abstract]. Presented at the VIIIth International Conference on AIDS, Amsterdam.

Underwood LG, Teresi JA (2002). The daily spiritual experience scale. *Ann Med* 24:22–33.

Valdez H, Chowdhry TK, Asaad R, Woolley IJ, Davis T, Davidson R, Beinker N, Gripshover BM, Salata RA, McComsey G, Weissman SB, Lederman MM (2001). Changing spectrum of mortality due to HIV: analysis of 260 deaths during 1995–1999. *Clin Infect Dis* 32:1487–1493.

Van Zyl LT, Seitz DP (2006). Delirium concisely: condition is associated with increased morbidity, mortality, and length of hospitalization. *Geriatrics* 61 (3):18–21.

Vincent B, Timsit JF, Auburtin M, Schortgen F, Bouadma L, Wolff M, Regnier B (2004). Characteristics and outcomes of HIV-infected patients in the ICU: impact of the highly active antiretroviral treatment era. *Intensive Care Med* 30:859–866.

Vogl D, Rosenfeld B, Breitbart W, Thaler H, Passik S, McDonald M, Portenoy RK (1999). Symptom prevalence, characteristics and distress in AIDS outpatients. *J Pain Symptom Manage* 18:253–262.

Welch K, Morse A (2002). The clinical profile of end-state AIDS in the era of highly active antiretroviral therapy. *AIDS Patient Care STDS* 16:75–81.

Wenger NS, Kanouse DE, Collins RL, Liu H, Schuster MA, Gifford AL, Bozzette SA, Shapiro MF (2001). End-of-life discussions and preferences among persons with HIV. *JAMA* 22:2880–2887.

Wood CG, Whittet S, Bradbeer CS (1997). ABC of palliative care: HIV infection and AIDS. *BMJ* 315:1433–1436.

World Health Organization (1986). *Cancer Pain Relief*. Geneva: World Health Organization.

World Health Organization (1990). *Cancer Pain Relief and Palliative Care: Report of a WHO Expert Committee* (Technical Bulletin 804). Geneva: World Health Organization.

World Health Organization (1998). *Symptom Relief in Terminal Illness*. Geneva: World Health Organization.

13

ETHICAL AND LEGAL ASPECTS
OF AIDS PSYCHIATRY

Mary Ann Cohen and Sharon M. Batista

From confidentiality, contact notification, and disclosure to decisional capacity, advance directives, and end-of-life care, AIDS presents special bioethical challenges to caregivers. Stigma, fear of rejection, and discrimination play significant roles in the bioethical aspects of the care of persons with HIV and AIDS. As a consequence, caregivers are often faced with bioethical dilemmas and conflicts. While many persons with HIV and AIDS are comfortable with disclosure to partners and family members, some persons with HIV refuse to disclose their serostatus even to sexual partners. Many persons with HIV and AIDS are able, especially with support, to come to safer and healthier decisions about disclosure and about their health and medical care. In this chapter, we will explore these dilemmas and provide suggestions on how to deal with them. Strategies for dealing with ethical dilemmas, determining decisional capacity, addressing end-of-life issues, and maintaining confidentiality in the care of persons with HIV and AIDS are also presented.

RELEVANT CONCEPTS AND TERMS

To begin a discussion of ethics as applied to clinical care, it is important to define the terms used in this context. The definitions of the terms used in this chapter are based not only on formal definitions as published in bioethics texts and articles but also their use in common medical practice. Table 13.1 provides definitions of some of the bioethics terms that are relevant to this discussion.

TABLE 13.1 Ethical Terms

Term	Definition
Advance directives	Specific wishes about medical care and decision-making that have been laid out in a formal process. One commonality for advance directives is that they all entail documentation. Examples of advance directives include living will, health-care proxy, DNR/DNI, and medical durable power of attorney.
Autonomy	Ethical concept referring to an individual's inherent right and ability to make his own decisions
Beneficence	The ethical duty to seek to "do good" or to bring about benefit in caring for the patient. This is sometimes referred to as *nonmaleficence* or *nonmalfeasance*.
Maleficence	The ethical duty to "do no harm" in patient care.
	These two concepts may be in conflict when a patient with problems with swallowing and recurrent aspiration pneumonia wants to eat and refuses to adhere to a regimen of percutaneous gastrostomy feedings.
Competence	The ability to make decisions; often refers to capacity determinations conducted in a court of law
	In the health-care setting, *competence* and *capacity* are often used interchangeably; the nuanced difference between the two concepts is not clinically relevant to our discussion in this chapter. Only the concept of capacity is used in this chapter.
Decisional capacity	The ability to make a specific decision as it relates to medical care, which can also be interpreted to apply more globally to extend as far as general health and safety
Guardian	Court-appointed individual who makes decisions for a person who is determined to lack capacity to make their own decisions
Substituted judgment	Describes the process by which a surrogate decision-maker makes decisions regarding the care of a patient based on the surrogate's perception of what the patient would have wanted or valued
Surrogate	Person who makes decisions for a patient who lacks the capacity to do so

DNI, do not intubate; DNR, do not resuscitate.

CAPACITY ASSESSMENT

Within the doctor–patient relationship, physicians are expected to understand and relate to their patients as their own primary decision-makers. Patients are presumed to be autonomous and to have decisional capacity. However, at times, decisional capacity can be called into question, such as when a medical condition impairs the patient's capacity to understand the illness or results in impaired judgment. Since autonomy is such a protected right, multiple criteria must be fulfilled in order to substitute another person's judgment for that of the patient in cases where the patient is unable to make an appropriate decision for him- or herself. This assessment is called an *assessment for capacity* and is specific for each decision— a separate assessment must be performed for each decision to be made if the patient's decision-making ability is under question.

Most commonly, the capacity of a patient is called into question when a patient demonstrates deficits in manipulating information to make a decision, as may appear with cognitive deficits; cannot explain the reasons for their decision; or makes a medical decision that appears not to be in the patient's best interests or may be dangerous to the patient's health or safety.

Steps to assess for capacity to make a specific decision

Frequently, and especially in the acute medical setting, a psychiatric consultation is requested to assess the ability of a patient to make a decision. A capacity assessment can be performed by any physician, provided that attention is paid to fulfillment of the specific criteria that are necessary. The following case is provided to illustrate a challenging capacity determination in the context of complicated HIV-related illness and the considerations relevant to determination of decisional capacity. After presentation of this case, we will delineate the criteria for assessing capacity and provide examples.

Case vignette: Specificity in determination of decisional capacity

Mr. A is a 42-year-old nurse anesthetist with end-stage AIDS and disseminated Kaposi's sarcoma who was admitted to the acute general-care hospital inpatient unit with hemoptysis, severe anemia (hematocrit 18), and severe weight loss (current weight 67 pounds) and CD4 of 40. He is alert but extremely weak. When Mr. A refused nursing home placement, his HIV clinician requested a consultation from the AIDS psychiatrist to determine whether his patient had decisional capacity to participate in discharge planning. The psychiatric consultant determined that Mr. A had a clear understanding of the nature, severity, and implications of his medical condition. He also understood that he had become too weak to care for himself but did not want to be placed in a skilled nursing facility. He opted for home hospice care. He was found to have the capacity to participate in discharge planning. However, a second consultation was requested to determine if the patient had the capacity to give informed consent for placement of a percutaneous gastrostomy prior to his discharge to home hospice care.

The medical team felt that this relatively invasive treatment did not seem to be consistent with the patient's values and his desire to be on home hospice. The patient was seen again in consultation. He felt that for comfort care, a percutaneous gastrostomy was preferable because his chewing and swallowing functions were impaired and he had a history of aspirating. He did not want to die of aspiration pneumonia, and he felt that the gastrostomy would make it easier for others to care for him and would support his nutrition at the end of life. The patient was found to have capacity to give informed consent for the procedure and was discharged to home hospice care.

The criteria for establishing capacity, typical questions that can be used to elicit the necessary information, and some examples of typical acceptable answers that would fulfill these criteria are provided in Table 13.2.

TABLE 13.2 Capacity Assessment: Criteria

Criteria*	Relevant Questions That May Be Used for Assessment
1. Acknowledgement and understanding of medical illness	• What is the reason you are in the hospital? • What illness(es) are the doctors treating you for? • What is your understanding of your illness? • What does having [X illness] mean to you?
2. Consistent ability to evidence a clear choice	• Your told me that you need ___ (a specific) treatment (or a specific diagnostic procedure). What do you think about that? • What is your decision? • What is your preference?
3. Ability to manipulate relevant information	• What leads to you make that particular decision? • On what basis did your doctors recommend that you do that? • Or that you not do that? • What could happen if you do not have that treatment (or diagnostic procedure)?
4. Ability to reiterate in the patient's own words the risks and benefits of the treatment compared to its alternatives	• What are the risks of your treatment options? • What are the benefits of each option? • If you do not accept this treatment, what other options are there? • Do you have other choices?

*Criteria based on Appelbaum and Grisso (1988).

Etiology: Factors That May Lead to Impairments in a Person's Decisional Capacity

Common conditions that may interfere with a person's ability to make a decision can include dementia, psychiatric illness—especially but not limited to mood or psychotic disorders—and the person's previous level of education. Cognitive impairment can be one of the more subtle features to detect because of the varying nature of deficits and varying levels of impairment that can be manifested. Similarly, education level can impact the assessment for capacity; thus the clinicians should take this into consideration when performing a cognitive assessment or assessing an individual's ability to manipulate information. Someone with a second-grade education level may have less sophisticated modes of communication, have trouble understanding certain words, or have difficulty with the reading, writing, and calculating tasks of a cognitive examination. That said, it is also important to recognize that persons with dementia, other psychiatric disorders, or lack of formal education may still have the capacity for medical decision-making.

Similarly, depressive or psychotic illness can be a barrier to the capacity for decision-making if the illness is so severe that it distorts the person's understanding of their illness (such as with delusional ideas related to the cause or meaning of the illness in question) or if the person is so distressed that he or she has lost interest in physical health and is no longer able to provide self-care. A common scenario encountered at the bedside is that of a person with major depressive disorder who is so depressed that they do not wish to live and therefore might refuse a life-saving procedure because of a wish to die; if the person were not depressed they would make a different choice. Therefore, it is essential to perform a mental status examination including a careful cognitive evaluation whenever assessing a patient for decisional capacity. Psychiatric symptoms such as depression or psychosis can impair judgment and should prompt deferral of final conclusions regarding decisional capacity until psychiatric treatment of the underlying disorders has been attempted.

Surrogate Decision-Making and Substituted Judgment

Much debate has arisen concerning the ethics of surrogate decision-making, especially as highlighted in the high-profile cases covered by the media in recent years. Surrogates must make decisions on the basis of three principles: known wishes, substituted judgment, and best interests (Berger et al., 2008).

Berger and colleagues (2008) clarify that surrogate decision-making occurs along a continuum. Surrogates base their decisions either on the known values and preferences of the patient, which may be explicitly known as delineated in a prior conversation, or on a general understanding of the patient's values or perceived best interests of the patient. In either case, such a decision made by a surrogate in the place of the incapacitated patient is referred to as *substituted judgment* (Jonsen et al., 2006).

In the case of a person lacking in capacity without advance directives, there are several legally established frameworks in place to determine who should make the decision in the place of the patient. These frameworks vary according to state, thus it is important to familiarize oneself with the standards according to the state in which one practices. Generally speaking, if next of kin or a spouse can be identified, the decision-making role transfers to the family members according to state-determined order of priority. This applies to medical treatment only. Typically, priority is first given to a partner, spouse, or first-degree relative. If neither of these is available, decision-making falls to second-degree relatives, and so on. If no surrogate can be identified, or if there are no family members willing to take on this responsibility, the treatment team must seek legal intervention for a guardian to be appointed to make decisions in the perceived best interests of the patient.

ISSUES IN SEVERE ILLNESS AND AT THE END OF LIFE

Care of persons with HIV presents specific challenges as the illness progresses. During care at the end of life, a period of time that is difficult even for palliative care physicians to define, it is most helpful to get a sense of the patient's values and treatment goals as early and often as possible, with the expectation that these may fluctuate at times with changes in diagnosis and prognosis. Open discussions with a patient can lay the groundwork for a well-rounded palliative experience that eliminates the patient's physical and emotional suffering. Similarly, discussions of values and priorities set the stage for establishing advance directives, if a patient desires them. Advance directives will be discussed extensively in this section. For more a more detailed discussion of some of the ethical dimensions of palliative care for the person with end-stage AIDS, please refer to Chapter 12 of this handbook. For resources to assist patients in establishing advance directives please refer to Chapter 14.

Advance directives

Increasingly, medical professionals are encouraging patients to consider making advance directives. Unfortunately, the urgency for patients to establish advance directives has been misconstrued in the popular media through their coverage of several high-profile cases; many people believe that opting for advance directives will result in conflicts between family members or withdrawal of care when care is desired, while the intention is indeed the contrary. The misconstruing of advance directives occurred long before these high-profile cases, as doctors seldom brought up advance directives until the very end of life. "The patient is crashing—Let's get a health-care proxy" was the hue and cry, and, of course, families and patients balked. A common response might be, "You mean, you are not giving my (wife, child, brother, sister, mother, father, husband, aunt) any more care?? You are letting my [loved one] die!" Advance directives, including do no resuscitate (DNR) or do not intubate (DNI) orders, as well as a living will and health-care proxy (HCP) enable individuals to delineate in written documents their wishes regarding their medical care should they become unable to make their own decisions. The official documents vary by state, but all have similar phrasing and intent. Often, much consideration goes into the writing of these documents.

Advance directives are a powerful means by which people can designate individuals that they trust and establish guidelines for their care when they no longer have the capacity to make decisions for themselves. In providing loved ones with advance directives, a person suffering from a serious illness or approaching the end of life is better able to address some of the loss of autonomy that many patients experience as they lose control over bodily functions lose ability to perform activities of daily living. From the surrogate decision-maker's perspective, taking over the care of a loved one can be overwhelming and stressful. Advance directives can lessen this stress and perceived burden by providing the surrogate decision-maker with an understanding of the wishes for directing the care of their loved one. Advance directives are empowering to the individuals who have them and to those whom they trust to make decisions for them.

Advance directives provide a systematic way of describing a patient's philosophy of medical care and what medical procedures or treatments they would or would not wish to undergo should they become more ill and unable to make decisions for themselves. Advance directives can do the following:

- Provide information about a person's values, such as the preference not to be dependent on machines to sustain their life
- Designate a trusted individual to make decisions if and when a patient no longer has the capacity to make them
- Help identify specific decisions to be made

Regardless of whether a patient is interested or not in creating written advanced directives, it is always helpful to encourage patients to discuss their wishes with their loved ones or significant others. Many patients feel comforted by their doctors' and family's interests in having this discussion. By having a discussion of their wishes for end-of-life care prior to or during the process of constructing advance directives, both the patient and family member(s) can come to better understand the intent of the document and the scope of the decisions, and avoid the shock of being contacted by medical personnel requesting assistance during a potential time of crisis.

There are several types of advance directives, each with different purposes and scope. Several common forms of advance directives are described in Table 13.3.

Table 13.3 Types of Advance Directives*

Name	Description	Advantages and Disadvantages
Consent for do not resuscitate (DNR)	A document stating that no emergency CPR should be performed in the event of a cardiac arrest or respiratory failure	*Advantages*: Legally binding *Disadvantages*: Narrow in scope
Consent for do not intubate (DNI)	A document stating that no emergency intubation should be performed if in the event of respiratory arrest	*Advantages*: Legally binding; often included in the same consent for DNR *Disadvantages*: Narrow in scope; often included in the same consent for DNR
Living will	A document that codifies advance directives and can provide explicit instructions about any type of health care, such as medical procedures and treatments. The living will can list as many instructions as an individual desires.	*Advantages*: The best possible advance directive when an individual cannot identify anyone he or she trusts, or when an individual has no remaining significant others or next of kin. Legally binding (may need a lawyer involved in creation of the document to be certain that it will withstand being challenged in a court of law). Limited in scope, since this document enumerates specific treatments and decisions. It may be of help particularly regarding difficult decisions that the patient has strong opinions about. *Disadvantages*: Cannot be all-inclusive. Limited in scope, since this document enumerates specific treatments and decisions. Given the limited scope or changing health status of the patient, it also needs to be updated periodically according to evolving preferences of the patient.

Health-care proxy (HCP)	A document that designates a person whom the patient trusts to make health-care decisions when he or she is unable to do so. The patient must have capacity at the time this document is created.	*Advantages*: Broad in scope; legally binding; the health-care agent (person selected by the patient to make decisions on his or her behalf if or when he or she loses decisional capacity) has flexibility to make numerous decisions on behalf of the patient based on their understanding of the patient's preferences and values. The HCP does not require an attorney and can be filled out at home, in a hospital, or at a doctor's office. It requires that two individuals serve as witnesses to signing of the document, to attest that designation of the health-care agent was not coerced. The HCP enables a person to discuss his or her health-care preferences over many years and enables the agent to get familiar with these preferences.
		Disadvantages: Requires that the individual have someone he or she trusts with decision-making and that the individual discuss his or her wishes in advance. An HCP can place a great deal of stress on the agent, depending on the level of understanding of the patient's values and desires.
Medical durable power of attorney	A form similar to a health-care proxy, in which the principal (the patient who is electing to make the advance directive) designates an agent to make decisions on their behalf should they become incompetent in the future	*Advantages*: Similar to health-care proxy. No hearings or court proceedings are necessary to set up a power of attorney
		Disadvantages: Special form required. There are some treatments that the agent cannot elect, which are specific to the state in which the person resides. Unlike the health care proxy, the medical durable power of attorney has multiple legal caveats.

*Berger et al. (2008); Martin et al. (2007).

Facts about advance directives include the following:

- A photocopy is just as valid as the original document.
- The patient may amend the advance directives at any time.
- The patient may change the designated health-care agent or revoke the advance directive completely at any time.

- They should not be kept in a safe but should be easily accessible.
- They can be miniaturized to wallet size and carried on the person.
- Copies should be provided to physicians and to the health-care agent and alternate agent or other designees.

Characteristics of useful advance directives include the following:

- They are written in consideration of specifically what kind of decisions will be made.
- They are informative of the patient's values.
- They may bind the treatment team to a particular action if it is desired by the patient.

Surrogate Decision-Making and Same-Sex Partners

The bioethical challenges of HIV and AIDS are considerably magnified in same-sex partnerships. Severe, complex illness is a universal stressor for patients, loved ones, partners, families, and friends. When same-sex partnerships are involved, anxiety can be magnified by homophobia and discrimination. Early in the epidemic, conflicts frequently arose between patients, parents, and partners in same-sex partnerships. Parents sometimes learned for the first time and on the same day that a son had AIDS and was dying and that he was gay. This "forced disclosure" led to conflicts. Often, the son was alienated from parents or had lived a double life since adulthood began. Parents experienced strong feelings, including ambivalence, with love, rage, guilt, and shock. In these situations, given the lack of communication, parents may not have known their son's philosophy of life and death, nor his wishes for medical care. A loving partner, by contrast, who may have nursed their son through the illness, may have had a clear understanding of the son's wishes. Conflicts heightened at the bedside, where some parents insisted on keeping their son alive at all cost regardless of the partner's perception of the son's wishes.

To address these dilemmas, the New York State Task Force on Life and the Law was established. It enabled a gay man to empower his partner, regardless of whether the union was considered legal or not in the state of residence, to carry out his wishes for medical care. The Task Force led the way to the enactment of the Health Care Proxy Law that was then adopted in many other states.

At the time of this writing, the law is in flux with regard to recognition of same-sex partnerships and it varies by state, with most states not recognizing the unions of same-sex couples. It is not at all unusual for the partner of a person with a complex, severe medical illness to experience a great deal of anxiety about their loved one's illness and about their role, if any, in providing care. For a same-sex partner, this anxiety can be heightened by the lack of legal protection of spousal rights and the knowledge that if their loved one should lose the capacity to make medical decisions (or designate a significant other as decision-maker), the partner might be unable to participate in decision-making simply because they are not in a legally recognized union. Numerous times, same-sex partners have approached the authors in a panic because they were worried that they would lose their right to participate in the care of their partner or treatments would be imposed because they were not married. Often, because of misperceptions about the law and about the ethics of decision-making in medicine, it is not uncommon for such partners to insist either with their doctors or loved ones that they be made health-care proxy or power of attorney in a time of crisis so that they can maintain some sort of control and involvement at all times and help the medical team carry out the patient's previously expressed wishes.

CONFIDENTIALITY

Because of concerns about stigma and discrimination when the first tests became available to detect the HIV virus in the mid-1980s, many states passed laws granting special protection to HIV-related health information. Although laws vary from state to state, types of laws that emerged included a subset requiring written informed consent for HIV testing and another subset requiring specific, written informed consent for release of HIV-related records to third parties (Brendel and Cohen, 2008). These laws specify a structure for obtaining informed consent for HIV testing and access to medical records as well as formalize the solution to a common concern for persons with HIV that access to their medical information be protected.

U.S. LAW: HEALTH INSURANCE PORTABILITY AND ACCOUNTABILITY ACT (HIPAA)

In 2003, privacy regulations established by the Health Insurance Portability and Accountability Act (HIPAA) went into effect (Schouten and Brendel, 2004). These broad regulations affect the management of health information by providers and other entities such as health plans. HIPAA can be difficult to understand in the context of its effects on confidentiality, and at times it is erroneously evoked to block access to patient information. While HIPAA is generally thought of as increasing privacy for medical record information, its effect is actually to increase the number of situations in which patient medical information may be shared without the patient's express, written, and informed consent (Brendel and Bryan, 2004). Specifically, HIPAA permits the disclosure of otherwise protected private health information, without specific consent, for treatment, payment, and health-care operations, as long as the patient has signed a privacy notice (Brendel and Bryan, 2004).

However, HIPAA is not the final determinant of what medical information can be released without specific consent. HIPAA explicitly states that specific state and federal laws that are more protective of patient privacy than HIPAA itself should prevail. In the case of persons with HIV/AIDS, state laws that require specific, written, informed consent prior to the release of HIV/AIDS records prevail over HIPAA and must be followed. In addition, federal legislation offers an added degree of protection over what HIPAA requires for substance abuse treatment records, a provision that also arises frequently in treating patients with HIV/AIDS. Specifically, written and specific consent is required for the release of these records (Brendel and Bryan, 2004).

Finally, psychotherapy records may also have added protections that require specific, written consent for their release, but these records must either meet narrowly defined criteria under HIPAA or be protected by state laws that supersede HIPAA regulations (Brendel and Bryan, 2004). It is critical for physicians to be aware of the relevant law in the jurisdiction(s) in which they practice in order to treat patient information confidentially within the confines of the law.

DISCLOSURE AND RELATED ISSUES

Although many ethicists hold that a person has the "right to know" if they are infected or at risk for HIV infection, this issue remains under debate (Dixon-Mueller, 2007). Similarly, it is widely understood that health professionals have a duty to warn persons at risk, since HIV infection is lethal and can be spread to others if left untreated. On the basis of this principle, it is common practice to encourage patients to disclose their HIV infection to others, especially first to the persons they may have put at risk of infection, including sexual partners or persons that have shared drug paraphernalia.

Partner notification

The general default is that physicians must safeguard information related to patients' HIV status and may not release it without consent, except in limited circumstances, such as mandated reporting. But what happens when a physician becomes aware that a patient has exposed or continues to expose another person or persons to HIV? This leaves the physician in a difficult ethical and legal position.

Nearly 20 years ago, the Council on Ethics and Judicial Affairs of the American Medical Association (AMA) called for the drafting of specific laws that balanced the protection of confidential patient information with the need to provide a method of warning unsuspecting sexual partners of HIV-positive individuals. Specific issues that were highlighted included the need to provide physicians with protection from liability for failure to warn at-risk contacts, the establishment of clear standards for when a physician should inform public health authorities, and the provision of clear guidelines for public health authorities who may need to trace the at-risk contacts (AMA, 1987). Physicians in these situations are still often left without legal direction, however. Currently, the AMA is continuing to address confidentiality and ethical issues raised by HIV-positive individuals who do not inform their partners or change their behavior that puts others at risk (AMA, 2003). In addition, because some states impose on mental health professionals a duty to warn that is not required of general medical practitioners, psychiatrists may face an even more complex ethical–legal dilemma about how to handle such situations.

Little progress has been made regarding mechanisms of disclosure to partners at risk. Many states offer third-party partner notification for a person who identifies specific persons at risk but feels unable to disclose to them on their own. It is unclear how frequently patients take advantage of this service.

Mandatory reporting

Currently, reporting of HIV-positive cases is legally mandated and centralized nationwide; the federal government requires that new diagnoses of HIV infection be reported to the Centers for Disease Control and Prevention (CDC). Ethically, disclosure of risk of HIV infection is mandatory only in situations where there is a risk of exposure of another person to HIV infection, but the legal specifics vary by state. From a public health perspective, there is a framework to ensure disclosure to those at risk of exposure: mandatory reporting to the state of new diagnoses of HIV infection (which exists in all states and details vary by state) in persons who identify specific persons at risk but are unable to disclose to them on their own. This means that a letter can be sent to a person to inform them that may have been exposed to HIV infection (without naming the person who might have exposed them) and that they should get counseled and tested.

Many states have laws that criminalize the behavior of people who put others at risk of HIV infection without warning in advance, for example, through unprotected intercourse or needle-sharing when one of the partners is aware of their positive serostatus. Intense debate has arisen not only in the United States but in other countries, such as the United Kingdom, regarding these laws, because it is possible that the legal consequences might not actually result in reduced transmission but rather increased stigmatization and incarceration of HIV-infected persons (Gable et al., 2009).

The clinician's obligations

Regardless of opinion regarding the fairness of the law, it is essential that clinicians understand the laws regarding disclosure, if any, as well as the laws regarding their own responsibilities to warn or advise others of HIV exposure risk, as these policies vary by state. Some states have no such policies whereas others are very stringent. Some states can hold both clinicians and patients at risk should a patient place another person at risk of infection without necessary precautions. It remains to be seen whether a consistent nationwide policy will arise.

Disclosure to primary support system and children

Disclosure to one's primary support group is typically a decision that involves significant consideration. HIV disclosure is a process, not an event. Many patients carry their illness as a secret and bear the weight of this burden on a daily basis. Disclosure can lighten the load by decreasing the anxiety of having to maintain such a secret, but it can also lead to stigmatization if the patient is consequently rejected by their loved ones. Please refer to Chapter 4 for a detailed discussion of this topic. Some individuals choose to tell only a small circle of family and friends, whereas others choose to tell no one, leaving their primary care providers as their only supports in illness. Disclosure is a stressful and sometimes painful process; regardless of the results, patients often will need extensive preparation before and during the process of disclosure, as well as assistance with coping with its effects.

There is generally no ethical framework for obligating a patient to reveal serostatus to social contacts who are not at risk for HIV transmission, such as family members, including both adults and children, if they are not interested in or prepared for disclosure. Although this stance is controversial, it applies to children of persons with HIV as well as to HIV-infected children, who may not have knowledge of their own serostatus. In 1999, the American Academy of Pediatrics issued a statement recommending disclosure to adolescents and children as early as possible in the lifespan to promote emotional adjustment and participation in their own care and to reduce the likelihood of HIV transmission via unprotected sex (American Academy of Pediatrics Committee on Pediatric AIDS, 1999). A recent article outlines a suggested 10-step process for disclosure of HIV serostatus to HIV-positive children (Barfield and Kane, 2008). Wiener and Lyon (2006) have developed a thoughtful guideline for disclosure to children, which explains that disclosure is a process and that a great deal of preparation goes into each step of this process. While their disclosure model refers to a parent or guardian disclosing to a child, much of this model can be generalized to other relationships in which disclosure takes place.

HIV TESTING

At the time of this publication, approximately 21% of persons in the United States who are infected with HIV do not know their serostatus (CDC, 2008). The CDC recommends routine testing for HIV in the primary care setting. Polymerase chain reaction (PCR) testing for diagnosis of HIV infection is one of the few clinical laboratory evaluations for which explicit informed consent is required in order to pursue testing, even if it is suspected that a specific person may have been put at risk by an exposure that could promote HIV infection, for example, in the case of an accidental needlestick or a high-risk sexual encounter. Given the complicated issues of stigmatization, readiness to accept the results of the test, and impact on psychological well-being, patients must be advised of what the test entails and what results mean in advance of the testing.

Particularly in developing countries that have communities with a high incidence of new infections, there is public debate over making HIV testing a more routine clinical practice. Patients would still be able to opt out if they do not wish to be tested (rather than opt in, as is currently the case), but by making the practice more routine, treatment could be initiated earlier in more patients and prevalence rates calculated more accurately (Dixon-Mueller, 2007; Yeatman, 2007).

CONCLUSIONS

In summary, there are a multitude of ethical concerns in common clinical practice that relate to the patient with HIV. Confusion and conflicts at the bedside can be minimized through attention to a patient's values. Advance directives exist within our ethical and legal framework as a means to strengthen the patient's control over their care. Although not highlighted extensively in this chapter, ample communication and rapport with the patient and family can help foster a therapeutic relationship and enable patients and their clinicians to discuss advance directives early in the course of illness and ensure that autonomy is preserved if or when capacity is lost. Through providing a supportive environment and open communication with the patient and his or her loved ones, health-care providers convey understanding of the patient's values and beliefs and can thus be of maximum assistance to the patient in times of need.

REFERENCES

American Academy of Pediatrics Committee on Pediatric AIDS (1999). Disclosure of illness status to children and adolescents with HIV infection. *Pediatrics* 103(1):164–166.

American Medical Association Council on Ethical and Judicial Affairs (1987). Ethical issues involved in the growing AIDS crisis, Report A–I-87, American Medical Association 1987–1988. Retrieved April 9, 2006, from www.ama-assn.org.

[AMA] American Medical Association (2003). Policy H-20-915: HIV/AIDS Reporting, Confidentiality, and Notification, American Medical Association 2003. Retrieved April 9, 2006, from www.ama-assn.org.

Applebaum PA, Grisso T (1998). Assessing patients' capacities to consent to treatment. *N Engl J Med* 319:1635–1638.

Barfield RC, Kane JR (2008). Balancing disclosure of diagnosis and assent for research in children with HIV. *JAMA* 300(5):576–578.

Berger JT, DeRenzo EG, Schwartz J (2008). Surrogate decision-making: reconciling ethical theory and clinical practice. *Ann Intern Med* 149:48–53.

Brendel RW, Bryan E (2004). HIPAA for psychiatrists. *Harv Rev Psychiatry* 12 (3):177–183.

Brendel R, Cohen MA (2008). Ethical issues, advance directives, and surrogate decision-making. In MA Cohen and JM Gorman (eds.), *Comprehensive Textbook of AIDS Psychiatry*. New York: Oxford University Press.

[CDC] Centers for Disease Control and Prevention (2008). HIV prevalence estimates—United States, 2006. *MMWR Morb Mortal Wkly Rep* 57 (39):1073–1076.

Dixon-Mueller R (2007). The sexual ethics of HIV testing and the rights and responsibilities of partners. *Stud Fam Plann* 38(4):284–296.

Gable L, Gostin L, Hodge JG Jr (2009). A global assessment of the role of law in the HIV/AIDS pandemic. *Public Health* 123(3):260–264.

Jonsen AR, Siegler M, Winslade WJ (2006). Preferences of patients. In *Clinical Ethics: A Practical Approach to Ethical Decisions in Clinical Medicine*, sixth edition. New York: McGraw Hill.

Martin RD, Cohen MA, Weiss Roberts L, Batista SM, Hicks D, Bourgeois J (2007). DNR versus DNT: clinical implications of a conceptual ambiguity: a case analysis. *Psychosomatics* 48(1):10–15.

Schouten R, Brendel RW (2004). Legal aspects of consultation. In TA Stern, GL Fricchione, NH Cassem, MS Jellinek, and JF Rosenbaum (eds.),

Massachusetts General Hospital Handbook of General Hospital Psychiatry, fifth edition (pp. 349–364). Philadelphia: Mosby.

Wiener L, Lyon M (2006). HIV disclosure: who knows? Who needs to know? Clinical and ethical considerations. In HJ Makadon, KH Mayer, J Goldhammer, and H Potter (eds.), *The Fenway Guide to Lesbian, Gay, Bisexual, and Transgender Health*. Philadelphia: American College of Physicians.

Yeatman S (2007). Ethical and public health considerations in HIV counseling and testing: policy implications. *Stud Fam Plann* 38(4):271–278.

14

Resources for Persons with AIDS and their Caregivers

Sharon M. Batista and Kelly L. Cozza

This chapter was developed as a basic reference list of resources for HIV clinicians to help them meet the various needs of persons with AIDS throughout the lifespan. The resources listed are by no means exhaustive or comprehensive, as there is a plethora of relevant literature, Web sites, and interest groups—too many to fit into a single chapter! Instead, this is a set of resources that the authors have found particularly useful when seeking answers to treatment- and social services–related questions at the bedside as well as in ambulatory and community settings. At the time of publication, these resources had been updated regularly and consistently; technology related to HIV evolves on an almost daily basis. A mixture of print and Internet-based resources is provided here—some will be useful to keep in the office setting for perusal or for patients, and some can be obtained on the Internet at a moment's notice when the need arises.

Many of the listings are for Web sites that can aid clinicians in accessing the most current information available on the Internet, which can change almost daily. The sites listed were current as of April 28, 2009.

Resources for Providers

The resources in this section are intended primarily to aid health-care providers in accessing up-to-date answers to questions regarding diagnoses and treatments as well as ethical and legal issues. There are also several sources for patient education materials. While many of these resources are from U.S.-based organizations, much of the information contained within them is applicable in international practice settings. There is also a section related exclusively to population-based and international resources, pertaining to specific ethnic groups or areas outside of the United States.

HIV disease and management information

Print materials

> A primary care guideline for the care of persons with HIV is available in print (Aberg et al., 2009) and online and is updated regularly at: http://www.journals.uchicago.edu/page/cid/IDSAguidelines.html.

Conferences and meetings

> National AIDS Treatment Advocacy Project: http://www.natap.org/
> This organization lists upcoming conference and events, articles, and publications.

Psychiatric information

Books and print materials

> *Comprehensive Textbook of AIDS Psychiatry*, by Mary Ann Cohen and Jack Gorman, Eds. New York: Oxford University Press, 2008.
> *Psychiatric Aspects of HIV/AIDS*, by Francisco Fernandez and Pedro Ruiz, Eds. Philadelphia: Lippincott Williams & Wilkins, 2006.

General medical information

Books and print materials

> *The Fenway Guide to Lesbian, Gay, Bisexual, and Transgender Health*, by HJ Makadon, KH Mayer, J Potter, and H Goldhammer, Eds. Philadelphia: American College of Physicians, 2007.
> *HIV/AIDS, Stigma and Children: A Literature Review*, by Harriet Deacon and Inez Stephney. Human Sciences Research Council, 2008.
> *Teenagers, HIV, and AIDS: Insights from Youths Living with the Virus*, by Maureen Lyons and Lawrence D'Angelo, Eds. Westport, CT: Praeger/Greenwood Publishing Group, 2007.

Web sites

> U.S. government HIV/AIDS Web site: www.aids.gov
> University of California, San Francisco (UCSF) Web site: www.hivinsite.org
> Clinical guidelines from the New York State Department of Health AIDS Institute: www.hivguidelines.org

These clinical guidelines concern management of mental illness, including substance abuse, in persons with HIV and AIDS across the lifespan. The site (hivguidelines.org) contains recommendations for treatment of depression in pregnant women.

> Johns Hopkins Web site: http://hopkins-aids.edu
> NY/NJ AIDS Education Training Center: www.nynjaetc.org

The NY/NJ AIDS Education Training Center provides curriculum, slide sets, guides, trainings, and resources.

> American Psychiatric Association (APA) AIDS Resource Database Search page www.psych.org/aids

General-interest listservs, periodicals, and interest groups

> Organization of AIDS Psychiatry (OAP)

OAP is a special interest group of the Academy of Psychosomatic Medicine that was founded by Dr. Mary Ann Cohen in 2004 to provide a support network for psychiatrists and other mental health clinicians who provide care for persons with HIV and AIDS. The OAP meets once a year at the annual meeting of the Academy of Psychosomatic Medicine (APM). OAP members have developed symposia for presentation at the APM meeting and joined the American Psychiatric Association Office of HIV Psychiatry in a collaborative symposium presentation in 2008. OAP members have participated in collaborative research in an online HIV psychiatry treatment consensus survey. As of October 26, 2009, the OAP has 220 national and international members.

To join the Organization of AIDS Psychiatry, write to the OAP, and get on the OAP Listserv, write to: http://www.apm.org/sigs/oap

There is no fee to be an OAP member or to be on the Listserv.

> HIV/AIDS Literature Listserv

This Listserv is maintained by Robert Malow, PhD, ABPP, director of the AIDS Prevention Program in the Stempel School of Public Health (Florida International University).

To subscribe to this Listserv, send your request via e-mail to Dr. Malow at RMalow@bellsouth.net and include your name and e-mail address. There is no fee to join the Listserv.

Palliative care and advanced directives

Articles

> Hurwitz CA, Duncan J, Wolfe J (2004). Caring for the child with cancer at the close of life. *JAMA* 292:2141–2149.

Web sites

> Center for Palliative Care Education:http://depts.washington.edu/
> pallcare/resources/resources.php?category=3

This site contains palliative care resources for print or download. It is for patients and providers.

> American Bar Association Consumer's Tool Kit for Health Care Advance
>   Planning: http://www.abanet.org/aging/toolkit/home.html
> Center to Advance Palliative Care: http://www.getpalliativecare.org

Patient handouts

> http://www.aidsinfonet.org/

Printable info sheets in English and Spanish about HIV and AIDS, medications, nutrition, and disclosure. Listings of some community resources can also be found at this site.

Pharmacology and drug–drug interactions

Books and print materials

> *Clinical Guide to Drug Interaction Principles for Medical Practice* by
>   GH Wynn, JR Oesterheld, KL Cozza, and SC Armstrong, Eds.
>   Washington, DC: American Psychiatric Press, 2009.
> *Psychiatric Medications and HIV Antiretrovirals: A Guide to
>   Interactions for Clinicians*, by ML Wainberg, J Faragon, F Cournos,
>   E Horwath, and A Castillo. New York: NY/NJ AIDS Education and
>   Training Center, 2008.
> *Recreational Drugs and HIV Antiretrovirals: A Guide to Interactions for
>   Clinicians*, by A Urbina, J Farragon, C Kubin, and A Castillo. New
>   York: NY/NJ AIDS Education and Training Center, 2008.

Articles

> de Leon J, Armstrong SC, Cozza KL (2006). Clinical guidelines for
>   psychiatrists for the use of pharmacogenetic testing for CYP450 2D6
>   and CYP450 2C19. *Psychosomatics* 47(1):75–85.
> Sandson NB, Armstrong SC, Cozza KL (2005). An overview of
>   psychotropic drug–drug interactions. *Psychosomatics*.46(5):464–494.
> Wynn GH, Cozza KL, Zapor MJ, Wortmann GW, Armstrong SC (2005).
>   Med-psych drug–drug interactions update. Antiretrovirals, part III:
>   antiretrovirals and drugs of abuse. *Psychosomatics* 46(1):79–87.

Wynn GH, Zapor MJ, Smith BH, Wortmann G, Oesterheld JR, Armstrong SC, Cozza KL (2004). Antiretrovirals, part 1: overview, history, and focus on protease inhibitors. *Psychosomatics*. 45(3):262–270.

Zapor MJ, Cozza KL, Wynn GH, Wortmann GW, Armstrong SC (2004). Antiretrovirals, Part II: focus on non-protease inhibitor antiretrovirals (NRTIs, NNRTIs, and fusion inhibitors). *Psychosomatics* 45 (6):524–535.

Web sites

Johns Hopkins Point of Care Information Technology Site: http://www. hopkins-hivguide.org/

University of Liverpool HIV Drug interactions list: http://www.hiv-druginteractions.org/

Medscape HIV/AIDS:

http://www.medscape.com/hiv?src=pdown%2520and%2520http:// hivinsite.ucsf.edu/

www.hiv-pharmcogenomics.org

New York Department of Health AIDS Institute HIV guidelines: http:// www.hivguidelines.org

The user may search for specific subgroups such as adolescent or geriatric as well as other topics.

http://www.tthhivclinic.com/interact_tables.html

REFERRAL AND RESOURCES FOR PATIENT CARE

Caregiver resources

National Family Caregiver's Association: https://www.thefamilycaregiver. org/caregiving_resources/agencies_and_organizations.cfm

Family Caregiver Newsmagazine: http://www.thefamilycaregiver.com

Miscellaneous resources

Articles and curricula

Ethical Issues and HIV/AIDS: A Multi-Disciplinary Mental Health Services Curriculum (Jue et al., 2000) from the American Psychological Association (APA) curricula.

Gostin LO, Hodge JG (2002). HIV partner counseling and referral services—handling cases of willful exposure. *Georgetown/Johns Hopkins Program on Law & Public Health*.

Web sites

Harm Reduction Coalition: www.harmreduction.org

The Harm Reduction Coalition (HRC) is a national advocacy and capacity-building organization that promotes the health and dignity of individuals and communities affected by drug use. HRC advances policies and programs that help people address the adverse effects of drug use, including overdose, HIV, hepatitis C, addiction, and incarceration.

Kaiser Family Foundation: http://www.kff.org/hivaids/index.cfm AIDS Community Research Initiative of America: http://www.acria.org/index.html

AIDS Community Research Initiative of America (ACRIA) is a non-profit community-based AIDS research and treatment education center.

International and population-based resources

Books and print materials

HIV/AIDS: Global Frontiers in Prevention/Intervention, by Cynthia Pope, Renee T. White, and Robert Malow, Eds. New York: Routledge, 2009.

Web sites

AIDS Alliance: http://www.aidsalliance.org/sw6876.asp?

This organization supports communities in reducing the spread of HIV and meeting the challenges of AIDS.

The Body: http://www.thebody.com/index/hotlines/internat.html

This online resource is useful for conducting searches for HIV/AIDS-related organizations and services in many countries around the world.

AIDS Map: www.aidsmap.com

This UK-based HIV/AIDS Web site has an international perspective and is in multiple languages.

United Nations' HIV/AIDS Web site: www.unaids.org
The National Minority AIDS Council: www.nmac.org

This Council has helped develop leadership in communities of color to address the challenges of HIV/AIDS since 1987.

The Latino Commission on AIDS: www.latinoaids.org

This nonprofit membership organization is dedicated to fighting the spread of HIV/AIDS in the Latino community.

The Asian and Pacific Islander's Coalition of HIV and AIDS: www.apicha.org

The Coalition's mission is to combat HIV/AIDS stigma and related discrimination, to prevent the spread of the HIV/AIDS pandemic in the Asian and Pacific Islander (A&PI) communities, and to provide care and treatment for A&PIs living with HIV/AIDS and for their families.

National Women's Health Information Center, U.S. Department of Health and Human Services: www.womenshealth.gov/hiv
Francois-Xavier Bagnoud Center: www.fxb.org

Further useful resources

University of Medicine & Dentistry of New Jersey
30 Bergen Street, ADMC 4
Newark, NJ 07107
Phone: 973-972-8393
Fax: 973-972-0399
Pamela Rothpletz-Puglia, PhD
rothplpm@umdnj.edu

HAB Project Officer
Helen Rovito
301-443-3286
hrovito@hrsa.gov

RESOURCES FOR PATIENTS AND FAMILIES

The resources listed below are not intended exclusively for the use of patients but are noteworthy for being directed at the interests, needs, and vantage point of the patient. Some patients will require assistance to access many of these resources, given that many are Internet-based or in publications that must be ordered. But a great many of the Web sites are user-friendly, worded simply and clearly, and well organized. The authors have included resources that communicate with patients at varied points of the lifespan and according to sexual orientation. Some resources provide public services, supply education regarding illness or the law, or are outreach efforts for persons in distress (such as hotlines).

General interest

Articles

> Davey MP, Foster J, Milton K, Duncan TM (2009). Collaborative approaches to increasing family support for HIV positive youth. *Fam Syst Health* 27(1):39–52.

Web sites

> The Body: http://www.thebody.com/index.html

Varied resources and contact information are available for nationwide organizations, by region within the United States, as well as some international resources. The site also has content in Spanish.

> American Social Health Organization: http://www.ashastd.org/nah/nah.html
> The Fenway Community Health Center: http://www.fenwayhealth.org/site/PageServer?pagename=FCHC_ins_fenway_ConsumerResources

This bisexual, gay, lesbian, and transgender (BGLT) health center in Boston, Massachusetts, has extensive online resources relating to HIV and BGLT issues. The Center serves medical and psychosocial needs of the Boston-area BGLT community.

Child and adolescent resources or resources geared toward parents

Books and print materials

> *Daddy and Me*, by Jeanne Moutoussamy-Ashe. Knopf Books for Young Readers, 2001.
> *Disclosing HIV/AIDS to Children: The Paths We Take*, by Dale DeMatteo and Jillian Roberts. Detselig Enterprises Ltd., 2001.
> *Someone at School Has AIDS: A Guide to Developing Policies for Student and School Staff Members Who are Infected with HIV*, by Katherine Fraser and James L. Bodgen. Alexandria, VA: National Association of State Boards of Education, 2001.
> *Teenagers, HIV, and AIDS: Insights From Youths Living With the Virus*, by Maureen Lyons and Lawrence D'Angelo, Eds. Westport, CT, Praeger/Greenwood Publishing Group, 2007.

Articles

> Barfield RC, Lane JR (2008). Balancing disclosure of diagnosis and assent for research in children with HIV. *JAMA* 300(5):576–578.

Web sites

> Advocates for Youth: http://www.advocatesforyouth.org/

This Web site focuses on adolescent reproductive and sexual health.

> Go Ask Alice: www.goaskalice.columbia.edu

This Columbia University Internet question-and-answer service is where teens can find answers to health questions.

> Sex, etc.: http://sexetc.org/

This Web site is for teens, by teens. It emphasizes sexual health.

> Planned Parenthood: http://www.plannedparenthood.org/
> National Association of School Psychologists (2005). Position Statement on HIV/AIDS. http://www.nasponline.org/information/pospaper_aids.html
> Interagency Youth Working Group: http://www.infoforhealth.org/youthwg/prog_areas/index.shtml
> http://www.infoforhealth.org/youthwg/pubs/YouthInfoNet/YIN52.shtml
> Make a Wish Foundation: http://www.wish.org/

The online directory can be used to locate a chapter in your area.
Make-A-Wish Foundation® of America
3550 North Central Avenue, Suite 300
Phoenix, Arizona 85012-2127
Monday–Friday, 7 A.M. to 4 P.M. MST
Phone: (602) 279-WISH (9474)
Toll-free: 1-800-722-WISH (9474)
Fax: (602) 279-0855

> Children's Hospice International: http://www.chionline.org/
> http://www.talkingwithkids.org/

This site provides information on talking with children about difficult issues. It is available in Spanish.

Bereavement

Compassionate Friends: http://compassionatefriends.org/

This site was developed for bereaved parents, grandparents, and siblings.

The Sibling Connection: http://www.counselingstlouis.net/

Bereavement information is provided for children who have lost a sibling.

Summer camps

Please refer to the list at the end of this chapter for a nationwide summer camp directory including location by state and contact information.

LGBT

Web sites

Fenway Health Center Resources Page: http://www.fenwayhealth.org/
site/PageServer?pagename=FCHC_ins_fenway_ConsumerResources
National Coalition for LGBT Health: http://www.lgbthealth.net/index.
shtml
Gay Men's Health Crisis: gmhc.org

Geriatric

Web sites and organizations by geographic location

Chicago
Howard Brown Health Center: howardbrown.org

This center has LGBT elder services. Call Rebecca Finer at (773) 388–8901.

Los Angeles
AIDS Project Los Angeles: apla.org; (213) 201–1621

Support is provided for those over 50 through support groups.

New York
Iris House's Divas: irishouse.org; (646) 548–0100
Gay Men's Heath Crisis 50+ Life-Long program: gmhc.org; (212)
367–1000

Gay Men of African Descent Seniors Program: gmad.org; (212) 828–1697

GRIOT Circle: griotcircle.org; (718) 246–2775

This Brooklyn-based support group is for persons with HIV who are over 50.

San Francisco
New Leaf Services: newleafservices.org; (415) 626–7000

New Leaf Services offers programs including home visits.

Washington, DC
Whitman-Walker Clinic: wwc.org; (202) 939–7690

The Clinic hosts an over-50 support group.

Via telephone Project LinkAge: A conference-call support group for HIV-positive people over 501-877-665-0288

Any location
HIV Over Fifty is the longest-running organization for those aging with HIV. It can be contacted at any time at (617) 233–7107. It will provide support and connect you with resources (including support groups and phone buddies) in your area.

Services and advocacy for gay, lesbian, bisexual, and transgender elders (SAGE): sageusa.org; (212) 741–2247

SAGE provides aid for BGLT HIV-positive people over 50.

BGLT

Books and print materials

The Fenway Guide to Lesbian, Gay, Bisexual, and Transgender Health, by HJ Makadon, KH Mayer, J Potter, and H Goldhammer, Eds. Philadelphia: American College of Physicians, 2007.

Periodicals

Poz Magazine and Web site

Available by mail subscription as well as on the Internet.

Web sites

Poz Magazine: www.poz.com

There is also a Spanish-language version at http://amigos.poz.com/

Gay Men's Health Crisis: www.ghmc.org

Ethnic groups and language groups

Books and print materials

HIV and Me: An African American's Guide to Living with HIV. Provided by The Body, 2009.

Web sites

Poz.com (see above for description) has some Spanish-language content.

Caregiver resources and palliative care

Web sites

National Family Caregivers Association: https://www.thefamilycaregiver.org/caregiving_resources/agencies_and_organizations.cfm
Center to Advance Palliative Care: http://www.getpalliativecare.org

Social networking

Web sites

www.poz.com

Community and public service resources

Web sites

Several organizations in New York City have Web sites with details of their services and contact information; please see Web sites for more information. These organizations offer support groups, food pantries, hospital visitation services, and pastoral care.

Together Our Unity Can Heal: An HIV/AIDS Support Organization: http://www.touch-ny.org
AIDS Council of Northeastern New York: http://www.aidscouncil.org/client-services/

http://www.themomentumproject.org/index.htm
God's Love We Deliver: http://www.glwd.org/
Gay Men's Health Crisis: http://www.gmhc.org/
Praxis Housing Initiatives: http://www.praxishousing.org/

General legal resources

Web sites

The Center for HIV Law and Policy: http://www.hivlawandpolicy.org/
cake/resourceCategories/view/23

Lambda Legal, The nation's oldest and largest legal organization
working for the civil rights of lesbians, gay men, and people with
HIV/AIDS: http://www.lambdalegal.org//.html

The HIV Law Project: www.hivlawproject.org

Nationwide Directory of Legal Resources: http://www.abanet.org/AIDS/
publications/aidsdirectory.pdf

LawHelp: http://lawhelp.org/

State criminal statutes on HIV transmission: http://www.thebody.com/
content/legal/art6936.html

Local legal resources

AIDS Law: http://www.aidslaw.org/

This organization is based in Louisiana.

Information about disclosure

The Well Project: http://www.thewellproject.org/en_US/Womens_Center/
HIV_and_Disclosure.jsp

This Web site addresses the ramifications of disclosure and how to decide to
whom and when to disclose.

The Disclosure Initiative: ask.tell@sfdph.org
http://www.hivdisclosure.org/

This information line is aimed at helping to disclose to partners and others
at risk.

Hotlines

Local

New York Lifenet Hotline

Residents throughout New York City can call for help at any time on any day, at 1-800-LIFENET (1-800-543-3638). This 24-hour hotline assists callers seeking help for emotional or substance abuse problems. Spanish-speaking callers can contact 1-877-AYUDESE ("Help Yourself"), a recently established "Spanish LifeNet" with bilingual workers who can link callers to available treatment services. In 1997, the service received the William Charet Award, the City Department of Mental Health's award for excellence in mental health programming.

1-800-LIFENET (1-800-543-3638)
1-877-AYUDESE (Spanish)
1-877-990-8585 (Asian LifeNet)
(212) 982-5284 (TTY)

> GMHC Hotline at (212) 807-6655 or 1-800-AIDS-NYC (1-800-243-7692)

Hours: open Monday through Friday 10:00 A.M. to 9:00 P.M. and Saturday 12:00 to 3:00 P.M. (Eastern Time; GMT minus 5 hours).

> For Spanish-speakers: GMHC Hotline at 1-800-AIDS-NYC (1-800-243-7692) or in New York City: (212) 807-6655

TTY: (212) 645-7470 (para personas con deficiencias auditivas)
Lunes a viernes
10:00 A.M. a 9:00 P.M. (ET)
Sábado, 12:00 a 3:00 P.M. (ET)

> San Francisco AIDS Foundation: http://sfaf.org/

California AIDS Hotline
(415) 863-AIDS (2437)

Nationwide

> AIDS hotline in Washington, DC

The hotline operates 24 hours a day, 7 days a week. It offers general information and referrals to resources in your area.

1-800-CDC-INFO
1-800-342-AIDS
1-800-344-7432 for Spanish
1-800-243-7889 (TTY)
E-mail: hiv@ashastd.org

Web site: http://www.ashastd.org/nah/nah.html

AIDS/HIV Nightline: http://www.hivnightline.org/; (415) 434-2437 San
  Francisco or 1-800-628-9240 nationwide
HIV Over Fifty: (617) 233-7107
National Suicide Prevention Lifeline: 1-800-273-TALK
National Drug and Alcohol Treatment Hotline: 1-800-662-HELP
National Domestic Violence Hotline: 1-800-799-7233 OR 1-800-787-
  3224
National Child Abuse Hotline: 1-800-4-A-CHILD
National Youth Crisis Hotline: 1-800-442-HOPE (4673)
National Runaway Switchboard: 1-800-621-4000
Panic Disorder Information Line: 1-800-64-PANIC
Project Inform HIV/AIDS Treatment Hotline: 1-800-822-7422

SUMMER CAMPS

Arizona

Camp Hakuna Matata
Contact: AIDS Project Arizona
Phoenix, AZ
Phone: (602) 253-2437

California

Camp Arroyo: year-round camp serving children with life-threatening
  diseases and disabilities
Contact: Camp Arroyo, Taylor Family Foundation
5555 Arroyo Rd.
Livermore, CA 94550
Phone: (925) 455-5118

Camp Care: support for women, children, and families infected and affected
  by HIV/AIDS
Contact: All About Care
4974 Fresno Street, PMB #156
Fresno, CA 93726
Phone: (559) 222-9471

Camp Dream Street: serves children with cancer, blood disorders, and other
  life-threatening illnesses
Contact: Dream Street Foundation
9536 Wilshire Blvd. Suite 310

Beverly Hills, CA 90212
Phone (310) 274-7227

Camp Pacific Heartland: full-service summer camp for children and adolescents infected and affected by HIV/AIDS; partner camp to Camp Hollywood Heart
Contact: Hollywood Heart
3310 W Vanowen St.
Burbank, CA 91505
Phone: (818) 260-0372

Camp Kindle: summer camp serving children infected and affected by HIV/AIDS
Contact: PO Box 803220
Santa Clarita, CA 91380
Phone: 1-877-800-CAMP (2267)

Camp Laurel: serves children infected and affected HIV/AIDS
Contact: 75 South Grand Avenue
Pasadena, CA 91105
Phone: (626) 683-0800

Camp Sunburst: long-term residential camp for children living with HIV/AIDS
Contact: Sunburst Projects
2 Padre Parkway, Suite 106
Rohert Park, CA 94928
Phone: (707) 588-9477

Colorado

Camp Ray-Ray: short-term residential camp for families affected by AIDS
Contact: Angels Unaware
6370 Union Street
Arvada, CO 80004
Phone: (303) 420-6370

Connecticut

Association of Hole in the Wall Camps: serves children with cancer and other serious blood conditions who, because of their disease, its treatment, or its complications, cannot attend an ordinary summer camp. They have a special immunology session. They offer a 1-week session for brothers and sisters.
Contact: The Hole In The Wall Gang Camp
565 Ashford Center Road

Ashford, CT 06278
Phone (860) 429-3444

Camp AmeriKids: serves children ages 7–15 infected and affected with HIV/
AIDS
Contact: 88 Hamilton Avenue
Stamford, CT 06902
Phone: 1-800-486 HELP (4357)

Camp Meechimuk: long-term residential camp for children affected by HIV/
AIDS
Contact: Hispanos-Unidos
116 Sherman Avenue, 1st floor
New Haven, CT 06511
Phone: (203) 781-0226

Camp Totokett: nondenominational summer camp for children ages 5–16
whose families are affected by HIV/AIDS
Contact: First Congregational Church of Branford
1009 Main Street
Branford, CT
Phone: (203) 481-4339

Florida

The Boggy Creek Gang: part of the Association of Hole in the Wall Camps
Contact: 30500 Brantley Branch Road
Eustis, FL 32736
Phone: (352) 483-4200

Georgia

Camp High Five: serving children infected and affected by HIV/AIDS
www.camphighfive.org
Contact: Camp High Five
3130 Vista Brook Drive
Decator, GA 30033
Phone: (404) 616-9809

Illinois

Camp Getaway: long-term residential camp for families affected by HIV/
AIDS
Contact: Access Community Health Network
1501 South California Ave.

Chicago, IL 60608
Phone: (773) 394-7063

Children's Place: serves children and families affected by HIV with a variety
of programming
Contact: The Children's Place Association
3059 West Agusta Blvd.
Chicago, IL 60622
Phone: (773) 826-1230

Indiana

Tataya Mato: long-term residential camp for children infected or affected by
HIV/AIDS
Contact: Jameson, Inc.
PO Box 31156
2001 S. Bridgeport, RD
Indianapolis, IN 46231
Phone: (317) 241-2661

Kentucky

Camp Heart to Heart: free summer camp for children (ages 5–12) living with
HIV/AIDS
Contact: Lions Camp Crescendo, Inc.
PO Box 607
Lebanon Junction, KY 40150
Phone: Daniel Coe (502) 969-0336, Teresa Davis (502) 456-6385

Massachusetts

Camp Safe Haven: serves children infected and affected by HIV/AIDS.
Family events, community-based camps, and retreat experiences and
year-long programs are held.
Contact: The Safe Haven Project, Inc.
PO Box 24
Vineyard Haven, MA 02568
Phone: (508) 693-1767

Michigan

Camp Rainbear: short-term residential camp for families affected by HIV/
AIDS

Contact: Rainbow Alliance, Inc.
8569 Stonegate Dr.
Northville, MI 48167
Phone: (248) 486-3872

Minnesota

Camp Knutson: serves families in which any member is infected with HIV/
   AIDS, at a 1-week residential camp
Contact: Camp Knutson and Knutson Point Retreat Center
11169 Whitefish Ave.
Crosslake, MN 56442
Phone: (218) 543-4232

Camp Heartland: serves children infected and affected by HIV/AIDS
Contact: One Heartland
1221 Nicollet Ave. Suite #501
Minneapolis, MN 55403
Phone: 1-888-216-2028

Missouri

Camp Hope: weekend-long camp for HIV-infected children and their
   families
Contact: Project Ark (AIDS/HIV Resources & Knowledge)
4169 Laclede Avenue
St. Louis, MO 63108
Phone: (314) 535-7275

Nebraska

Camp Knutson: serves families in which any member is infected with HIV/
   AIDS, at a 1-week residential camp.
Contact: Camp Knutson and Knutson Point Retreat Center
Nebraska Address
PO Box 81147
Lincoln, NE 68501
Phone: 1-877-800-CAMP (2267)

New Jersey

Camp Bright Feathers: long-term residential camp for children affected by
   HIV/AIDS

Contact: YMCA Camp Ockanickon, Inc.
1303 Stokes Rd.
Medford, NJ 08055
Phone: (856) 428-5688

New York

The Birch Family Camp
Contact: Herbert G. Birch Services
275 Seventh Ave, Nineteenth Floor
New York, NY 10001
Phone: (212) 741-6522, ext. 208

The Double "H"–Hole in the Woods Ranch
Part of the Association of Hole in the Wall Camps
Contact: 97 Hidden Valley Road
Lake Luzerne, NY 12846
Phone (518) 696-5676

Camp Courage: serves children between the ages of 7 and 17 who are living
   with AIDS. The sister camp, TLC, serves children who have a parent or
   sibling who has AIDS or who has died from the disease.
Contact: Camp Good Days and Special Times, Inc.
1332 Pittsford-Mendon Road
Mendon, NY 14506-9732
Phone: (585) 624-5555

Camp S.O.A.R.: camping and recreational activities for children infected or
   affected by HIV/AIDS
Contact: Catholic Charities Community Services
1945 E. Ridge Rd., Suite 24
Rochester, NY 14622
Phone: (585) 339-9800

Camp Viva: 1-week camp and after-camp follow-up program serving
   children and families with HIV/AIDS
Contact: Family Services of Westchester, White Plains Office
One Summit Avenue
White Plains, NY 10606
Phone: (914) 948-8004
Pact Weekend Camp
Contact: Children's Hospital of Buffalo, PACT Program
218 Bryant Street
Buffalo, NY 14222
Phone: (716) 878-7666

North Carolina

Agape Summer Camp: day camp for children affected by AIDS
Contact: Agape Family Center, Metrolina AIDS Project
PO Box 32662
Charlotte, NC 28232
Phone: (704) 333-1435

Camp Kaleidoscope: summer program open to all Duke University Medical
   Center pediatric patients ages 7–16
Contact: Box 3417
DUMC
Durham, NC 27710
Phone (919) 681-4349

Victory Junction Camp: year-round camp for children (ages 8–13) living
with HIV/AIDS. Includes disease-specific summer camp sessions, family
retreat weekends, specialized programs, sibling weekends, and camper
reunion. This is a sister camp to the Hole in the Wall Gang Association.
Contact: 4500 Adam's Way
Randleman, NC 27317
Phone: (336) 498-9055

Ohio

Camp Sunrise: residential camp for children impacted by HIV/AIDS
1160 N. High Street
Columbus, OH 43201
Phone: (614) 297-8404

Oregon

Camp Starlight
Program of the Cascade AIDS Project
Contact: 620 SW 5th Ave, Suite 300
Portland, OR 97204
Phone: (503) 238-4420

Pennsylvania

Camp Dreamcatcher: year-round programs for children infected or affected
   by HIV/AIDS
Contact: 110 East State Street, Suite C
Kennett Square, PA 19348
Phone: (610) 925-2998

South Carolina

Camp for Kids: short-tern camp for children living with HIV/AIDS
Contact: Sue Kulen Camp for Kids, Inc.
Columbia, SC
Phone: (803) 957-7814

Texas

Camp Firelight: day camp for children affected by HIV/AIDS
Contact: AIDS Outreach Center
Fort Worth, TX
Phone: (817) 335–1994

Camp Hope: serving children ages 6–15 with HIV/AIDS
Contact: AIDS Foundation Houston, Inc.
3202 Weslayan Annex
Houston, TX 77027
Phone: (713) 623-6796

Camp H.U.G. (Hope, Understanding, Giving): weekend camp for families
and children with HIV/AIDS
Contact: AIDS Foundation Houston, Inc.
3202 Weslayan Annex
Houston, TX 77027
Phone: (713)-623-6796

Jennifer's Camp: long-term residential camp for children infected and
affected by HIV/AIDS
www.aarcsa.com
Contact: Alamo Area Resource Center
527 N. Leona, Bldg A, 3rd Floor
P.O. Box 7160
San Antonio, TX 78207
Phone: (210) 358-9995

Virginia

Camp Funshine: serves children with HIV/AIDS and their families for a
weekend camping program
Contact: Special Love
117 Youth Development Court
Winchester, VA 22602
Phone: (540) 667-3774

Camp Wakonda: serves children and families infected and affected by HIV/AIDS in a day-camp environment
Contact: Diocesan Center, Frances Barber
600 Talbot Hall Road
Norfolk, VA 23505
Phone: (757) 461-3595

Vermont

Twin States Kids Camp: short-term residential camp for children infected and affected by HIV/AIDS
Contact: Twin States Network
PO Box 2606
W. Brattleboro, VT 05303
Phone: (888) 338-8796

Washington

Northwest Reach Camp: long-term residential camp for children and families infected and affected by HIV/AIDS
Contact: REACH Ministries
419 Martin Luther King Jr. Way
Tacoma, WA 98405
Phone: (253) 383-7616

Rise N' Shine Camp: long-term residential camp for children infected and affected by HIV/AIDS
Contact: Rise N' Shine Foundation, Inc.
417 23rd Avenue South
Seattle, WA 98144
Phone: (206) 628-8949

Washington, DC

Camp Safe Haven: Maryland long-term residential camp for children infected or affected by HIV/AIDS
Contact: Lutheran Social Services of the National Capitol Area
4406 Georgia Ave, N.W.
Washington, DC 20011
Phone: (202) 723-3000

Wisconsin

One Heartland: Responsible for Camp Heartland, which serves children
   infected and affected by HIV/AIDS
Corporate Headquarters
Contact: 1845 North Farwell Ave., Suite 310
Milwaukee, WI 53202
Phone: 1-800-724-4673

ACKNOWLEDGMENTS

The authors would like to thank the following persons for their contributions
of resources to this chapter:

Kenneth B. Ashley, MD (personal communications)
Director, Mental Health Services
Peter Krueger Clinic, Beth Israel Medical Center
Assistant Professor of Psychiatry & Behavioral Sciences
Albert Einstein College of Medicine of Yeshiva University
kashley@chpnet.org

Robert M. Malow, Ph.D., ABPP (personal communications)
Health Promotion and Disease Prevention
Research Professor
Stempel School of Public Health, Florida International University
RMalow@bellsouth.net

INDEX